THERMAL AGENTS IN REHABILITATION

THERMAL AGENTS IN REHABILITATION

SUSAN L. MICHLOVITZ, M.S., P.T.
EDITOR

ASSISTANT PROFESSOR OF ORTHOPEDIC SURGERY
AND REHABILITATION
PROGRAMS IN PHYSICAL THERAPY
HAHNEMANN UNIVERSITY
PHILADELPHIA, PENNSYLVANIA

STEVEN L. WOLF, Ph.D., P.T.
EDITOR-IN-CHIEF

ASSOCIATE PROFESSOR
DEPARTMENT OF REHABILITATION MEDICINE
EMORY UNIVERSITY SCHOOL OF MEDICINE
ATLANTA, GEORGIA

F. A. DAVIS COMPANY Philadelphia

CONTEMPORARY PERSPECTIVES IN REHABILITATION
VOLUME 1, THERMAL AGENTS IN REHABILITATION

Second printing, 1986
Third printing, 1987

Printed in the United States of America

The authors and the editors of this book have made every effort to ensure that all heat, cold, and laser agents that are recommended are in accordance with accepted standards at the time of publication. The agents specified within this book may not have specific approval by the Food and Drug Administration (FDA) in regard to the indications and dosages that are recommended by the editors and/or the authors. The manufacturers' product literature and the FDA are the best sources of current usage information.

Library of Congress Cataloging-in-Publication Data
Main entry under title:

Thermal agents in rehabilitation.

(Contemporary perspectives in rehabilitation; v. 1)
Includes bibliographies and index.
1. Cold—Therapeutic use. 2. Thermotherapy.
3. Physical therapy. I. Michlovitz, Susan L. II. Wolf, Steven L. III. Series. [DNLM: 1. Cold—therapeutic use. 2. Heat—therapeutic use. 3. Rehabilitation—methods. WB 469 T411]
RM863.T48 1986 615.8'329 85-16122
ISBN 0-8036-6164-9

TO ELEANOR JANE CARLIN FOR PROVIDING ME WITH
MY FIRST OPPORTUNITY AS A P.T. STUDENT
AND AS A FACULTY MEMBER

FOREWORD

Over 2 years ago, Sue Michlovitz shared with me her concerns about allied health care curricula. In particular, she was distressed about the uncritical manner in which topics such as "thermal agents" were taught and about the counterproductive effect such instruction might have on clinical decision making. Sue worried that students were not urged to appreciate the need for formulating sound reasons for using thermal agents, and stated her belief that clinicians usually made a limp appeal to tradition, patient/physician expectations, or simply expedience when asked to justify these modalities. Our discussion also touched on the fear that the health care community might develop a general perception of physical therapy as a "shake and bake" approach to patient treatment, indifferent to careful assessment of the indications or contraindications for these treatments. We agreed that such an attitude could not be allowed to develop, because it would retard any progress among clinicians toward independent clinical decision making.

At the same time, the text *Clinical Decision Making in Physical Therapy* had become a reality, and the development of a *Contemporary Perspectives in Rehabilitation (CPR)* series was well beyond the planning stages. *Clinical Decision Making* emphasized the need for developing sound treatment rationales in physical therapy, while *CPR* was to be an ongoing series of books focusing on using documentation and problem solving formats in rehabilitation. A logical union existed, therefore, between the *CPR* concept and Sue Michlovitz's concern that traditional instruction on thermal agents centered on action and psychomotor performance without due consideration for treatment rationale. Vigor, unabated enthusiasm and persistence subsequently characterized her preparation of this book and marks it as the first volume in the CPR series.

Indeed, this text occupies a unique place in the realm of information on thermal agents. The presentations are contemporary, explaining novel as well as traditional equipment in such a way that the reader is addressed as both a service provider and purchaser. Readers are urged to think and problem solve, and, unlike other texts on this subject, this book stresses the importance and relevance of thermal applications within a framework of documented findings.

The contributions are remarkably sensitive to this book's potentially large body of readers; for example, generalists, sports physical therapists, orthopedic specialists, and home health providers. Throughout, the presentation of data and problem-solving formats address the reader as someone who will resist an indiscriminate application of a thermal agent or device.

Most notably, this text will find a secured place among physical therapy educational programs. The format is well within the grasp of undergraduate physical therapy students, but the content is geared to focus on the direction taken by the professional—problem-solving integrated with supportive documentation.

Therefore, this text is intended for conscientious allied health students and clinicians who believe that the use of thermal agents is predicated on sound judgment, demonstrated efficiency, and quantitative documentation. There is little doubt that the professional seeking these components for supportive rationales in the application of thermal agents will find this book a source of enlightenment.

Steven L. Wolf, PhD, PT
Series Editor

PREFACE

Thermal agents are used in physical therapy and rehabilitation to reduce pain, to enhance healing, and to improve motion. The physical therapist should have a solid foundation in the normal physiologic control of the cardiovascular and neuromuscular systems prior to using an agent that can alter the function of these structures. In addition, a background in the physiology of healing mechanisms and of pain serves as a basis for the rationale of using thermal agents.

Often, the decision to include a thermal agent in a therapy plan or to have the thermal agent *be* the sole treatment rendered (as in the case of the frequently used "hot packs and ultrasound combination" for back pain) is based on empirical evidence. The purpose of this book is to provide the reader with the underlying rationale for selection of an agent to be included in a therapy program, based on (1) the known physiologic and physical effects of that agent; (2) the safety and use of the heat/cold agent, given the conditions and limitations of the patient's dysfunction; and (3) the therapeutic goals for that particular patient. The authors have been asked to review critically the literature available that documents efficacy and effectiveness of each thermal agent. A problem-solving approach to the use of thermal agents is stressed throughout the text.

The primary audience for this text is the physical therapist. The student will gain a solid foundation in thermal agents, the clinician will strengthen his or her perspective of thermal agents, and the researcher is given information that will provide ideas for clinical studies on thermal agents. Athletic trainers and other professionals who use thermal agents in their practice should find this text of value.

The text is in three parts. Part I, Foundations for the Use of Thermal Agents, includes information from basic and medical sciences that can serve as a framework for the choice to include thermal agents in a rehabilitation program. A discussion of the proposed mechanisms by which heat and cold can alter inflammation, healing, and pain is included in these chapters.

Part II of the text, Instrumentation: Methods and Application, incorporates concepts of equipment selection, operation and maintenance, and clinical application. The leading chapter in this part is on instrumentation principles and serves to introduce concepts of electrical circuitry and safety as applied to equipment used for thermal therapy. Physical therapists have become responsible for product purchase and making recommendations about products through the expansion of consultation services, private practices, sports medicine clinics, extended care facilities, and home health care. Therefore, we must be prepared to engage in dialogue with manufacturers, product distributors, and other colleagues about the safety and quality of these products. To this end, some practical suggestions are provided in Chapter 3, intended to assist with purchase decisions.

Chapters 4 through 8 discuss the operation and application of heat and cold agents. Numerous principles of clinical decision making are included within each chapter. There are certain principles that are inherent to all agent applications: (1) The patient must be evaluated and treatment goals established; (2) contraindications to treatment must be known; and (3) the safe and effective use of equipment must be understood.

Chapter 9, on low-power laser, deviates somewhat from the overall theme of thermal agents. Low-power laser is not expected to produce an increase in tissue temperature, so its effects could not be attributed to thermal mechanisms. Therefore, this cannot be categorized as a thermal agent. However, I believe this topic is worthy of inclusion in this text because (1) the indications for its use overlap those of thermal agents; (2) laser is a form of non-ionizing radiation as are diathermy and ultrasound, which are used for pain reduction and tissue healing; and (3) laser would most likely be included in a physical therapy student curriculum in the coursework that includes thermal agents. At the time of this writing (Summer 1985), low-power laser is still considered by the U.S. Food and Drug Administration as an investigational device. Only carefully designed clinical studies will help determine the laser's clinical efficacy—perhaps contributing to the body of knowledge needed to change the laser's status from an investigational to an accepted therapeutic product.

Part III, Clinical Decision Making, is designed to assist the student and clinician in integrating basic concepts that have been presented throughout the entire book, emphasizing problem solving and evaluation.

Much information has been published in the medical literature on the effects or clinical results of heat and cold application. Oftentimes, the therapist is called upon to justify the use of a certain modality. A careful review of the research literature may be necessary to provide an explanation for treatment.

There are many areas that require further investigation. For example, contrast baths (alternating heat and cold) are often used in sports medicine clinics. But a careful review of the literature reveals that only scanty information supports the use of contrast baths for any patient population. It is important for the clinician to be able to interpret accurately and to apply the methods and results that are presented in the literature. The inclusion of a chapter (Chapter 10) on techniques for reviewing the literature and establishing a paradigm for clinical studies of thermal agents provides the clinician with such a background on which to build.

Chapters 11 and 12 are devoted to specific patient populations in which thermal agents are commonly used. The chapter on sports medicine is representative of a population with a known cause of injury and predictable course of recovery. The majority of these patients are otherwise healthy. On the other hand, the chapter on rheumatic disease presents a model for a patient population that can be expected to have chronic recurrent—sometimes progressive—dysfunction associated with systemic manifestations.

Two appendices are included—temperature conversion scales (this text uses the centigrade scale); and a list of some of the manufacturers of thermotherapy products in the United States.

SLM
Editor

ACKNOWLEDGMENTS

The completion of a multi-author text requires the hard work, dedication, and coordination of many people. I would like to thank the following people for contributing to this project and for assisting me through its completion:

Each of the 10 contributing authors.

Steve Wolf and Mary Watkins for their encouragement, support, and editorial assistance from the conception through the completion of this text.

The students I have taught at both Hahnemann University and Temple University, whose questions and concerns regarding thermal agents we have addressed. A special thanks to Dorsett Edmunds for her assistance with the literature search for Chapters 4 and 5.

Dean Currier and John Barr for their careful reviews and suggestions of portions of the manuscript.

Wesley L. Nyborg for his corrections and suggestions on therapeutic ultrasound.

Sue Giangrasso for her endless typing and retyping of the manuscript at all hours of the day and night.

Bill McBeth and Bill Holl for photography of some of the clinical pictures in Chapters 3 through 7.

The staff at F. A. Davis for their support. Another special thanks to Phyllis Spagnolo for her careful and precise artwork.

My colleagues at Hahnemann University—especially our Program Director, Risa Granick—for their encouragement during the time I worked on this book.

SLM
Editor

CONTRIBUTORS

JOSEPH A. KLEINKORT, M.A., P.T.

President, Chronic Pain Associates, P.C.
4499 Medical Drive, Suite 380
San Antonio, Texas

LUTHER C. KLOTH, P.T., M.S.

Associate Professor
Program in Physical Therapy
Marquette University
Milwaukee, Wisconsin

SUSAN L. MICHLOVITZ, M.S., P.T.—EDITOR

Assistant Professor of Orthopedic Surgery and Rehabilitation
Programs in Physical Therapy
Hahnemann University
Philadelphia, Pennsylvania

ROBERTA A. NEWTON, Ph.D., P.T.

Associate Professor
Department of Physical Therapy
Medical College of Virginia/VCU
Richmond, Virginia

H. T. M. RITTER, III, B.A., C.B.E.T.

Project Engineer
ECRI
Plymouth Meeting, Pennsylvania

LAURENCE M. SEITZ, M.S., R.P.T.

President
Rehabilitation Performance Center
Elizabeth, New Jersey

WAYNE S. SMITH, M.Ed., R.P.T., A.T.C.

U.S. Public Health Service
Currently Chief Therapist–Athletic Trainer, USCG
Alameda, California

MARK T. WALSH, P.T., M.S.

Director Hand and Orthopedic Rehabilitation Services
"A physical therapy practice"
Levittown, Pennsylvania

MARY P. WATKINS, M.S., P.T.

Assistant Professor of Orthopedic Surgery and Rehabilitation
Programs in Physical Therapy
Hahnemann University
Philadelphia, Pennsylvania

STEVEN L. WOLF, Ph.D., P.T.—EDITOR-IN-CHIEF

Associate Professor
Department of Rehabilitation Medicine
Emory University School of Medicine
Atlanta, Georgia

VINCENT J. ZARRO, M.D., Ph.D

Associate Professor of Pharmacology and Medicine
Hahnemann University
Philadelphia, Pennsylvania

MARVIN C. ZISKIN, M.D., M.S., Bm.E.

Professor of Radiology and Medical Physics
Temple University Medical School
Philadelphia, Pennsylvania

CONTENTS

PART 1

FOUNDATIONS FOR THE USE OF THERMAL AGENTS

CHAPTER 1

MECHANISMS OF INFLAMMATION AND REPAIR

VINCENT ZARRO, M.D., PH.D.

Inflammation is the term applied to a series of reactions by vascularized tissue in response to an injury. The purpose of the inflammatory reaction is to attempt to control the effects of the injurious agent and return the tissue to a normal state. Obviously, such a reaction in itself is not a disease and in fact is necessary for survival.

Healing of an accidental laceration of the skin or of a surgical incision is an example of the beneficial effects of the inflammatory reaction. In some cases, however, inflammation is part of a disease process without apparent benefit. Rheumatoid arthritis is an example of such a disease in which there is an inflammatory state causing injury to joints. In this disease, the synovial membrane lining the joint becomes inflamed. As the disease progresses, the inflamed synovium causes destruction of the articular cartilage (Fig. 1–1). In cases when inflammation is harmful, therapy such as thermal agents or medications is used to control the process, thus facilitating return of function.

Nearly 2000 years ago, Celsius first described the four signs associated with inflammation: swelling, heat, redness, and pain. Later another characteristic, loss of function, was added and these five signs came to be called the "cardinal signs of inflammation." A carbuncle or "boil" occurring in the skin as a reaction to invasion by bacteria is a good example of the cardinal signs of inflammation.

Once the inflammatory reaction has stopped, or at least has sealed off the injurious agent, it attempts to repair the injured tissue and return it to its normal state. This latter part of the reaction is known as healing or repair. Unfortunately, not all repair ends in restoration of normal tissue. If the injury is large or occurs in certain tissues, such as the brain, scar replaces normal tissue and loss of function occurs.

Inflammation then includes all the steps involved from injury to repair or healing. In this chapter, these various steps causing inflammation, as well as factors modifying this process, are discussed.

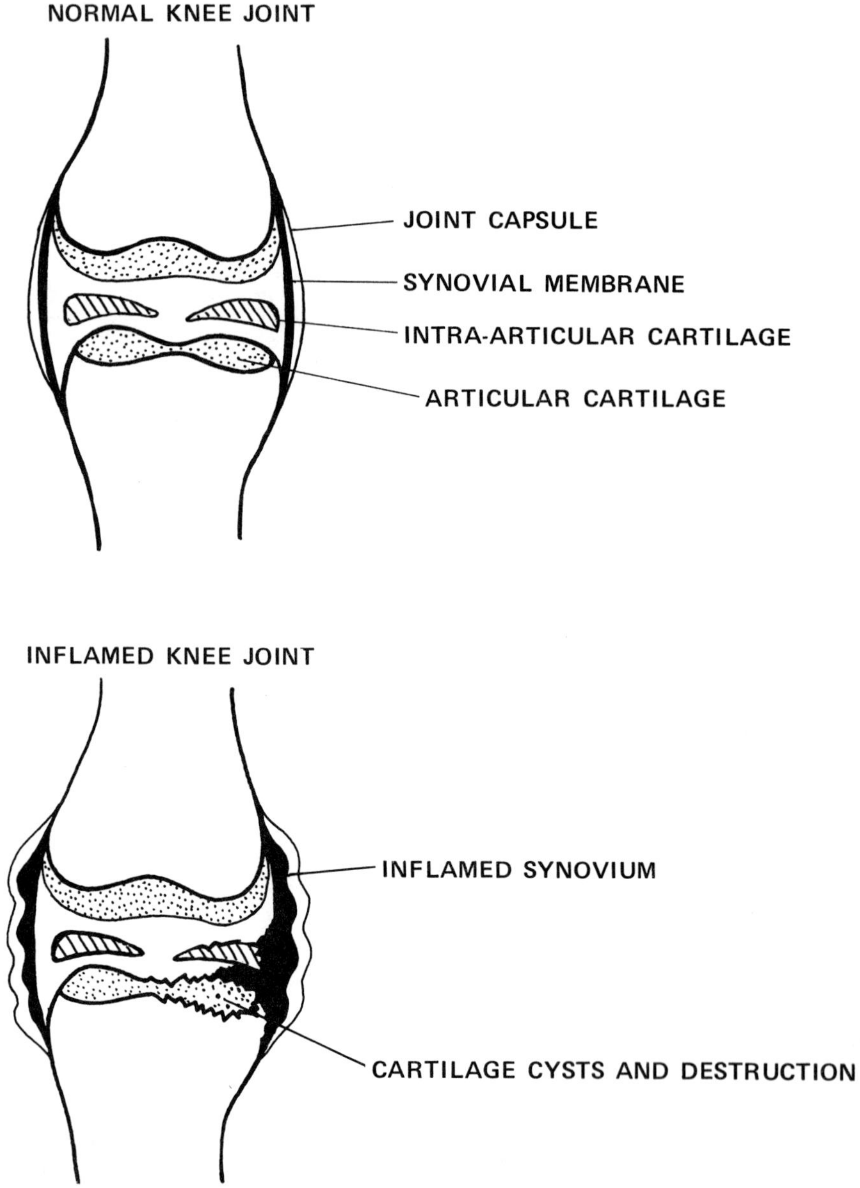

FIGURE 1–1

Comparison of inflamed and normal synovial membrane. Ongoing chronic inflammation of the synovial membrane grows over the articular cartilage in rheumatoid arthritis and causes destruction of the joint.

THE INFLAMMATORY PROCESS

The inflammatory process involves two large series of events. The first events are changes in the local circulation of blood, known as hemodynamic changes, and the second events occur at various cellular levels.[1] In recent years, there has been a focus of research activity on substances involved in initiating and controlling the inflammatory process. These substances are collectively called mediators.[2]

For purposes of discussion, the hemodynamic events, cellular events, and mediators will be considered under separate headings. In reality, however, no clear separation can be made between the hemodynamic and cellular events as the inflammatory process proceeds. The mediators are involved in virtually all the stages.

Hemodynamic Events

Inflammation begins when an agent (injury) causes a disruption in the normal physiology of a tissue. Table 1–1 lists some common causes of injury that will trigger inflammation. Although the inflammatory reaction follows the same pathway regardless of the etiology of the injury, some causes will tend to emphasize certain events. For example, anoxia (such as occurs in peripheral vascular disease) tends to form dry necrotic tissues, whereas bacterial invasion causes pus formation.

Once injury occurs, there is a rapid vasoconstriction of arterioles lasting a few seconds, followed by vasodilation. The vasodilation causes an increase in the amount of blood that accumulates in capillaries and a rise in mean intercapillary pressure.

Mediators have a profound effect on arteriolar caliber as well as a direct effect on the capillary wall. In general, norepinephrine causes vasoconstriction; histamine, bradykinin, and prostaglandins cause vasodilation. The study of the effects of mediators on the circulation, however, is complex because of the interactions with each other as well as reflex changes.[3] It is clear, though, that the first event to occur in inflammation is arteriolar dilation with a resultant increase in intercapillary volume and pressure. This, together with a direct effect of some mediators on the capillary wall, leads to extravasation of fluid into the interstitial tissue.

At this relatively early point, however, the permeability of the capillary membrane remains only slightly altered and therefore no protein or cells escape. This edema fluid, which collects in the extravascular space, is called a *transudate* and consists mainly of water and dissolved electrolytes. It is clear in appearance, contains very few cells, and has a specific gravity under 1.012.

TABLE 1–1
Some Common Causes of Injury Producing Inflammation

Trauma (e.g., sprains)	Burns
Bone fractures	Autoimmune diseases
Foreign bodies	Rheumatoid arthritis
Bacterial invasion	Systemic lupus erythematosus
Decreased blood supply	Polymyositis
Bacteria and fungi	

As the capillaries remain dilated, with an increase in the volume of blood and an increase in the intercapillary pressure, a series of events occurs involving blood cells. The blood cells flow at a slower rate and have a tendency to move toward and adhere to the capillary walls, a process called *margination.* At the same time, mediators released into the area cause an increase in the permeability of the capillary walls. The combination of margination of the white blood cells and increased capillary permeability causes the cells to migrate through the opened capillary pores into the surrounding tissue. This outflow of cells from the intravascular to the extravascular space is called *emigration.*

Another factor favoring the movement of leukocytes is the secretion of chemical substances with the ability to attract them. These chemicals, known as *chemotactic factors,* are discussed in the section on mediators. The increase in capillary permeability also causes the lower molecular weight proteins of the blood to escape into the tissue. The edema fluid, which was at first clear, now becomes more viscous (owing to the protein) and cloudy (owing to the leukocytes). The specific gravity rises to over 1.012 and the fluid is called an *exudate.* When an exudate contains considerable numbers of leukocytes, it is commonly called *pus.* A diagrammatic representation of these events is presented in Figure 1–2.

Usually, only leukocytes are seen in an exudate, but if the inflammatory reaction is very intense, red blood cells may also emigrate. The amount of fluid escaping from the capillaries into the surrounding tissue is dependent on differences in pressure between the intravascular (capillary) hydrostatic pressure and the intravascular oncotic pressure. Physiologically, the intravascular pressure at the arteriolar end of the capillary is greater than the tissue pressure, so fluid, nutrients, and oxygen pass into the tissue. At the venule end, the oncotic pressure in the capillary is higher than the intravascular hydrostatic pressure, so fluid and waste products enter the capillary. Any upset in the integrity of the capillary or any pressure changes will produce edema. For example, in congestive heart failure there is an increase in systemic venous pressure. This increased pressure is reflected back into venules, thereby increasing capillary pressure. Less fluid is reabsorbed from the tissue into the capillary, and edema results. In the inflammatory reaction, a series of events occur leading to edema.

The presence of edema for long periods, especially if it occurs in an area of poor circulation such as in peripheral vascular disease, will interfere with proper oxygenation. The so-called stasis ulcers, common in peripheral vascular disease, heal poorly in the presence of persistent edema.

Cellular Events

The names and quantities of circulating blood cells are listed in Table 1–2. Leukocytes are involved in all types of inflammation. Monocytes, when they emigrate from the capillary into the tissue, have the ability to transform themselves into large cells called *macrophages.* These cells have a remarkable phagocytic potential and can engulf large amounts of bacterial and cellular

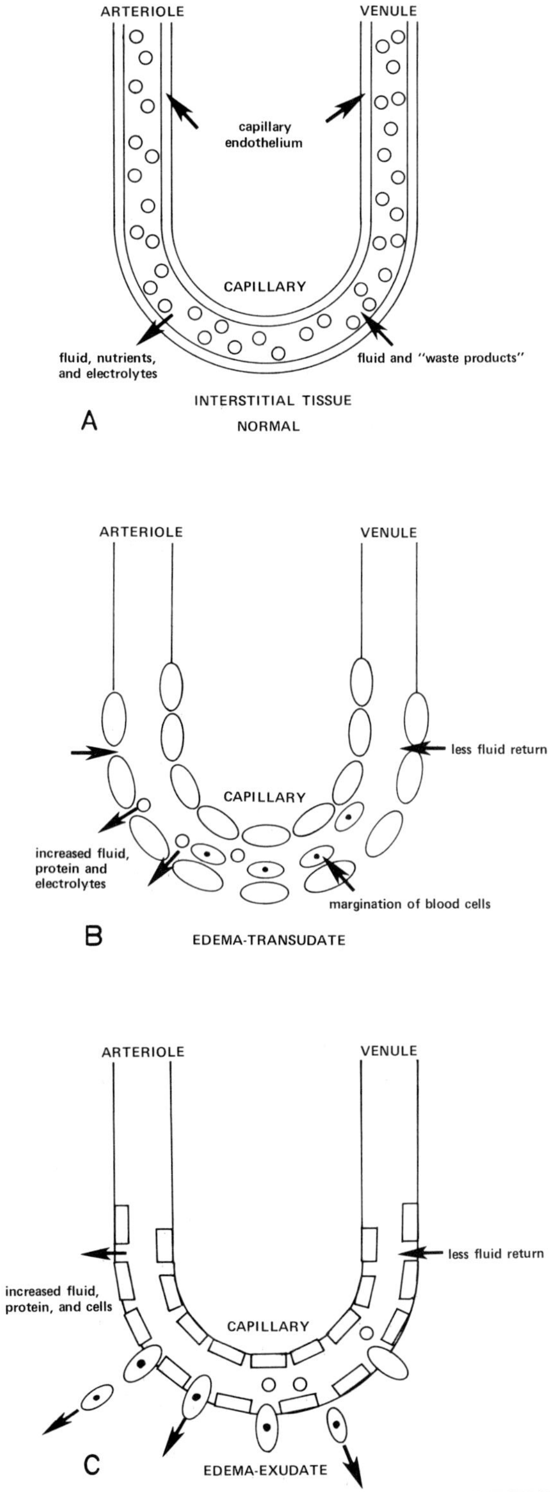

FIGURE 1–2

Diagrammatic representation of the production of edema. *A, Normal:* The intravascular and extravascular (tissue) pressures are such that there is an outward movement at the arteriolar end and inward movement at the venule end. *B, Transudate:* In response to injury, mediators are produced, arterioles dilate, blood volume and pressure in the capillaries increases, outward filtration increases, and edema forms. Blood cells marginate. *C, Exudate:* As inflammation becomes more intense, neutrophils and other blood cells emigrate into the surrounding tissue to form thick edema fluid (pus).

TABLE 1–2
Circulating Blood Cells and Approximate Number Per Cubic Millimeter*

	Approximate Number of Cells Per mm^3	Approximate Percentage
Red blood cells	5,000,000	—
Total leukocytes	6,000	100
Neutrophil	3,300	55
Lymphocyte	2,100	35
Monocyte	420	7
Basophil	60	1
Eosinophil	120	2

* Leukocytes are also given as percentage of each type cell.

debris. Macrophages are formed only in the tissue and do not circulate freely in the blood.

Once the neutrophil leaves the bloodstream and arrives at the site of injury, it begins its action immediately. This cell is mobile and phagocytizes bacterial and other debris. It contains granules rich in a variety of enzymes called *lysozymes,* which function to digest engulfed particles. As some neutrophils disintegrate, the enzymes are released into the tissue. These chemicals perpetuate the inflammatory reaction by acting as irritants, and they also have chemotactic activity, attracting other leukocytes into the area of inflammation. The monocytes and macrophages engulf large quantities of debris and are known as *scavenger cells.* By and large, the basophil and eosinophil are mostly involved only in certain types of inflammation.

The lymphocytes play the largest role in inflammation involving the immune reaction. This is a more sustained type of reaction known as chronic inflammation. For example, an inflammation of the liver (hepatitis) caused by sensitivity to a drug is characterized by large numbers of eosinophils in the liver biopsy. Systemic lupus erythematosus is a disorder characterized by chronic inflammation in various organs, caused by an antigen-antibody reaction. The characteristic cell type in tissue biopsy in this disease is the lymphocyte.

Mediators of Inflammation

In general, the body controls all physiologic functions either by nerve stimulation (for example, walking) or by release of a chemical substance (for example, control of metabolism by thyroid hormone). Ultimately, even nervous system control involves chemicals (release of acetylcholine at the neuromuscular junction). It is not surprising then that a variety of chemical substances is involved in initiating and controlling the inflammatory reaction.

PROSTAGLANDINS. Starting with the observation in 1930 that human semen will cause contractions of the uterus, experiments over the years have clarified the role of a group of chemicals called prostaglandins. Originally thought to be produced only by the prostate gland (thus the name, prostaglandins), it is now known that these chemicals are produced by virtually all the cells of the body.

Prostaglandins are produced by a complex series of reactions initiated when the integrity of the cell membrane is altered by an injury. When this occurs, the phospholipid of the cell membrane releases a substance called arachidonic acid. The arachidonic acid is converted by enzymes called cyclo-oxygenases to intermediary compounds, which then form prostaglandins. In addition, chemically related compounds called thromboxanes are formed.

In a similar manner, arachidonic acid may be acted on by another enzyme, lipoxygenase, to form another series of compounds called leukotrienes. The various prostaglandins, thromboxanes, and leukotrienes are all chemically related. They are identified by letters and numbers and are involved in a variety of physiologic functions. For example, prostaglandin E_2 (PGE_2) causes fever, thromboxane A_2 (TXA_2) causes aggregation of platelets, and so forth.

The role of prostaglandins in pain production seems to be more indirect. Prostaglandin I_2 (PGI_2) and PGE_2 in themselves do not cause pain but are synergistic with bradykinin and probably histamine when injected together; that is, the pain produced by a certain dose of bradykinin is more intense in the presence of the prostaglandins. A summary of prostaglandin production is given in Figure 1–3.

In summary, the prostaglandins and related thromboxanes and leukotrienes formed in response to cell injury are involved in virtually all steps of inflammation. It is interesting to note that both the anti-inflammatory steroids such as prednisone and the nonsteroidal anti-inflammatory agents (for example, aspirin) affect the production of prostaglandins. The steroids stabilize cell membranes and the nonsteroidal anti-inflammatory drugs inhibit cyclo-oxygenase activity.

Not all prostaglandins produce inflammation. Some are involved physiologically in maintaining organ integrity. Prostaglandins, for example, are necessary for proper kidney function and for normal mucus production in the stomach. Interference with their action, such as occurs with the use of nonsteroidal anti-inflammatory drugs, may cause renal insufficiency or gastric ulcer formation.

COMPLEMENT. Complement, or more accurately the complement system, consists of a series of proteins that are activated by either immune complexes or a variety of chemicals, such as bacterial endotoxins. The activated components are involved in many steps of the inflammatory reaction. For example, one activated component increases vascular permeability, another attracts white blood cells, another causes cell lysis, and so forth.

BLOOD COAGULATION. At least two components in the blood coagulation scheme are involved in inflammation. Activation of factor XII (Hageman factor) through the fibrinolytic system produces plasmin, which can activate certain complement components. Activation of factor XII by the kinin sys-

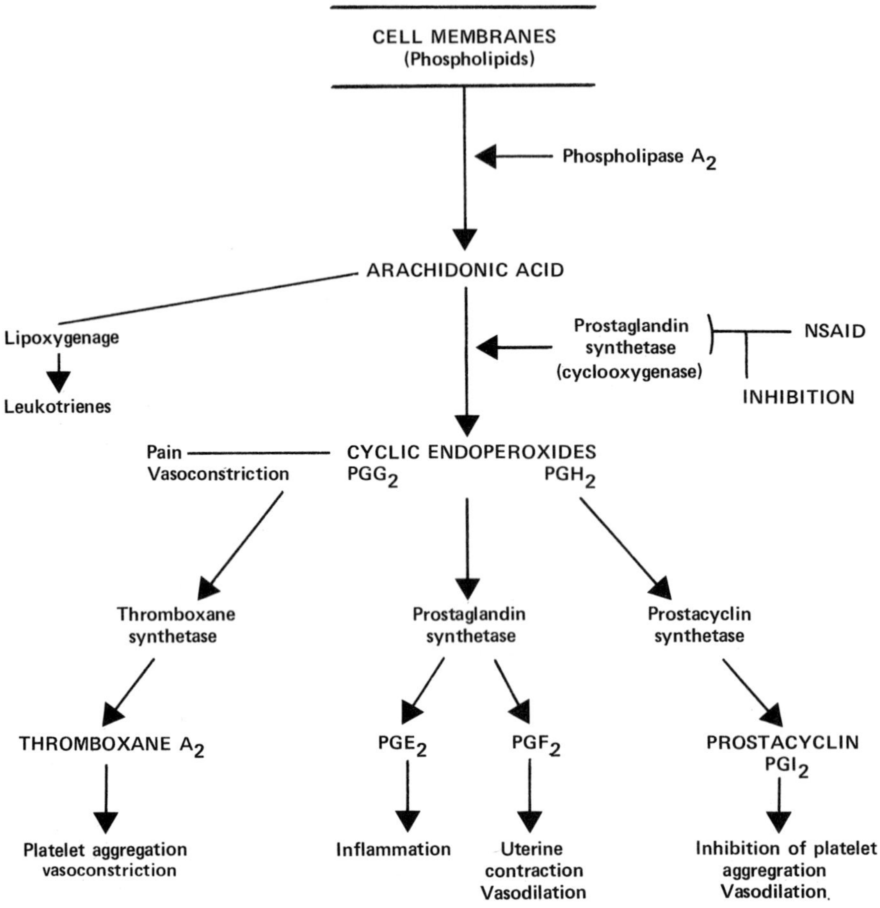

FIGURE 1–3

Pathway of synthesis of prostaglandins and site of NSAID inhibition of cyclooxygenase. (Adapted from Nikander, McMahoon, and Ridolfo: *Non-steroidal anti-inflammatory agents.* Ann Rev Pharmacol Toxicol 19:469, 1979.)

tem produces bradykinin. As mentioned earlier, bradykinin is probably the most important mediator in pain production.

OTHERS. Histamine and serotonin are stored in a variety of cells in the body. When released in response to injury, they have a profound effect on the microcirculation. Histamine causes a profound dilation of arterioles and also an increase in capillary permeability.

Chemicals within the neutrophil (proteases) and the lymphocyte (lymphokines), released when the cell disintegrates, have effects on the microcirculation and migration of cells.

In summary, many chemical substances formed in the body are involved in initiating and controlling the inflammatory reaction. Their roles are interrelated and vary according to the etiology and intensity of the reaction. Their study is important because potentially their action may be altered by drugs or thermal agents.

HEALING OR REPAIR

Theoretically, the endpoint of the inflammatory reaction is to return the injured tissue to its former state. In reality, this rarely occurs completely. Two tissues are involved in repair. The first is the characteristic cell of the injured tissue and the second is the connective tissue cell. Cells may be classified according to their ability to regenerate. Those with the greatest potential are called *labile cells.* These include cells of the skin, lining of the gastrointestinal tract, and blood. The next group, called *stabile cells,* has the ability to regenerate but to a lesser extent and more slowly than the labile cells. In this group are cells of the liver, bones, and kidney. *Permanent cells* have no regenerative ability. The nerve cells and cells of skeletal and cardiac muscle are in this group. Current thought suggests that these cells may be suppressed by certain factors, rather than possessing an intrinsic inability to regenerate. From a clinical point of view, however, it is true that nervous tissue and cardiac and skeletal muscle do not regenerate. In reference to skeletal muscle, dramatic changes in size may be seen. Atrophy occurs with decreased use, and hypertrophy occurs with exercise. These changes, however, are due to the size of each cell and not to a change in the number of cells.

Connective Tissue

Connective tissue consists of cells and the proteins they synthesize. In effect, it is the "cement" substance of the body, occupying all spaces not occupied by other tissue. The characteristic cell of connective tissue is the *fibroblast.* Other more specialized cells, such as the *osteoblast* and *chondroblast,* are also connective tissue cells. The proteins of connective tissue are collagen, elastin, and reticulin. Collagen is the most abundant protein in the body. Collagen fibers consist of many long collagen molecules having a molecular weight of 285,000. There are at least three different types of collagen, depending on the amino acid content of the molecule. The collagen in bone, tendon, and cartilage differ, depending on the quantity of the different types of amino acids in the molecule.

Although not classified as a connective tissue cell, the capillary endothelial cell is also very important in the healing and repair stages of inflammation. Especially in chronic inflammation, there is a proliferation of endothelial cells that, when extensive, is referred to as *neovascularization.* This process may serve to perpetuate inflammation. If it interferes with the integrity of normal tissue, function is markedly affected. Neovascularization of the retina of the eye in diabetic retinopathy, for example, may lead to blindness.

When healing occurs, fibroblasts of connective tissue "fill in" where the primary tissue cells cannot. Fibroblasts grow into the area of injury and produce collagen. As the collagen contracts, a scar is produced. Full contraction of the scar may take several months. How much of the final result of the healing process will consist of normal cells and how much will consist of scar depends on a variety of factors. A small skin laceration will have virtually no scar, because the cells have excellent regenerative potential. An inflammation in the liver (hepatitis) will result in good regeneration of liver cells and some scar tissue (fibrosis). If the insult was very great, however, the amount of fibrosis will interfere with liver function.

Finally, injury to nervous tissue (such as occurs in a stroke), to heart muscle (myocardial infarction), or to skeletal muscle is totally repaired with scar tissue. This scar tissue, of course, is devoid of any normal function.

STAGES OF INFLAMMATION AND REPAIR

As was stated earlier, the inflammatory reaction consists of various stages, each blending into the next. It is important, however, from a physical therapy point of view, to make a judgment about the predominant event that is occurring at a particular time. One can consider three stages of inflammation and repair. Stage 1 begins with microvascular dilation and neutrophilic infiltration and continues with macrophagic formation and capillary endothelial proliferation. This stage begins immediately and lasts 1 to 2 weeks. Stage 2 begins in the middle of the first week and is greatest during the second week. This stage is characterized by fibroblastic infiltration and collagen formation; the tissue produced at this stage is called granulation tissue, or scar. Stage 3 begins at the end of the second week and is characterized by the start of contraction of the scar. During this stage, the vascularity becomes less and the tensile strength of the collagen increases. The process may continue for a year or more.

The preceding time sequence is accurate for clean wounds in which the edges are in good contact—for example, a surgical incision. If the wound is infected or is due to a crush injury, or if the edges of the wound are separated, the process takes considerably longer. In addition, the scar (granulation tissue) in these wounds is greater, and contraction may not result in a small scar with good tensile strength. There are considerable individual differences in the degree of scar tissue formed. Younger people have a tendency to form more scar than do elderly people. Formation of a large hypertrophic scar is called a *keloid.*

Normally, contraction of the scar does not produce deleterious effects. In certain surgical procedures or wounds (ligaments), severe contraction may interfere with function. If splints are applied to skin-grafted wounds for the first 14 days postsurgically, considerably less scar contraction occurs.[4]

Chronic Inflammation

Except for contraction of the scar, the acute inflammation reaction is virtually complete in 2 weeks. If the reaction continues for 1 month, it is called subacute inflammation. If it continues for months or years, it is called chronic inflammation. Chronic inflammation may occur as an extension of acute inflammation such as may occur if a joint is repeatedly traumatized.

More often, however, chronic inflammation represents a reaction to certain stimuli and differs considerably from acute inflammation. Invasion of lung tissue by the tuberculosis organism does not cause the reaction characterized by the cardinal signs of inflammation. Instead, the body reacts to the hard coating of the organism by surrounding it with lymphocytes and monocytes. Macrophages are formed, and these cells with ingested debris attempt to seal off the organism and confine it to one area. The predominant cells involved in chronic inflammation are the lymphocyte, monocyte, and macrophage. This difference is profound compared with acute inflammation, where the major cell type is the neutrophil.

Another major difference between acute and chronic inflammation is fibroblastic proliferation. As the chronic process continues, more fibroblasts are formed, more collagen is produced, and scar formation becomes extensive. In chronic inflammation, therefore, the usual result is replacement of normal tissue with scar even in organs that have the ability to regenerate. Rheumatoid arthritis is a dramatic example of chronic inflammation. In this disorder, for unknown reasons, the synovial membrane becomes inflamed and causes repeated damage to the cartilage lining of the bone. In contrast, gout is an acute synovitis caused by the deposition of sodium urate crystals in a joint. Although producing an intense inflammation, the joint returns to normal in about 3 weeks even with no treatment. Little, if any, permanent damage occurs.

In summary, chronic inflammation differs dramatically from acute inflammation in that in the former, the process continues for months or years. In chronic inflammation, the predominant cell types are the monocyte, lymphocyte, and macrophage, and fibroblastic proliferation and scar formation are greater.

FACTORS MODIFYING INFLAMMATION AND REPAIR

A number of factors may modify all or some of the steps in the inflammatory reaction. Table 1–3 lists some of the common factors that may affect inflammation. Some have a profound effect. For example, inadequate blood

TABLE 1–3
Factors Modifying Inflammation

Age
Nutritional status
Anemia
Hormone deficiencies
Diabetes
Peripheral vascular disease
Drugs (glucocorticoids)
Presence of foreign bodies
Extent of wound
Type of injury
Tissue injured
Thermal agents (heat, cold)

supply such as occurs in peripheral vascular disease may prevent any wound healing from taking place.

As stated in the beginning of this chapter, the inflammatory reaction is necessary for survival but, as part of a disease process, it may produce disability. When the inflammatory reaction is harmful, therapy is aimed at stopping or at least minimizing it. Two physical agents that can modify the inflammatory reaction are heat and cold.

Thermal Agents

The experimental study of the effects of heat and cold on the inflammatory reaction has yielded conflicting data. At this time it is not possible to extrapolate the experimental results to clinical states.

The effects of heat and cold in experimentally induced inflammation were extensively studied by Schmidt and co-workers and summarized in a review article.[5] Edema was induced by the established experimental methods of injecting substances into rat paws and measuring the degree of swelling. Dextran, carrageenan, kaolin, and formalin were used. Each represents a somewhat different type of inflammation, but carrageenan correlates best with human inflammatory arthritis disease. In addition, adjuvant arthritis, tuberculin reaction, and granuloma ring test were studied as representatives of more chronic arthritis involving antigen-antibody reaction.

Heat was either administered as whole body hyperthermia or applied to the paws and tail only. This local application, however, also caused a rise in the body temperature of the animals. Cold was applied as whole body hypothermia. Results are summarized in Figure 1–4. It is obvious that the effects of heat or cold vary according not only to the agent used but also to the various stages in the production of inflammation. This may certainly explain the conflicting clinical data on the value of heat or cold. Outcomes may vary according to the method of application, time, disease state, stage of disease, and many other factors.

TYPE OF INFLAMMATION	HEAT	COLD
ACUTE	AGGRAVATED	DEPRESSED
CHRONIC	DEPRESSED	—
PROSTAGLANDIN PRODUCTION	—	AGGRAVATED

FIGURE 1–4
The effects of heat and cold on inflammation.

From the preceding experiments, one can conclude that cold or heat can either inhibit or enhance inflammation. Heat inhibits experimental inflammation, which is a model of chronic inflammation. Cold acts to inhibit mainly the more acute types of inflammation.

In contrast, studies of the effect of cold on prostaglandin production showed an enhancement of production and action.[6]

In other types of inflammation, such as sodium urate crystal deposition in the dog knee, heat had a beneficial effect.[7] Sodium urate crystals cause acute gout, and the inflammation produced is a good example of acute inflammation. On the other hand, Harris and McCroskery studied the effect of temperature on degradation of cartilage by rheumatoid synovium and found a marked increase in damage with elevated temperature.[8,9] It would seem that any increase in joint temperature would increase cartilage destruction in patients with rheumatoid arthritis.[10]

In a histologic study, Farry and co-workers[11] applied cold to radiocarpal ligament injuries in the pig. Whereas there was an increase in edema (swelling) of the treated area, there was a decrease in the number of polymorphonuclear cells and lymphocytes. This study gives good experimental reasons for the common clinical practice following ice treatment with elevation and a compression bandage.

In summary, experimental studies of the effects of heat and cold on inflammation have yielded conflicting results. This is not surprising, considering the complexity of the inflammatory reaction and inability to design accurate experiments to quantitate a particular step.

Immobilization

In contrast to heat and cold, there is good experimental evidence that immobilization, especially when combined with good surgical repair, produces faster healing with a better end result. Frank and associates[12] showed that injury to the medial collateral ligament in rabbit knees, allowed to heal without repair or immobilization, healed much more slowly than did those of control subjects.

The best healing in complete Achilles tendon lacerations in rabbits occurred when the ends were sutured and immobilization with splints was continued for at least 7 days.[13]

However, immobilization does not always produce a good result when applied indiscriminately. In dogs with tendon lacerations, immobilization only, compared with immobilization and early controlled passive motion, produced poorer end results. This was especially true if immobilization was carried out for 12 weeks or more.[14,15]

Position of a limb during immobilization also affects the end result. In a study of Colles' fractures, application of a cast with the forearm in pronation produced better results than other positions of rotation.

It also cannot be assumed that immobilization is good for all injuries. In fractures of the ulnar shaft the application of a cast produced healing in 10.5 weeks, whereas no cast or a splint for only 2 weeks produced healing in 6.7 weeks.[16]

Changes in the biochemistry of connective tissue also occur with immobilization. Since fibroblast activity and connective tissue are so intimately involved in the healing process, it is logical to believe that these changes will also affect wound healing. In studies on synovial joints of various animal species, immobilization for up to 9 weeks materially affected the biochemistry of connective tissue. Grossly, there was excessive deposition of tissue in all areas of the joint. With time, this tissue formed scar and produced adhesions.

Biochemically, there is a decrease in the water, hyaluronic acid, and glycosaminoglycans content of the connective tissue. These changes lead to an abnormal cross-linking of collagen fibers and decrease in elasticity. Therefore, immobilization causes an increased amount of abnormal collagen with poor function.[17,18]

In summary, there is good experimental evidence that *in general* immobilization produces faster healing with a better end result. Length of time over which immobilization is beneficial varies according to the type of injury.

SUMMARY

The inflammatory process is a complex event involving local hemodynamic changes, as well as profound cellular events. In addition, mediators are involved in all stages of inflammation.

In cases when inflammation becomes part of a disease process, therapy is directed at attenuating it as much as possible. A variety of physical therapy measures will affect experimental inflammation, but extrapolation of beneficial effects in a particular clinical state is not always possible.

REFERENCES

1. Robbins, LR and Cotran, RS: *Pathologic Basis of Disease.* WB Saunders, Philadelphia, 1978, pp 55–140.
2. Moncada, S, Flower, RJ, and Vane, JR: *Prostaglandins, prostacyclin, and thromboxane* A_2. In Gilman, AG, Goodman, ES, and Gilman, A (eds): *The Pharmacological Basis of Therapeutics.* Macmillan, New York, 1980.
3. Haddy, FJ, Scott, JB, and Grega, GJ: *Peripheral circulation: Fluid transfer across the microcirculation.* Int Rev Pharm 9:63, 1976.
4. Peacock, EE: *Wound Repair,* ed 3. WB Saunders, Philadelphia, 1984.
5. Schmidt, KL, et al: *Heat, cold and inflammation.* Rheumatology 38:391, 1979.
6. Chavis, R, Vygantas, AN, and Vygantas, CM: *Experimental inhibition of prostaglandin-like response after cryotherapy.* Am J Ophthalmol 82:310, 1976.
7. Dorwart, BB, Hansell, JR, and Schumacher, HR: *Effects of heat, cold and mechanical agitation of crystal induced arthritis in the dog.* Arthritis Rheum 16:540, 1973.
8. Harris, ED and McCroskery, PA: *The influence of temperature and fibril stability on degradation of cartilage collagen by rheumatoid synovial collagenase.* N Engl J Med 290:1, 1974.
9. Hollander, JL: *Collagenase, cartilage and cortisol.* N Engl J Med 290:50, 1974.
10. Feibel, A and Fast, A: *Deep heating of joints: A Reconsideration.* Arch Phys Med Rehabil 57:513, 1976.
11. Farry, PJ, et al: *Ice treatment of injured ligaments: An experimental model.* New Zealand Med J 12:12, 1980.

12. Frank, C, Amiel, D, and Akesow, WH: *Healing of the medial collateral ligament of the knee. A morphological and biochemical assessment in rabbits.* Acta Orthop Scand 54:1917, 1983.

13. Nystrom, B and Holmlund, D: *Experimental evaluation of immobilization in operative and nonoperative treatment of Achilles tendon rupture. A radiographic study in the rabbit.* Acta Chir Scand 149:669, 1983.

14. Gelberman, RH, et al: *Effects of early intermittent passive immobilization on healing canine flexor tendons.* J Hand Surg 7:170, 1982.

15. Wood, SL, et al: *The importance of controlled passive mobilization on flexor tendon healing. A biochemical study.* Acta Orthop Scand 52:615, 1981.

16. Pollock, FH, et al: *The isolated fracture of the ulnar shaft. Treatment without immobilization.* J Bone Joint Surg 65:339, 1983.

17. Donatelli, R and Owens-Burhart, H: *Effects of immobilization on the extensibility of periarticular connective tissue.* Journal of Orthopaedic and Sports Physical Therapy 3:67, 1981.

18. Akeson, WH, et al: *The connective tissue response to immobility: An accelerated ageing response?* Exp Gerontol 3:289, 1968.

CHAPTER 2

CONTEMPORARY VIEWS ON PAIN AND THE ROLE PLAYED BY THERMAL AGENTS IN MANAGING PAIN SYMPTOMS

ROBERTA A. NEWTON, PH.D., P.T.

Pain is a protective mechanism that alerts the individual to make an appropriate response to prevent further tissue damage. Pain is defined as an unpleasant sensory and emotional experience that is associated with actual or potential tissue damage; or pain may be described in terms of such tissue damage.[1] It is a sensory experience described in quite different terms than other sensory modalities. For example, touch is a peripheral stimulus perceived as a touch sensation, whereas pain is a complex phenomenon described in terms of a pluridimensional theory encompassing a sensory component, emotional component, motor component, and cultural component.

One of every four people in the United States is affected by pain each year. When the pain state outlasts the initial trauma and subsequent recovery period, then the pluridimensional aspect of the pain experience is quite evident. The chronic pain state not only affects the individual experiencing pain but is also physiologically and psychologically draining to the individual's family and close associates. Total cost for treatment of the chronic pain patient and work days lost is tremendous.[2] Estimates in dollars and day loss at work pertain only to those individuals with chronic pain conditions and do not include the acute pain state—that is, headaches, injuries, or the postoperative period. With the increasing cost to remediate pain and the gap in the understanding of normal and chronic pain mechanisms, an Interagency Committee of the United States Government was established to address these issues. Since 1978 the interdisciplinary investigation of pain mechanisms and its remediation has proliferated.

The ability of the clinician to treat appropriately a painful condition is dependent upon a sound clinical problem-solving approach. Such an approach includes an understanding of the normal neurophysiologic mechanisms of pain; knowledge of mechanisms associated with acute, chronic, and referred pain; appropriate assessment techniques; and rationale for the selection of a particular therapy. Furthermore, the clinician needs to analyze critically the literature and use only those reports that have appropriate research design, which includes good documentation of methodology and results. Caution should be taken when extrapolating data from laboratory research to direct patient care.

The purposes of this chapter are (1) to present the current concepts of pain theory; (2) to present theories relating to acute, chronic, and referred pain; (3) to discuss methods for assessing pain; and (4) to provide an overview of the role of thermal agents in pain management. The theories on pain will provide the student and clinician with a basic foundation necessary for those who desire to pursue the literature further. Both review articles and original research articles are included in the reference list.

PAIN THEORIES

Pain theories to date are pluridimensional and multidisciplinary. They can be categorized into three major areas. The sensory-discriminative component serves to analyze the noxious stimulus in terms of its location and intensity. The affective-motivational component includes the emotional responses, goals, desires, and expectations of the individual. The cognitive-evaluative component refers to the process by which the noxious sensation is examined, compared with past experiences, and given meaning in relation to the present and future implications of the pain experience. An individual's reaction to the noxious stimulus is also influenced by cultural connotations. Thus, the response to a noxious stimulus may range from a simple flexion response to more complex escape plans to a very complex psychophysiologic behavior pattern seen in the chronic pain patient.[3]

Early pain theories were based upon simple neuroanatomic circuitry or a single neurophysiologic concept. As technology advanced, pain theory became more sophisticated. The impetus to examine the pain mechanism was a new theory, the Gate Control Theory of Melzack and Wall.[6] Since that time (1965) neurophysiologic, neuroanatomic, and neurochemical approaches have begun to delineate the peripheral and central mechanisms of pain. Furthermore, the mechanisms involved in the centrifugal (descending) control of pain are being identified. New hypotheses are being developed and tested. Successful testing of these hypotheses adds new pieces to the puzzle or revises already established pieces. Many gaps in the pain puzzle still exist. As a result, the pain theories are dynamic and constantly changing. This section provides the reader with a historic perspective of pain theories and the theories currently utilized.

Specificity and Pattern Theory

Two traditional and opposing theories for pain evolved during the late 1800s. Both theories use concepts of sensory physiology that were developed by von Frey[4] and Goldscheider.[5] These theories are the specificity theory and the pattern theory, respectively.

The specificity theory proposed that a specific pain system existed. When pain receptors located in the skin were stimulated, the impulses were transmitted via a direct pathway to the pain center located in the brain. Von Frey utilized the Müller doctrine of specific nerve energies, anatomic evidence, and scientific deductive reasoning to develop his theory. The Müller principle stated that a stimulus applied to a receptor would provide the same sensation in the brain center regardless of the type of stimulus. Müller further concluded that a receptor had a low threshold of activation for a particular stimulus (adequate stimulus) but could respond to other stimuli if the intensity was sufficient. Von Frey also expanded another Müller concept by stating that four major categories of cutaneous sensations existed—that is, warm, cold, touch, and pain. Each category had a separate projection system (Fig. 2–1).

Anatomic evidence utilized by von Frey was histologic identification of specialized receptors and free nerve endings. Since free nerve endings were located in skin throughout the entire body and an intense stimulus applied anywhere on the skin resulted in a pain sensation, he logically reasoned that free nerve endings were pain receptors. Thus, the specificity theory states that any noxious or potentially tissue-damaging stimulus applied to the surface of the skin would result in a pain sensation.

The pattern theory also contains a peripheral and central component. As is evident by its name, the pattern or coding of sensory information is the key element. The coding is the temporal and spatial sequencing of action potentials generated in the periphery. This theory negates the idea

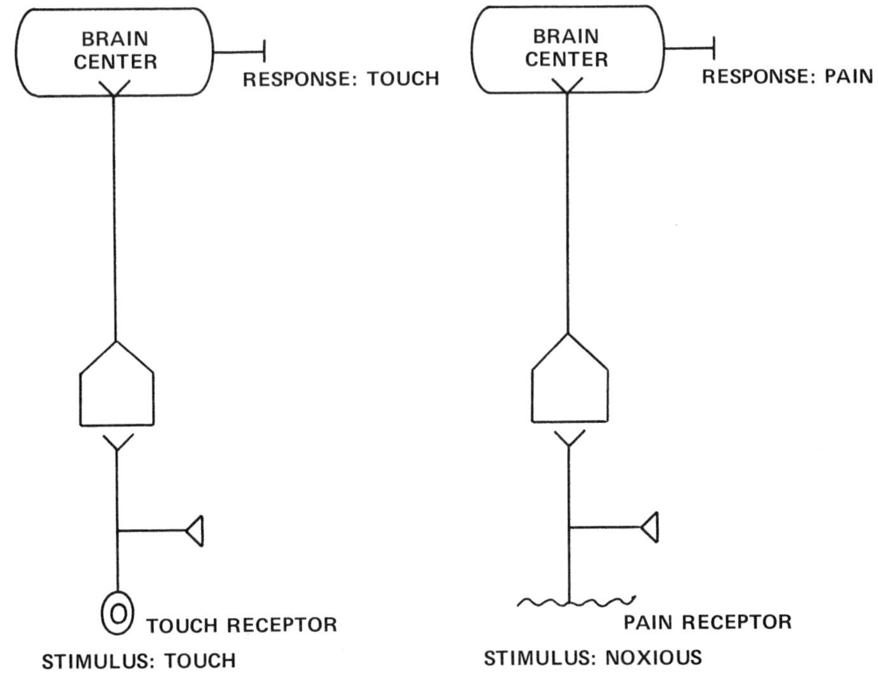

FIGURE 2–1
Specificity theory demonstrating separate systems for sensory modalities.

of a specific pain receptor, but rather considers the intense stimulation of nonspecific receptors as the adequate stimulus for eliciting the pain sensation. Figure 2–2 shows that if a touch stimulus was applied to a receptor, a particular pattern of action potentials could be produced in the sensory axon. The resultant sensation would be touch. If a more intense and potentially damaging touch stimulus was applied to the receptor, a different pattern of action potentials would be generated and the resultant sensation would be pain. One fallacy in this concept is that specific specialized receptors have been documented histologically.

A second portion of the pattern theory is central summation. A nonnoxious stimulus could result in an abnormal volley of action potentials that could be interpreted centrally as a pain experience. The underlying neurophysiologic mechanisms, to explain an abnormal discharge, including a self-sustaining reverberating circuit or a positive feed-forward circuit in which the inhibitory regulation has been removed, are not described.

Gate Control Theory

In 1965 Melzack and Wall[6] proposed a new theory relating to the pain experience. This theory represents a cornerstone in the development of neurophysiologic mechanisms that address the concept of peripheral and central gating. The gate theory incorporated the feature of receptor specialization from the specificity theory with spatiotemporal coding of action potentials from the pattern theory. To these two concepts Melzack and Wall added the interaction of peripheral afferents with a modulation system

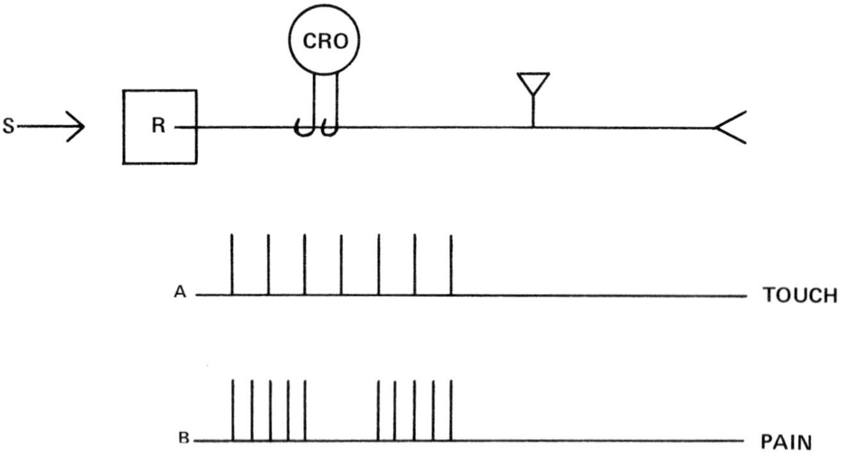

FIGURE 2–2

Schematic representation of the pattern theory.

A. Action potentials resulting from a touch stimulus(s) and recorded on a cathode ray oscilloscope (CRO). The resultant sensation is *touch*.
B. Action potentials resulting from a noxious stimulus and recorded on a cathode ray oscilloscope. The resultant sensation is *pain*.

Key: S = stimulus; R = receptor, CRO = cathode ray oscilloscope.

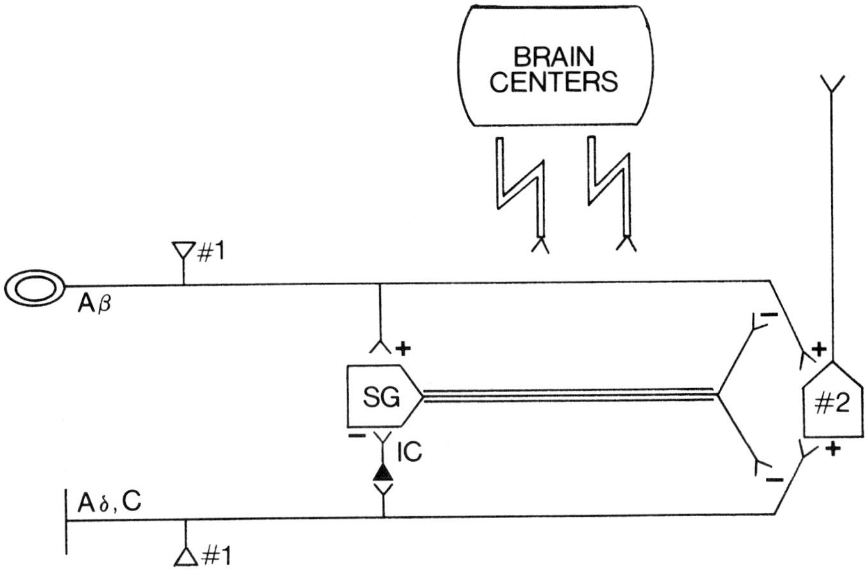

FIGURE 2–3

Schematic representation of the revised Melzack and Wall Gate Control Theory. Key: #1 = first-order neuron, either Aβ, Aδ, or C primary afferent; #2 = second-order neuron (T cell); SG = substantia gelatinosa; IC = inhibitory interneuron.

located in the substantia gelatinosa of the spinal gray matter.[7] Furthermore, they proposed a descending modulatory system. Figure 2–3 is a schematic representation of the gate control theory.

The neuroanatomic features of this circuit include large-diameter sensory neurons (Aβ); small-diameter sensory neurons (Aδ, C); the substantia gelatinosa that corresponds to Rexed's laminae II and III of the dorsal horn of the spinal gray matter; and a transmission cell (T cell), also known as a tract cell or second-order neuron. The A-beta, A-delta, and C neurons may also be termed first-order neurons or primary afferents. Both the large- and small-diameter primary afferents impinge upon the substantia gelatinosa cells and upon the second-order neuron. The substantia gelatinosa acts as a modulator (gate control) by terminating presynaptically upon the large- and small-diameter afferent neurons just prior to their termination upon the tract cell. The control was postulated to occur by the neurophysiologic mechanisms termed presynaptic inhibition.

When the substantia gelatinosa is active, an increase in presynaptic control on the first-order axons occurs and the "gate" is in the relatively closed position; that is, a decrease in the amount of sensory input to the transmission cell occurs. On the other hand, a reduction in substantia gelatinosa activity results in a decrease in the amount of presynaptic control on the first-order neuron, and the "gate" is considered to be in a relatively open position; that is, the amount of sensory information reaching the second-order neuron is relatively unaltered. The balance of activity in the large- and small-diameter sensory neurons determines the relative position of the "gate."

If the large-diameter afferents are activated, then an initial increase in T-cell activity occurs and is followed by a reduction of activity. The initial increase in T-cell activity would result from direct activation of the tract cell by the primary afferents, whereas the reduction is an indirect result of substantia gelatinosa activation leading to presynaptic inhibition of the primary afferents.

If, however, the small-diameter afferents are activated, then the initial increase in T-cell activity would be followed by maintained activity in the tract cell. The initial increase in T-cell activity is also caused by direct activation of primary afferents. However, the influence of the small-diameter primary afferents via an inhibitory interneuron depresses the activity of the substantia gelatinosa cells. The resultant would be a decrease in the amount of presynaptic control on the large- and small-diameter sensory neurons and a relatively open position of the "gate."

Melzack and Wall proposed that the predominant amount of ongoing activity occurred in the small-diameter sensory neurons. When the balance of small- to large-diameter neuronal input is no longer maintained and reaches a critical value, the T cells are activated. The activation of this ascending system leads to the perception of pain and behavioral responses.

One component of the system that was briefly described but not fully elucidated was the descending control system. These researchers proposed that central events such as emotion and past experience could evoke descending input, which would impinge upon the gating mechanism to block pain sensation at the spinal level.

As the various hypotheses were tested, the theory was revised.[8,9] Revisions of the gate lead to the realization that a more complex neural circuitry existed in the dorsal horn; to the consideration that postsynaptic connections could play a modulatory role in the gating mechanism; and to the idea that the concept of the gate theory is a balance between activity in non-nociceptive and nociceptive (Aδ, C) neurons rather than large- and small-diameter afferents. Furthermore, successful testing of the hypothesis that Aβ afferents could "close" the "gate" led to the use of transcutaneous electrical nerve stimulation for pain modulation in humans.[10]

Extensive clinical testing of externally applied electrical stimulators for pain relief in the chronic pain patient began in the early 1970s.[11] The Melzack and Wall gate control theory of pain, provides a partial neurophysiologic explanation for the use of transcutaneous electrical nerve stimulators (TENS) to relieve acute and chronic pain.

In summary, Melzack and Wall provided a theory that utilized an interaction of sensory input for modulation of pain sensation. Testing of the hypothesis has led to further delineation of pain mechanisms as well as the use of a clinical device for electrotherapeutic modulation of pain.

Peripheral and Central Nervous System Mechanisms Subserving Pain

When examining the current concepts of pain, neurophysiologic and neurochemical relationships need to be explored. The amount of knowledge gained in this area within the past two decades far exceeds knowledge accumulated in the other areas of neuroscience. As a result, theories are rapidly revised. Students and clinicians should be cognizant of the fact that no pain theory is engraved in stone. This is witnessed by continuing changes in the current pain literature and applications of pain theories in the justification of clinical procedures.

PERIPHERAL MECHANISMS

NOCICEPTORS. Receptors responsible for the transmission of pain impulses are described morphologically as free nerve endings. The best-studied nociceptors, primarily by single-fiber electrophysiologic techniques in both animals and humans, are the nociceptors located in the skin.[12–15] Nociceptors found in the viscera and in the cardiac and skeletal muscle are less well understood.[16] The adequate stimuli for excitation of nociceptors includes intense heat, intense cold, strong mechanical deformation, and chemical substances. Those receptors that respond to only one noxious stimulant are termed *specific nociceptors,* whereas those nociceptors that respond to several noxious stimuli are termed *polymodal nociceptors.* The transducer mechanism used by the nociceptor to change the stimulus to the energy form used by the nervous system (action potentials, impulses) is not completely understood.

Antidromic activation of the primary afferents by an electrical stimulus results in the release of a substance at the receptor ending. This substance is assumed to be substance P.[17] If this assumption is successfully tested, it would provide a peripheral hyperalgesic mechanism. Furthermore, chemical substances such as prostaglandin E, bradykinin, and serotonin are released in the skin near nociceptors when trauma or inflammation occurs.[18] These or similar substances may be released in muscle upon injury to the muscle.[19] The role of these substances in the alteration of the responsiveness (i.e., increased sensitivity or sensitization) of the nociceptor is currently being investigated.

PRIMARY AFFERENT NEURONS. The use of electrical stimulation with preferential blockade of peripheral nerves in man has revealed two distinct populations of primary afferent neurons subserving pain.[15,20,21] One group when preferentially stimulated evoked a sharp and pricking pain sensation of short duration. This group of afferents was identified as the myelinated A-delta (Aδ) or group III primary neurons. Conduction velocities of this population range between 4 and 30 m/sec. The second group when activated produced a longer-lasting burning sensation that was dull and more diffusely localized. The population of primary afferents that gives rise to these sensations is the unmyelinated C or group IV afferents. Conduction velocities of C afferents ranges between 0.5 and 2 m/sec. (These two pain sensations are also termed first and second pain, respectively.)

Primary afferent neurons may also be classified according to the type of stimulus that activates the nociceptor or its associated neuron or both. Three types of nociceptive afferents have been identified. One major type of nociceptive afferent is the A-delta high-threshold mechanoreceptor afferent, which responds exclusively to noxious mechanical stimulation. After repeated exposure to an intense thermal stimulus, other mechanoreceptors become activated. This second type was identified as the A-delta heat nociceptive afferent but is currently termed mechanothermal nociceptor.[22] A third major type of afferents is the C polymodal nociceptive afferent, which responds to noxious heat in the 45°C to 51°C range, to noxious mechanical stimulation, and to noxious chemical stimulation. Approximately one third of the C afferents respond to intense cold; however, their activation does not contribute to the perception of pain.[23] Approximately 85 to 90 percent of the C nociceptor afferents identified in primates are C polymodal afferents; and to date, all identified C neurons in human beings are C polymodal afferents. In humans, the relationships between activation of A-delta mechanothermal afferents and perception of first pain, and between activation of C polymodal afferents and perception of second pain have been established.[24]

Electrophysiologic studies on the cat saphenous nerve demonstrate that the A-delta afferents exhibit excitation failure when stimulated at 20 to 30 Hz.[25] On the other hand, C afferents exhibit excitation failure at stimulation rates of 5 to 10 Hz. Excitation failure is the process by which an action potential is not generated each time the nerve fiber is externally stimulated.

TERMINATION OF NOCICEPTIVE AFFERENTS IN THE DORSAL HORN. The majority of the primary afferents course through the dorsal root and terminate on cells located in the dorsal horn of the spinal gray matter. Just prior to entry into the spinal cord, similar types of afferents begin to group together. Those signaling pain (Aδ, C) travel through the lateral division of the dorsal root and may travel several spinal segments within Lissauer's tract before entering the spinal gray matter. The larger primary afferents travel through the medial division of the dorsal horn and penetrate directly into the dorsal horn.[26] Although the majority of the afferents enter the spinal cord through the dorsal root, a significant population (20 percent of the unmyelinated neurons) enters the spinal cord through the ventral root.[27,28] This latter population is of particular clinical interest when considering reasons for the return of pain in those patients having undergone dorsal rhizotomies for pain relief.

Both histochemical and electrophysiologic studies demonstrate termination of C afferents in lamina I (marginal layer) and lamina II of the spinal cord. Termination of C afferents in lamina III is questionable.[7] A-delta mechanonociceptive afferents have been identified in laminae I, III, and layers IV to VI. Large-diameter A-beta afferents have a few direct connections in laminae I, II, and most extensively terminate in laminae III, IV, and V. Termination of these afferents in lamina V is questionable.

CENTRAL MECHANISMS OF PAIN

TRACT CELLS. The details of the neuronal circuitry of those cells that lie within the confines of the dorsal horn are complex and not within the scope of this chapter. Such detailed descriptions may be found elsewhere.[7,27] Two categories of second-order neurons that warrant discussion are those that form the ascending projection system, the spinothalamic and trigeminothalamic tracts. These neurons receive both direct and indirect connections from the nociceptive afferents. These classes of neurons are the wide–dynamic range neuron and the nociceptive-specific neuron.

The wide–dynamic range neuron has been extensively studied and is considered to be the candidate for the T cell described in the gate control theory. The cell body of this neuron is located in lamina V of the dorsal horn of the spinal gray matter as well as in the magnocellular layer of the trigeminal nucleus caudalis. This region in the trigeminal nucleus is considered a homologue of lamina V.

These neurons are termed wide–dynamic range because they receive input from multiple sources (Fig. 2–4*A*). A-beta mechanoreceptive, A-delta, and C nociceptive afferents impinge upon the wide–dynamic range neurons. The receptive field for these tract cells is larger than the receptive field for a primary afferent neuron. Furthermore, the receptive field of the tract cell is arranged in such a manner that stimuli based on a continuum from touch to noxious pinch would produce an increase in the frequency of neuronal discharge dependent upon the stimulus.[29] For example, a low frequency of action potentials would be elicited from a touch stimulus, whereas a higher frequency of action potentials would result from a noxious pinch. These neurons also have a large subliminal fringe associated with the receptive field. Subliminal fringe is an area that, when stimulated, produces local neuronal membrane changes and not an action potential.

The second class of tract cells is the nociceptive-specific neurons, which respond exclusively to noxious mechanical or thermal stimuli or both (Fig. 2–4*B*). In contrast to the wide–dynamic range neuron, these neurons have a small receptive field, generally less than 2 cm^2. These cells are concentrated in lamina I, but some neurons have been identified in lamina V and in the trigeminal nucleus. As evidenced by their name, these neurons receive input from high-threshold A-delta mechanosensitive afferents and C polymodal nociceptive afferents. The nociceptive-specific neurons may be further subdivided into a group that responds only to noxious mechanical stimulation carried exclusively by the A-delta high-threshold mechanosensitive afferents. The second subclass of nociceptive-specific neurons responds to intense, nonpainful pressure and to noxious stimuli. The response of the nociceptive-specific neuron to a stimulus is frequency dependent; that is, the frequency of action potentials generated by the neurons will increase in response to the intensity of the stimulus.

The neuronal contributions of these tract cells to pain are fairly well substantiated. The wide–dynamic range neuron could contribute to the localization aspect of pain as well as modality discrimination (i.e., touch to mechanical pinch). Furthermore, activation of these neurons in humans leads to reports of burning or needle-like sensations that are confined to a specific area of the body.[30] On the other hand, the nociceptive-specific neurons tend to be more modality specific; that is, they are more suited to provide information to the central nervous system regarding the specific type and location of the noxious stimulus.

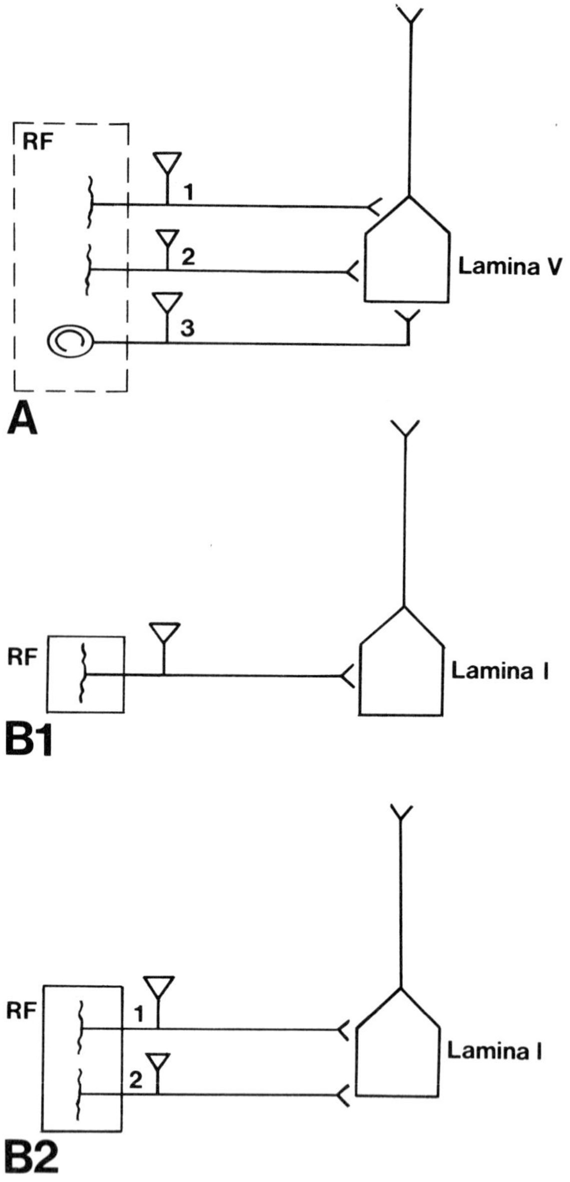

FIGURE 2–4

Schematic representation of categories of second-order neurons.

A. Wide–dynamic range neuron with convergent input from primary neurons: #1 = C polymodal afferent; #2 A = Aδ nociceptive afferent; #3 = Aβ mechanoreceptive afferent.

B1. Nociceptive specific neuron with input exclusively from Aδ high-threshold mechanoreceptive afferent.

B2. Nociceptive specific neuron with convergent input from primary neurons: #1 = C polymodal afferent; #2 = Aδ nociceptive afferent.

RF = receptive field.

Both the nociceptive-specific and wide–dynamic range neurons signal intensity. Furthermore, a prolonged discharge lasting several hundred milliseconds occurs in the cells. This after-discharge has been noted following electrical stimulation of C fibers and radiant heating of skin at temperatures above 45°C.[16] The prolonged discharge would suggest temporal facilitation at the synaptic level, primarily associated with the wide–dynamic range neuron. Substance P located in the terminals of the small primary afferents is the putative neurochemical substance implicated to produce the prolonged after-discharge.[31] This finding, when substantiated, would provide one possible mechanism for second pain, and one possible mechanism for continued pain perception in various painful conditions.

In summary, this discussion of the second-order neuron was limited to a brief description of the neuronal characteristics and the primary afferent input. Convergence of known and postulated input from other sources will be described elsewhere (centrifugal control of pain). These two neuronal classes comply with other theories to fit the role of ascending neurons subserving pain. The nociceptive-specific neurons fit the specificity theory for permitting a pain input to reach higher centers in a relatively unaltered fashion. On the other hand, the wide–dynamic range nociceptors would fit the category of the T cell as described by the Melzack and Wall gate control theory.

Ascending Projections and Higher Centers Subserving Pain

Both laboratory and clinical evidence support the hypothesis that the wide–dynamic range neurons and the specific-nociceptive neurons are only two classes of neurons that compose the spinothalamic tract. Some second-order neurons that are activated by mechanical stimulation also need to be considered in the modulatory role for pain control.[29] Thus, the spinothalamic tract participates in many of the components of pain; that is, affective, arousal, sensory-discriminative, as well as other functions. To classify this tract in the older terminology of paleospinothalamic and neospinothalamic may now be an oversimplification.[32] This classical pain pathway, located in the ventrolateral quadrant of the spinal cord, not only terminates in the ventroposterolateralis nucleus (VPL) of the thalamus but also sends collaterals to the medial brainstem region.[33]

Many levels of the neuraxis have been examined in relation to a role in the pain process. Data implicating higher center processing of pain have been derived from a variety of techniques performed upon a variety of species, including humans.

MEDULLA AND PONS. Ascending fibers from the ventrolateral quadrant of the spinal cord send projections to (1) medial portion of the reticular formation, particularly the nucleus gigantocellularis; (2) the lateral pons; and (3) the central gray area. These collaterals are termed the spinoreticular projection.

White and Sweet[34] noted that stimulation of structures in the medulla of conscious humans produced both the sensory-discriminative and the affective-motivational components of the pain response. The sensory component corresponds to observations made in animals that show many neurons in this area responded to noxious stimuli;[35] however, these neurons have wide receptive fields. The affective-motivational component corresponds to the observation that electrical stimulation within the nucleus gigantocellularis (NGC) in animals produced escape behavior in cats,[36] whereas destruction of the NGC resulted in a deficit in escape behavior.[37]

The NGC is considered a relay in the spinoreticulothalamic system for pain transmission. Furthermore, the NGC has connections with the autonomic nuclei, which are also located within the reticular formation. These connections may play a role in autonomic responses to intense and noxious stimuli.[27] Since the reticular formation is lacking in somatotopic organization and has connections with the autonomic centers, the limbic forebrain structures and hypothalamus, this area may be more involved in the autonomic and affective components of pain rather than subserving a discriminatory function.

MESENCEPHALON. Mesencephalic structures also receive projections from a variety of areas including the spinoreticular projection. Electrical stimulation of the medial periaqueductal gray region in humans elicits emotional responses such as unpleasantness and fear. The pain tends to be deep, and confined to midline structures.[38] Destruction of these mesencephalic structures does not alter localization of acute noxious stimuli.[39] The midline structures are more allied with the emotional aspects of the pain process, whereas the lateral structures are more closely associated with the sensory-discriminative aspect; however, this is not a mutually exclusive relationship.

THALAMUS. Considerable evidence demonstrates that wide–dynamic range neurons and nociceptive-specific neurons of the spinal cord project to three main nuclei of the thalamus: the ventrobasal nuclei, the posterior nuclei, and the medial intralaminar nuclei. Few neurons in these groups respond exclusively to nociceptive input.[40]

Noxious input to the ventrobasal complex (nucleus ventralis posterior, nucleus ventralis lateralis) projects to discrete areas of the contralateral side of the body. Approximately 6 to 10 percent of the cells in this region respond to noxious stimuli.[41] In humans, lesioning in the ventrobasal complex produces deficits in somatosensory discrimination. Tingling in a specific location is a typically described sensation when these nuclei are stimulated.[38] This observation suggests a sensory-discriminative component of painful stimuli that has been supported by studies in the cat. This is further supported by anatomic evidence that these neurons project to both the primary (SI) and secondary (SII) areas of the somatosensory cortex.[27]

The role of the posterior thalamic nuclei in pain is conflicting. This region lacks somatotopic organization, and the neurons have wide receptive fields.[40] The majority of somatosensory input arises from the contralateral side of the body; some is ipsilateral. In humans, stimulation of this area also elicits pain sensation.

Cells of the medial and intralaminal thalamic nuclei have large receptive fields, lack somatotopic organization, and receive bilateral input. Nuclei forming the intralaminar complex include the nuclei paracentralis, centralis medialis, centralis lateralis, centromedian, and parafascicularis (Cm-Pf).[27] This complex responds to auditory, visual, and intense mechanical stimuli. They receive input from the ventrolateral quadrant of the spinal cord and indirect input from the nucleus gigantocellularis.

Electrical stimulation of the Cm-Pf complex in humans produces a burning or aching sensation referred from contralateral and some ipsilateral regions of the body. Recordings from some neurons in this area in humans demonstrate that these cells respond to pinprick.[42] Lesioning this area in the human has been somewhat effective in relieving intractable pain; the nondiscriminative quality of pain was removed while preserving the sensory-discriminative aspect. This observation provides a clue that these diffuse thalamic nuclei may be involved in the affective quality of pain. Further evidence is that these neurons project not only to the cerebral cortex but also to the limbic cortex and amygdala.

CORTEX. The role of the primary somatosensory area in pain perception is not clearly understood. Lesioning in this area has no effect on acute or chronic pain, and electrical stimulation does not produce pain.[34] Thus, the SI cortex, while serving an important function for spatiotemporal discrimination of sensation, is not an important region for perception of pain.

The secondary somatosensory area of the cerebral cortex has been more extensively studied. This area receives an extensive projection from the posterior thalamic nuclei. Furthermore, these neurons receive multisensory input. Although some researchers have reported no alteration in pain perception with lesions in this area,[34] others have reported hypalgesia.[30]

Recent studies in this region have performed neuronal recordings following electrical stimulation of tooth pulp afferents.[27,43] An increase in stimulus intensity produced an increase in the amplitude of activity recorded in SII region.

The cortex, then, may be involved with the pain mechanisms at two levels. The first level would be a system involved with sensory discrimination such as localization. A second level would be involved with a more complex system associated with complex behavioral responses that include affective and motivational responses and comparisons of pain sensation with past experiences.

In summary, the rostrad projections for pain involve many levels of the neuraxis. The interconnections of these various systems are complex and not completely understood. The use of electrical stimulation or lesioning studies provides some information about the function of a particular system but may not be a true representation of what actually occurs in the intact, awake animal.

Centrifugal Control of Pain

Although the ascending control for regulation of sensory input has been well established, the descending control system for modulation of pain has only been examined extensively since the late 1960s. The major impetus occurred in 1969 when Reynolds[44] noted that electrical stimulation of the periaqueductal gray (PAG) area produced analgesia in unanesthetized rats. Since that study, modulation of noxious input at the spinal level has been identified,[45] as well as descending control of pain at various levels of the neuraxis. A second major impetus was the isolation of an endogenous substance in neural tissue by Hughes in 1974.[46] This substance, enkephalin, fit the criteria for an endogenous substance that when released would inhibit pain.

Correlative evidence for centrifugal control of pain is based on studies using stimulation-produced analgesia (SPA) and microinjections of exogenous opiates. Naloxone has been used extensively in these studies. Naloxone is a morphine antagonist that competes for the same receptor site as the opiates (such as morphine), the enkephalins, and beta-endorphin (β-endorphin). A receptor site is a specialized region of the neuronal membrane. A neurochemical substance has a specific molecular configuration that matches a particular receptor site (Fig. 2–5). When the neurochemical substance attaches to the receptor, physiologic responses mediated by the chemical transmitter occur. For example, movement of specific ions results in depolarization or hyperpolarization of the nerve membrane. An antagonist has a similar molecular configuration that will permit the antagonist to attach to the receptor site and "tie up" available spaces. The effects of the neurochemical substance are blocked. In many instances, the antagonist has a greater affinity for the receptor site and can even reverse the effects of the agonist.[47] For example, naloxone can be used as an antidote in cases of morphine overdose or can be used in helping to elucidate the effects of a thermal agent in pain reduction.

Location and density of the opiates varies among species. The highest concentrations occur in the limbic cortex (most specifically, the anterior amygdala), the periaqueductal gray, the hypothalamus, the thalamus, and to a lesser degree the cortex, caudate nucleus, other midbrain structures, and the gray matter of the spinal cord.[48] Although many brain structures have opiate receptor areas, the question arises as to the importance of the opiate receptor in a particular region subserving pain inhibition.

The two most-studied endogenous opiates are β-endorphin and methionine enkephalin (met-enkephalin). β-endorphin is a 31–amino acid chain with a half-life of approximately 4 hours. Half-life refers to the time needed for inactivation of the substance by enzymes located in the tissue. β-endorphin has potent effects including catatonia with corresponding inhibition of neuronal cell activity in the caudate nucleus, cortex, brainstem and thalamus; analgesia; and behavioral disturbances. Due to the fact that β-endorphin is found in the pituitary and is long-lasting, it may be involved with whole animal responses associated with severe stress.[49]

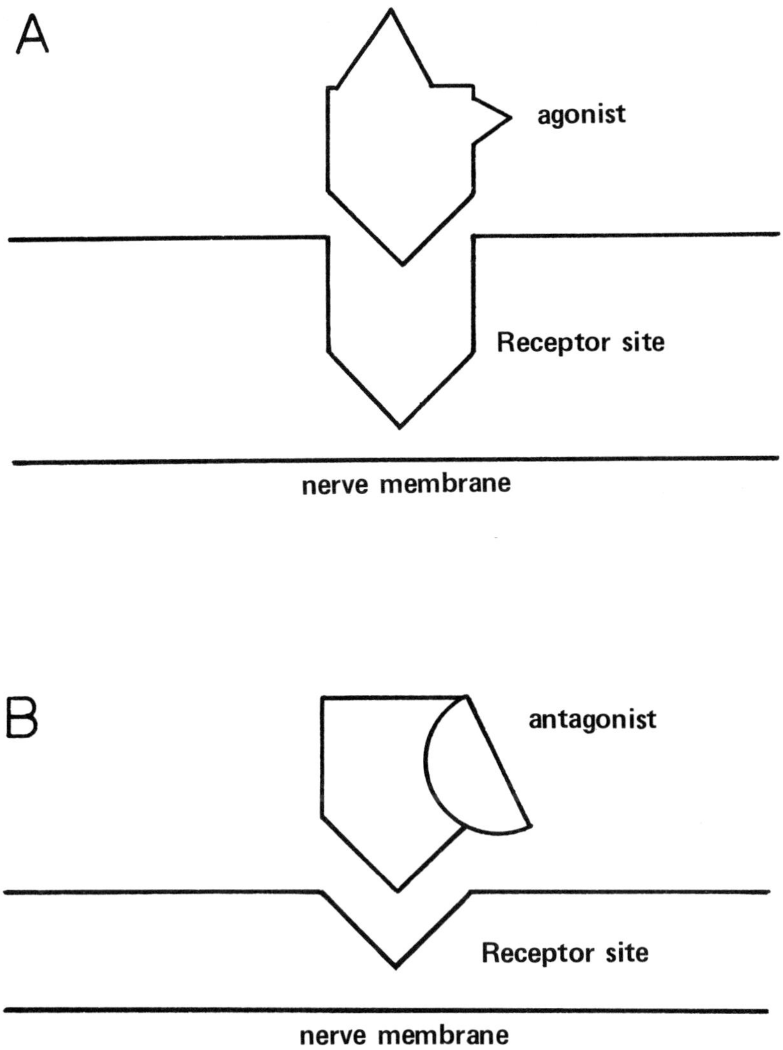

FIGURE 2–5

A. An agonist (e.g., morphine) approaching a receptor site located on the neuronal nerve membrane.
B. An antagonist (e.g., naloxone) approaching the same receptor site.

The enkephalins—met-enkephalin and leucine enkephalin—are 5–amino acid molecules with a half-life of 2 minutes. These peptides have been identified in many regions of the brain and in different concentrations. Many areas that have a high concentration of enkephalin also have an increased density of those neurons containing substance P or serotonin (5-HT). The *postulated* role of these neuropeptides in pain regulation will be discussed subsequently.

SPINAL LEVEL. The neuronal circuitry for pain regulation at the spinal level is not completely understood. One mechanism, primary afferent depolarization, was expanded by Wall[27] to include neurons in the substantia gelatinosa. When electrically stimulated, cells within the substantia gelatinosa produced a decrease in primary afferent activity and inhibited the neurons in lamina V that had been activated by noxious stimuli. The neurochemical transmitter implicated to mediate the presynaptic inhibition was gamma-aminobutyric acid (GABA). Microinjection of opiates into the spinal cord also inhibited activity of dorsal horn neurons elicited by noxious stimuli.[50] This observation was supported by the finding that neurons containing enkephalin existed in the substantia gelatinosa (Fig. 2–6).[51] These neurons are prominent in laminae I and II but are also found in laminae III and V. They may serve functions other than inhibitory functions and may therefore be activated independent of descending pain modulatory systems. Not only presynaptic inhibition but also postsynaptic inhibition should be considered in pain regulation at the spinal level.

PAIN INHIBITION FROM SUPRASPINAL LEVELS. This modulatory control not only occurs upon spinal neurons but also at other supraspinal sites. These systems include both neural opiate and nonopiate projections. Furthermore, humoral opiate and nonopiate pain modulatory systems exist.[45] These latter systems, no doubt, are activated in response to very stressful situations and are involved in systemic responses.

Since only sparse connections from the periaqueductal gray (PAG) area to the spinal level exist, pain regulation by this area is mediated via

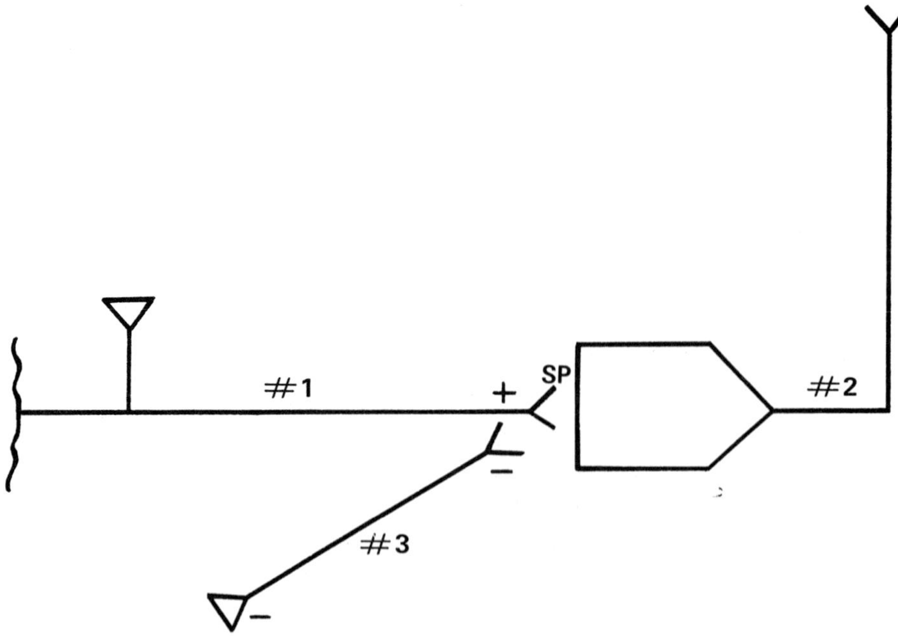

FIGURE 2–6

Schematic representation of presynaptic inhibition of an enkephalinergic neuron (#3) upon a primary afferent neuron (#1) containing substance P (SP). The primary afferent neuron is synapsing with a second-order neuron (#2).

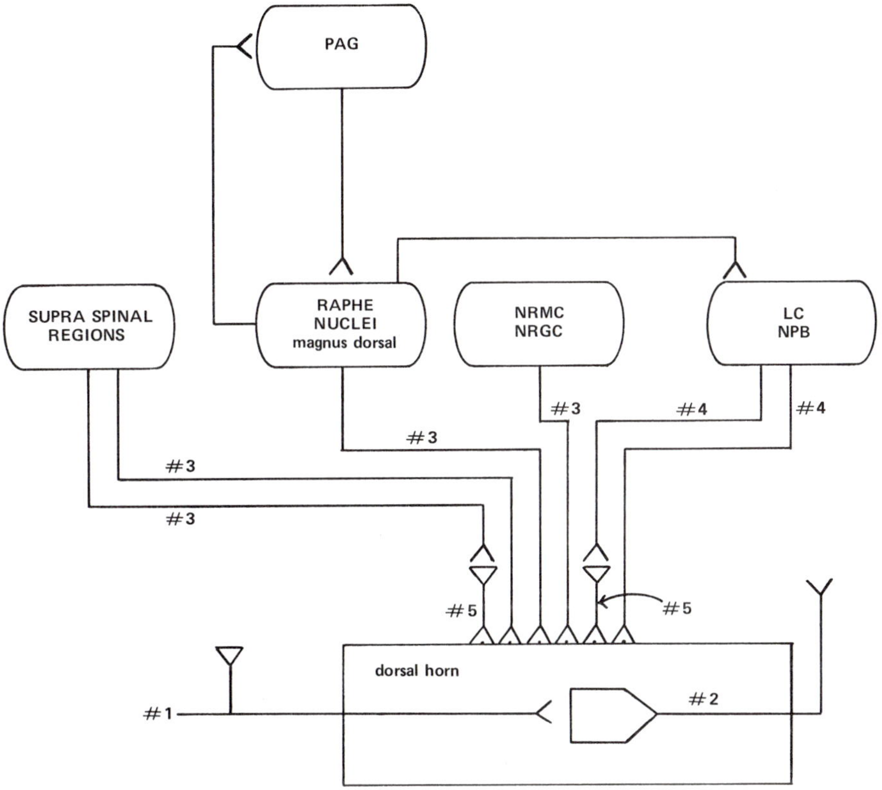

FIGURE 2–7

Schematic representation of centrifugal control of pain. Known and postulated pathways are drawn.

Key: PAG = periaqueductal gray; NRMC = nucleus reticularis magnocellularis; NRGC = nucleus reticularis gigantocellularis; LC = locus ceruleus; NPB = medial and lateral parabrachial nuclei; #1 = primary afferent neuron; #2 = second-order neuron; #3 = serotonin neuron; #4 = norepinephrine neuron; #5 = enkephalin neuron.

indirect pathways. The PAG projects to the nucleus raphe magnus, nucleus reticularis magnocellularis, and nucleus reticularis gigantocellularis (NRGC) (Fig. 2–7), which in turn projects to the dorsal horn of the spinal cord.[52] The nucleus raphe magnus, when stimulated, tends to inhibit the A-delta component of afferent input more than the A-beta component. This nucleus also contains serotonin-carrying neurons.

Studies indicate that descending serotonergic neurons are heavily concentrated in lamina I and are presumed to have a direct monosynaptic inhibitory effect on the second-order neuron (ascending tract neuron).[53] Although a serotonin-mediated descending pathway has been identified for pain inhibition, it may not be essential for the opiate or SPA pain mechanisms.[22] Furthermore, the raphe nucleus may utilize additional and yet unidentified pathways.

A second system, originating in the pons, also produces dorsal horn inhibition and analgesia. This system, postulated to be a norepinephrine

(NE)–mediated system, originates in the region of the ventral locus ceruleus, nucleus subceruleus, and medial and lateral parabrachial nuclei. The descending inhibitory system may terminate directly on second-order neurons or indirectly via an enkephalinergic interneuron.

Neuropharmacologic studies further complicate the puzzle by the identification of coexistence of several neurotransmitters within the same cell; for example, serotonin (5-HT) and substance P are found in cells in the spinal cord,[54] and enkephalin and substance P are found in descending brainstem neurons.[55] The functional significance of this coexistence is not known.

To summarize, at least two distinct descending systems for pain inhibition exist. One system, the opiate pathways utilizing the enkephalin interneuron, is dependent upon the norepinephrine system. A second system would entail those neuroanatomic pathways that do not use an opiate mediator interneuron.

The recent advances in the area of descending systems and dorsal horn circuitry have proliferated in recent years. Owing to the complexity of the system, many details are lacking and numerous hypotheses exist. The approach taken by researchers in this area is to identify the connections via neuroanatomic, neurophysiologic, and neurochemical means. By examining the interactions of the various components, a more sophisticated explanation of the system will be provided, rather than just considering the descending systems as filters for noxious input. Furthermore, the various motor and behavioral responses will be delineated.

PAIN CONDITIONS: ACUTE, CHRONIC, AND REFERRED

The underlying neurophysiologic mechanisms to explain acute, chronic, and referred pain are also incomplete. Complexity arises in the chronic pain condition, since the pain state outlasts the initial experience, and involves complex psychologic and physiologic responses. Each pain state, and the proposed mechanisms associated with each, will be explained.

Acute Pain

The acute pain experience may last a few minutes or several days. It has been defined as "pain of recent and sudden onset, usually, but not always, with demonstrable etiology and limited course."[56] Usually, the unpleasant experience is associated with autonomic and emotional responses. The primary function of acute pain is to alert the individual of potential tissue damage so that appropriate measures may be taken—that is, withdraw from the stimulus or seek medical assistance.

Generally, a noxious or potentially tissue-damaging stimulus activates nociceptors and the information is carried via A-delta or C afferents to the spinal cord. Upon reaching the spinal cord, several routes are available. The information is transmitted to the sympathetic preganglionic neuronal pool, whereby reflex responses in the peripheral vascular system and other visceral organs are elicited. Connections to the ventral horn upon the alpha and gamma motoneuronal pool evoke reflex responses including skeletal muscle contraction to escape the stimulus or muscle spasm. Nociceptive information transmitted to higher centers results in autonomic and emotional responses as well as pain perception.

Several mechanisms are proposed to explain the prolonged after-discharge noted with acute pain. Sensitization of nociceptors is a decrease in the threshold value of the receptor to additional stimuli, or enhancement of the response. The increase in sensitivity at the site of injury is termed primary hyperalgesia. The area surrounding the injury may also be sensitized and the patient experiences secondary hyperalgesia. Secondary hyperalgesia is believed to be due to antidromic activation of C primary afferents and release of substance P in the region.[22] A second postulate for after-discharge is the release of substance P from small primary afferents upon the second-order neuron.

Similar mechanisms can explain the pain-spasm-pain cycle in skeletal muscle. The initial injury produces an initial contraction for splinting or immobilization of the injured part. Continued muscle contraction leads to muscle ischemia and release of chemical substances that sensitize Aδ and C pain afferents in the muscle. By-products of metabolism alone do not produce nociceptive activation,[57] but factors such as bradykinin, serotonin, and histamine are implicated.[58] The heightened sensitivity of the nociceptors leads to additional reflexive contraction in the muscle; the result is a positive feedback loop. A similar loop can be established in the sympathetic reflex arc. Re-establishment of inhibitory mechanisms stops the pain-spasm-pain cycle.

Chronic Pain

Chronic pain is defined as a "pain of long duration, often associated with anguish, apprehension, depression, or hopelessness"[56] and extends months to years beyond the recovery period or recurs intermittently for years. Some clinicians use 6 months post-trauma or -disease as a basis to consider pain as chronic; others designate the length of time in accordance with a particular condition. Both environmental and psychologic factors are important considerations in the evolution of this type of pain.[59] The emotional, physiologic, and behavioral responses also differ from acute pain.

Underlying neurophysiologic mechanisms include positive-feedback loops as described earlier; that is, an increase in the sensitivity of the nociceptors leads to a maintained pain-spasm-pain cycle. The result is that semipermanent or permanent changes can occur at the spinal level to maintain these loops. A second mechanism involves long-lasting peripheral nerve compression.[27] Compression results in the destruction of large primary afferent neurons. As a result, an imbalance of large (tactile) and small (pain) fiber input occurs.

Chronic pain, however, extends beyond the neurophysiologic model, as is evidenced by Loser's schema.[60] The first level, nociception, refers to the application of a stimulus that activates A-delta and C primary afferents. The second level, pain, is the perception of the noxious stimulus. Suffering, the third level, is described as negative affective responses. This last level can be activated by pain perception, but also by stress and anxiety. Suffering can lead to the fourth level, pain behavior. The responses elicited by this level are evident in both verbal and nonverbal communication (i.e., posture, facial expressions, drug intake, continued seeking of medical attention, and becoming a nonfunctional member of society). In the evaluation and treatment of these patients, observational analysis should serve to measure pain relief rather than relying exclusively on verbal reports. Although chronic pain has a physiologic component, a multidimensional view is·needed to elucidate all components of this condition.

Referred Pain

Referred pain is "pain felt at a site in the body elsewhere from the source of disease or injury."[56] Thus, it can be considered an error in localization. Referred pain from the viscera to the body surface is projected upon the same dermatome. For example, myocardial pain afferents arise from T1 to T5, and pain associated with a myocardial infarction is felt at the T1 to T2 dermatomes, radiating down the arm. Furthermore, referred pain is not exclusively unique to visceral afferents.[61]

Two theories explain the concept of referred pain, and they are based on convergence of visceral and somatic terminations on higher-order neurons. Evidence is available for convergence on the same neuron in the deep layers of the dorsal horn.[62] The convergence-facilitation theory states that visceral afferents lower the threshold of the second-order neuron to incoming cutaneous input. Thus, only the cutaneous information reaches the higher centers of the nervous system.

The second theory, the convergence-projection theory, considers that the pain experienced at a particular site is learned by the association of multiple cues. This site, then, does not necessarily correspond to the site of injury.

Travell[63] has identified irritable points in the muscle (trigger points) that produce referred pain. Specific referred patterns elicited from trigger points are evidenced for each muscle. Recent publications diagram muscles of the trunk and extremities with their referred pain profile.[64,65] Therefore, in order to evaluate and select appropriate treatment for the pain patient, an understanding of the known and theorized mechanisms underlying various painful states is needed.

ASSESSMENT OF PAIN

A comprehensive assessment of the pain experience should provide the clinician with an indication of the source(s) of pain so that the cause of the pain is treated and not just the symptomatology. Furthermore, the assessment should assist in the selection of the appropriate thermal agent and provide a baseline so that documentation of improvement can be assessed. Not only verbal descriptions of pain but also nonverbal clues (including facial expressions and posture) should be recorded.

Pain Scales

The most commonly used pain assessment is a rating scale. A 10-centimeter scale can be marked in several formats: (1) a series of numbers from 0 to 10 marked on the scale; (2) verbal rating scale (VRS), with a series of descriptors; or (3) a visual analog scale (VAS), with only the ends of the scale marked.[66] Depending upon the word choice of the latter two scales, intensity or the affective quality of pain can be assessed. For example, the word choice of "strong" or "intense" can be used to evaluate the intensity of the pain, whereas phrases such as "bad as it can be" or "as unpleasant as it can be" can provide some indication of the affective quality.

When designing such a test, the following points should be considered. The scale should be drawn accurately. For example, if the horizontal line becomes thicker, then a cue concerning the intensity of pain could be transmitted to the patient. Only one pain scale should be drawn on the page, so that an accurate-as-possible measure can be obtained that is not biased by previously marked pain scales. Another manipulation of the pain scale is the reversal of the scale so that the most intense measure is on the left, or so that the scale is presented vertically. Whether these reversals of scale provide a better documentation of pain has not been examined. Scott and Huskisson[67] examined a vertical versus horizontal VAS and noted that although patients scored slightly lower using the horizontal scale, a significant difference was not noted between the two.

Both the VRS and VAS can be converted to a numerical format so that arithmetic manipulations can be performed. The scales have been shown to be correlated for pain measurement ($r = 0.84$, $p < 0.01$) and pain relief ($r = 0.81$, $p < 0.001$).[68] Although many researchers consider the VAS to be a more sensitive indicator, other studies do not lend support.

These scales are simple and quick to use, but some limitations need to be considered. First is the assumption that the categories of descriptors on the VRS or the numerical scale can be partitioned into equal psychologic units. Second is the assumption that a simple linear scale can assess one component in a very complex pain experience and that the patient can accurately remember pain intensity. These scales are also influenced by personal experience, culture, and expectations, including what the patient considers is expected of him or her by the therapist.

McGill Pain Questionnaire

In an attempt to assess the multidimensional aspects of pain, the McGill Pain Questionnaire (MPQ) was developed.[69,70] The researchers developed a pain assessment that included three classes of word choices to evaluate the sensory, evaluative, and affective components of pain. These descriptors were obtained with a high degree of agreement from subjects with different educational, socioeconomic, and cultural backgrounds. The questionnaire was also designed to describe pain in terms of quantitative measures. These measures are the total number of words chosen (NWC), the pain rating index (PRI), and the present pain intensity (PPI).

The word descriptors are divided into three categories and 20 subcategories. Each subcategory contains up to six words that are qualitatively similar and are ranked in descending order according to intensity. Each word, then, can be assigned a numerical value. The sensory category contains 13 subcategories that describe the main experience in terms of the spatiotemporal, pressure, thermal, and sharp-dull aspects of pain. Words such as "flickering" and "beating" describe the temporal aspect; "jumping" and "shooting" describe the spatial aspect; "stabbing," "cramping," and "tugging," the pressure aspect; and "burning" and "scalding," the thermal aspect of the pain experience. The affective category, divided into six subcategories, describes pain in terms of autonomic responses, fear, and tension. Pain descriptors such as "terrifying," "sickening," and "vicious" are included. The third category, evaluative, is a single category used to describe the intensity of the total pain experience. Words such as "annoying," "unbearable," and "troublesome" are used.

The patient is instructed to circle one word from each category that best describes his or her pain. If a category does not apply, it is left unmarked. Values for the NWC and PRI can be obtained from this list. NWC is the number of words (or categories) chosen. The PRI is obtained by assigning a numerical value to each word choice, then determining the mean. This value then provides an average value for the pain experience and has proven to be a sensitive indicator in pain assessment.

Melzack determined that the PRI correlated significantly with NWC ($p < 0.01$). Both the reliability and validity of the PRI scale have been tested on patients with a variety of painful conditions.[71–73] Unique profiles have been identified for chronic pain conditions, including, for instance, low back pain and arthritis.[74]

Another part of the pain questionnaire is the body diagram. A front and back view of a human is presented, and the patient marks the location of the pain on the diagram. The patient also marks "E" or "I" by the area where the pain is—"E" for external pain and "I" for internal pain.

Part three addresses pain in relation to duration and activities that influence the intensity. The patient describes the pain in terms of continuous, intermittent, or momentary, and then lists those activities that increase or decrease the pain. The patient may further describe the pain in accordance with the time of day the pain is better or worse. This latter information can be correlated with the type of activities that cause or reduce pain.

The fourth part of the evaluation relates to pain intensity. A five-point scale is marked with the terms mild, discomforting, distressing, horrible, and excruciating. The patient is asked to rate pain intensity at that moment: at the time when the pain is at its worst and at the time when the pain is at its least. This test is the present pain index (PPI), which gives an indication of pain during the administration of the questionnaire.

Additional information gathered on the MPQ includes a medical history, drug intake, and present treatments. If further information is needed, the patient is given a standardized home recording card.

The original questionnaire has been adapted to provide a shorter version (Fig. 2–8). The advantage of the MPQ is that it provides a greater sensitivity in assessing the painful experience than the analog scale does.

Other Assessments

Other testing methods have been used in the acute and, most particularly, in the chronic pain patient population. Two assessments deserve brief mention, but to provide details is beyond the scope of this text. The Sensory Decision, or Signal Detection Theory (SDT) is designed to discriminate among sensory stimuli (pain sensation) and is not a measure of the intensity of pain experienced. Controversy exists as to the use of this test in pain measure. Another commonly used test to assess the chronic pain patient is the Minnesota Multiphasic Personality Inventory (MMPI). Specific chronic pain personality profiles have been determined from the MMPI.

APPLICATION OF THERMAL AGENTS FOR PAIN RELIEF

Clinical rationale for pain relief is based primarily upon empirical observation and integration of information from basic and applied sciences. Although heat and cold are known to relieve pain in a variety of conditions, including tissue injuries and arthritis, the underlying mechanisms are unknown. Local neurologic and vascular changes in response to the thermal agent and the mechanisms accounting for such changes await systematic testing, evaluations, and elucidation.

Heat

Muscle spasm secondary to some type of muscle, joint, or neurologic trauma can be relieved by heat. Inhibition of pain may result from nervous system changes or vascular changes. Cosentino and colleagues[75] reported a decrease in sensory nerve conduction velocity following the application of ultrasound. They stated that the decrease was similar to that reported for motor nerve conduction velocity. This observed phenomenon may be related to the frequency component of ultrasound and not the thermal effects.

Mense[76] noted that direct warming of the cat muscle spindle decreased the neuronal activity of the secondary endings and increased the neuronal activity of the primary endings. The increase in primary afferent activity of the spindle could be postulated to "close" the "gate." Mense also observed

1. Where is your Pain?

Please mark, on the drawings below, the areas where you feel pain. Put E if external, or I if internal, near the areas which you mark. Put EI if both external and internal.

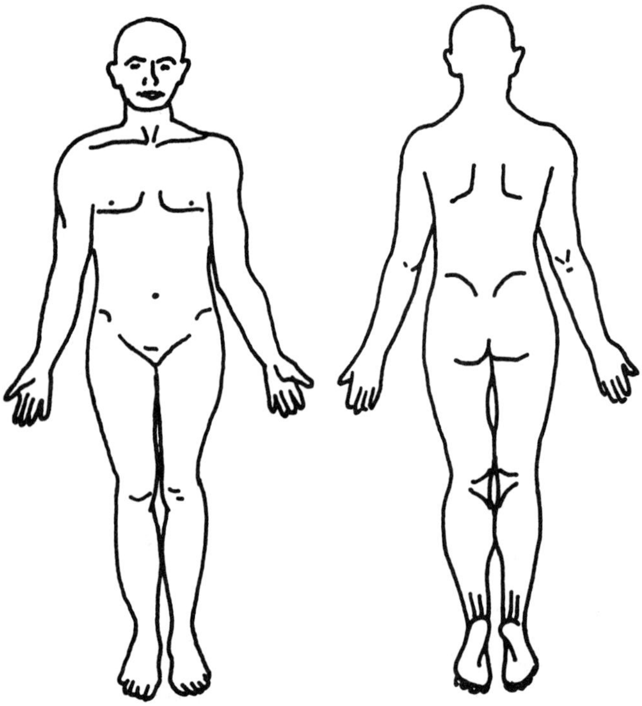

2. Please mark on the scale how much pain you have.

VISUAL ANALOGUE SCALE

PAIN AS BAD AS IT COULD BE ______________________________ NO PAIN

FIGURE 2–8

Adapted from parts 1, 2, and 3 of the McGill Pain Questionnaire.

3. Pain Rating Index

There are many words that describe pain. From the list below, select only those words that describe your pain as it feels right now. Only select one word in each column, and only if it applies to your pain. YOU DO NOT NEED TO MARK A WORD IN EVERY COLUMN—ONLY MARK THOSE WORDS THAT DESCRIBE YOUR PAIN!

1.	2.	3.	4.
Flickering	Jumping	Pricking	Sharp
Quivering	Flashing	Boring	Cutting
Pulsing	Shooting	Drilling	Lacerating
Throbbing		Stabbing	
Beating			
Pounding			

5.	6.	7.	8.
Pinching	Tugging	Hot	Tingling
Pressing	Pulling	Burning	Itchy
Gnawing	Wrenching	Scalding	Smarting
Cramping		Searing	Stinging
Crushing			

9.	10.	11.	12.
Dull	Tender	Tiring	Sickening
Sore	Taut	Exhausting	Suffocating
Hurting	Rasping		
Aching			
Heavy			

13.	14.	15.	16.
Fearful	Punishing	Wretched	Annoying
Frightful	Grueling	Blinding	Troublesome
Terrifying	Cruel		Miserable
	Vicious		Intense
	Killing		Unbearable

17.	18.	19.	20.
Spreading	Tight	Cool	Nagging
Radiating	Numb	Cold	Nauseating
Penetrating	Drawing	Freezing	Agonizing
Piercing	Squeezing		Dreadful
	Tearing		Torturing

FIGURE 2–8 *Continued*

increased Golgi tendon organ (GTO) activity upon warming. The GTOs provide an inhibitory influence to the homonymous motoneuronal pool. The GTO activity could possibly provide an inhibitory input to break up the pain-spasm-pain cycle. Caution should be used when extrapolating the data to clinical procedures, since the thermal agent was applied directly to exposed nerves of the cat.

The counterirritation theory can also be based on a gating mechanism.[77] Application of an external heat source produces a bombardment of activity from thermoreceptors. This increase in action potentials can block pain input. Melzack and Wall's gate theory provides the necessary circuitry for such blockage.[78] Another central nervous system phenomenon that occurs is generalized or whole body relaxation with heat. This relaxation can also produce pain relief, particularly if pain results from tension or skeletal muscle spasm. Activation of the descending pain inhibitory systems during thermal heating awaits justification.

Vascular changes in response to application of heat can also reduce pain. Vasodilatation and increase in blood flow up to 30 ml/100 g of tissue have been observed.[79] A greater blood flow increases the supply of nutrients to the area for repair process and removes by-products from the injured tissue. By-products include prostaglandins, bradykinin, and histamine, all implicated in receptor and afferent fiber sensitization that can cause a pain-spasm-pain cycle. Local heating also activates somatovisceral reflex arcs. Stimulation of cutaneous thermoreceptors decreases activity of the sympathetic nervous system and produces vasodilatation in deeper blood vessels.

Cold

The use of cold to decrease pain is through brief intense or prolonged cold. Both local and central nervous system mechanisms can be used to explain pain reduction.

Travell identified three possible mechanisms underlying the effects of brief intense cold: receptor adaptation; a counterirritant effect; and a neurogenic effect. A decrease in skin temperature following the application of a vapocoolant spray could produce cooling sufficient to cause receptor adaptation.[80] This idea was referenced to the findings of Cattell[81] whereby tactile receptors adapted in response to an intermittent stream of air. Whether the effects produced by these two dissimilar types of stimuli are equivalent or not is not known at this time.

The counterirritant effect was based on the research by Gammon and Starr[82] who observed that a 4°C to 10°C cold application to the skin was effective in relieving pain induced by a topical application of capsaicin. This observation and the neurogenic effect can be based on the gate theory; that is, an irritant can block pain fibers by activation of receptors that will ''close'' the ''gate.'' Furthermore, Iggo[27] noted that any intense stimuli that are noxious to the individual may also activate inhibitory processes, by a yet undefined mechanism. He does not advocate the use of noxious stimuli as a therapeutic means for pain reduction.

When cold is applied for a longer period of time, both local and central changes occur. One central nervous system model, the gate mechanism, has been described. Cooling of the skin (35°C to 24°C over a 7- to 10-second period) results in a rapid increase in the frequency of action potentials recorded on an afferent fiber.[83] This activity can be used to block pain input. To date, no evidence has supported the activation of the endorphin system by cold thermal agents.

Metabolic changes occur in both the receptor and afferent axons. Nerve conduction velocities have been examined in response to cooling longer than 5 minutes. For every 1°C decrease in intramuscular temperature, a decrease of 1.2 m/sec in motor conduction occurs,[79] and a corresponding 2 m/sec decrease has been noted for two sensory nerve conduction velocities.[84] The smaller-diameter afferents are more sensitive to cold than are the larger-diameter afferents. These observations, then, would decrease the probability of pain input to continue.

The local vasomotor response to cold is immediate vasoconstriction. This would result in an initial decrease in the amount of vasodilator substances released into the surrounding tissue. A decrease in the release of these substances could potentially decrease the degree of sensitization of the nociceptors.

SUMMARY

As is shown in this chapter, pain theories are dynamic and changing. What is postulated to date will be successfully defended or refuted. Current review articles are available to keep the clinician abreast of these changes. As the theories advance, so must the rationale for clinical treatment utilizing thermal modalities.

REFERENCES

1. Merskey, H and Able-Fessard, DG: *Pain terms: A list with definitions and notes on usage.* Pain 6:249, 1979.
2. Bonica, JJ: *Pain research and therapy: Past and current status and future needs.* In Ng, KY and Bonica, JJ (eds): *Pain, Discomfort and Humanitarian Care.* Elsevier, New York, 1979, pp 1–48.
3. Mayer, DJ and Price, DD: *A physiological and psychological analysis of pain: A potential model of motivation.* In Pfaff, D: *Physiological Mechanisms of Motivation.* Springer-Verlag, New York, 1982, pp 433–471.
4. von Frey, M: *Beitrage zur Physiologica des Schmerzsinns.* Ber kgl sachs Ges Wiss 46:185, 1894.
5. Goldscheider, A: *Veber den Schmerz in physiologischer und klinischer Hensicht.* Berlin, Hirschwald, 1894.
6. Melzack, R and Wall, PD: *Pain mechanisms: A new theory.* Science 150:971, 1965.
7. Wall, PD: *The role of substantia gelatinosa as a gate control.* In Bonica, JJ (ed): *Pain.* Raven Press, New York, 1980, pp 205–231.
8. Nathan, PW: *The gate-control theory of pain: A critical review.* Brain 99:123, 1976
9. Wall, PD: *The gate control theory of pain mechanisms: A re-examination and re-statement.* Brain 101:1, 1978.

10. Wall, PD and Sweet, WH: *Temporary abolition of pain in man.* Science 155:108, 1967.

11. Long, DM: *External electrical stimulation as a treatment of chronic pain.* Minnesota Medicine 57:195, 1974.

12. Georgopoulos, AP: *Functional properties of primary afferent units probably related to pain mechanisms in primate glabrous skin.* J Neurophysiol 39:79, 1976.

13. Burgess, PR and Perl, ER: *Myelinated afferent fibers responding specifical to noxious stimulation of the skin.* J Physiol (Lond) 190:541, 1967.

14. LaMotte, RH and Campbell, JN: *Comparison of responses of warm and nociceptive C-fiber afferents in monkey with human judgments of thermal pain.* J Neurophysiol 41:509, 1978.

15. Van Hees, J: *Human C-fiber input during painful and nonpainful skin stimulation with radiant heat.* In Bonica, JJ and Able-Fessard, D (eds): *Advances in Pain Research and Therapy,* Vol 1. Raven Press, New York, 1976, pp 35–40.

16. Zimmerman, M: *Peripheral and central nervous mechanisms of nociception, pain, and pain therapy: Facts and hypotheses.* In Bonica, JJ et al (eds): *Advances in Pain Research and Therapy,* Vol 3. Raven Press, New York, 1979, pp 3–32.

17. Lynn, B: *The detection of injury and tissue damage.* In Wall, PD and Melzack, R (eds): *Textbook of Pain.* Churchill-Livingstone, New York, 1984, pp 19–33.

18. Beck, PW, Handwerker, HO, et al: *Nervous outflow from the cat's foot during noxious radiant heat stimulation.* Brain Res 67:373, 1974.

19. Mense, S and Schmidt, RF: *Muscle pain: Which receptors are responsible for the transmission of noxious stimuli?* In Rose, FC (ed): *Psychological Aspects of Clinical Neurology.* Blackwell Scientific Publications, Oxford, 1977, pp 265–278.

20. Torebjörk, HE and Hallin, RG: *Perceptual changes accompanying controlled preferential blocking of A and C fibre responses in intact human skin nerves.* Exp Brain Res 16:321, 1973.

21. Kerr, FWL: *An overview of neural mechanisms of pain.* Neurosci Res Program Bull 16:30, 1978.

22. Dubner, R and Bennett, GJ: *Spinal and trigeminal mechanisms of nociception.* Ann Rev Neurosci 6:381, 1983.

23. LaMotte, RH, Ghalhammer, JG, et al: *Peripheral neural mechanisms of cutaneous hyperalgesia following mild injury by heat.* J Neurosci 2:765, 1982.

24. Price, DD, Hu, JW, Dubner, R, and Gracely, R: *Peripheral suppression of first pain and central summation of second pain evoked by noxious heat pulses.* Pain 3:57, 1977.

25. Torebjörk, HE and Hallin, RG: *Excitation failure in thin nerve fiber structure and accompanying hypalgesia during repetitive electrical skin stimulation.* In Bonica, JJ (ed): *Advances in Neurology,* Vol 4. Raven Press, New York, 1974, p 733.

26. Kerr, FWL: *Neuroanatomical substrates of nociception in the spinal cord.* Pain 1:325, 1975.

27. Yaksh, TL and Hammond, DL: *Peripheral and central substances involved in rostrad (ascending) transmission of nociceptive information.* Pain 13:1, 1982.

28. Kerr, FWL and Wilson, PR: *Pain.* Ann Rev Neurosci 1:83, 1978.

29. Price, DD and Dubner, R: *Neurons that subserve the sensory-discriminative aspects of pain.* Pain 3:307, 1977.

30. Mayer, DJ, Price, DD, and Becker, DP: *Neurophysiological characterization of the anterolateral spinal cord neurons contributing to pain perception in man.* Pain 1:59, 1975.

31. Hökfelt, T, Kellerth, J-O, Nilsson, G, and Plinow, B: *Experimental immunohistochemical studies on the localization and distribution of substance P in cat primary sensory neurons.* Brain Res 100:235, 1975.

32. Melzack, R: *The Puzzle of Pain.* Basic Books, New York, 1973.

33. Price, DD, Hayes, RL, Ruda, M, and Dubner, R: *Spatial and temporal transformation of input to spinothalamic tract neurons and their relation to somatic sensation.* J Neurophysiol 41:933, 1978.

34. White, JC and Sweet, WH: *Pain and the Neurosurgeon: A Forty-Year Experience.* Charles C Thomas, Springfield, 1969.

35. Pearl, GS and Anderson, KV: *Response patterns of cells in the feline caudal nucleus reticularis gigantocellularis after noxious trigeminal and spinal stimulation.* Exp Neurol 58:231, 1978.

36. Casey, KL: *Somatosensory responses of bulboreticular units in awake cat: Relation to escape-producing stimuli.* Science 173:77, 1971.

37. Anderson, KV and Pearl, GS: *Long term increases in nociceptive thresholds following lesions in feline nucleus reticularis gigantocellularis* (abstr). 1st World Congress on Pain 1:70, 1975.

38. Nashold, BS, Jr, Wilson, WP, and Slaughter, G: *The midbrain and pain.* In Bonica, JJ (ed): *Advances in Neurology,* Vol 4. Raven Press, New York, 1974, pp 69–169.

39. Schuarcz, JR: *Periaqueductal mesencephalotomy for facial central pain.* In Sweet, HW, Labrador, R, and Martin-Rodriguez, JG (eds): *Neurosurgical Treatment in Psychiatry, Pain and Epilepsy.* University Park Press, Baltimore, 1977, pp 661–667.

40. Casey, KL and Jones, EG: *Suprasegmental mechanisms: An overview of ascending pathways: Brain-stem and thalamus.* Neurosci Res Program Bull 16:103, 1978.

41. Nyquist, JK: *Somatosensory properties of neurons of thalamic nucleus ventralis lateralis.* Exp Neurol 48:123, 1975.

42. Ishijima, B, Yoshimasu, N, Fukushima, T, et al: *Nociceptive neurons in the human thalamus.* Confin Neurol 37:99, 1975.

43. Andersson, SA, Keller, O, and Vyklicky, I: *Cortical activity evoked from tooth pulp afferents.* Brain Res 50:473, 1973.

44. Reynolds, DV: *Surgery in the rat during electrical analgesia induced by focal brain stimulation.* Science 164:444, 1969.

45. Mayer, DJ: *The centrifugal control of pain.* In Ng, L and Bonica, JJ (eds): *Pain, Discomfort, and Humanitarian Care.* Elsevier, Amsterdam, 1980, pp 83–105.

46. Hughes, J: *Search for the endogenous legend of the opiate receptor.* Neurosci Res Program Bull 13:55, 1975.

47. Pert, C: *Opiate receptors and pain pathways.* Neurosci Res Program Bull 16:133, 1978.

48. Kuhar, MJ, Pert, CB, and Snyder, SH: *Regional distribution of opiate receptor binding in monkey and human brain.* Nature 245:447, 1973.

49. Hughes, J: *Intrinsic factors and the opiate receptor system.* Neurosci Res Program Bull 16:141, 1978.

50. Duggan, AW: *The differential sensitivity to L-glutamate and L-aspartate of spinal interneurons and Renshaw cells.* Exp Brain Res 19:522, 1974.

51. Elde, R, Hökfelt, T, Johansson, O, et al: *Immunohistochemical studies using antibodies to leucine-enkephalin: Initial observations on the nervous system of the rat.* Neuroscience 1:349, 1976.

52. Basbaum, AI, Clanton, CH, and Fields, HL: *Three bulbospinal pathways from the rostral medulla of the cat.* J Comp Neurol 178:209, 1978.

53. Hoffert, MS, Miletic, V, et al: *Immunocytochemical identification of serotonergic axonal contacts on characterized neurons in cat spinal dorsal horn.* Anat Rec 202:83A, 1982.

54. Pelletier, G, Steinbusch, HWM, et al: *Immunoreactive substance P and serotonin present in the same dense-core vesicles.* Nature 293:71, 1981.

55. Hökfelt, T, Terenius, L, et al: *Evidence for enkephalin immunoreactive neurons in the medulla oblongata projecting to the spinal cord.* Neurosci Lett 14:55, 1979.

56. *Report of the Panel on Pain to the National Advisory Neurological and Communicative Disorders and Stroke Council.* HEW, NIH Pub #79-1912, Bethesda, MD, 1979, p 201.

57. Kniffki, KD, Mense, S, et al: *Responses of group IV afferent units from skeletal muscle to stretch, contraction, and chemical stimulation.* Exp Brain Res 31:511, 1978.

58. Fock, S and Mense, S: *Excitatory effects of 5-hydroxytryptamine, histamine and potassium ions on muscular IV afferent units: A comparison with bradykinin.* Brain Res 105:459, 1976.

59. Fordyce, WE: *Behavioral Methods for Chronic Pain and Illness.* CV Mosby, St Louis, 1976.

60. Fordyce, WE: *A behavioral perspective on chronic pain.* In Ng, LKY and Bonica, JJ (eds): *Pain, Discomfort, and Humanitarian Care.* Elsevier/North-Holland, New York, 1980, pp 233–252.

61. Procacci, P and Zoppi, M: *Pathophysiology and clinical aspects of visceral and referred pain.* In Bonica, JJ, Lindblom, V, et al: *Advances in Pain Research and Therapy,* Vol 5. Raven Press, New York, pp 643–658.

62. Hancock, MB, Foreman, RD, et al: *Convergence of visceral and cutaneous input onto spinothalamic tract cells in the thoracic spinal cord of the cat.* Exp Neurol 47:240, 1975.

63. Travell, J: *Temporomandibular joint dysfunction.* J Prosthet Dent 10:745, 1960.

64. Travell, JG and Simons, DG: *Myofascial Trigger Point Manual.* Williams & Wilkins, Baltimore, 1982.

65. Simons, DG and Travell, JG: *Myofascial origins of low back pain.* Postgrad Med 73:66, 1983.

66. Gracely, RH: *Psychophysical assessment of human pain.* In Bonica, JJ (ed): *Advances in Pain Research and Therapy,* Vol 3. Raven Press, New York, 1979, pp 805–824.

67. Scott, J and Huskisson, EC: *Vertical and horizontal analogue scales.* Ann Rheum Dis 38:560, 1979.

68. Ohnhaus, EE and Adler, R: *Methodological problems in the measurement of pain: A comparison between the verbal rating scale and the visual analogue scale.* Pain 1:379, 1975.

69. Melzack, R and Törgerson, WS: On the language of pain. Anesthesiology 34:50, 1971.

70. Melzack, R: *The McGill Pain Questionnaire: Major properties and scoring methods.* Pain 1:277, 1975.

71. Klepac, RK, Dowling, J, et al: *Sensitivity of the McGill Pain Questionnaire to intensity and quality of laboratory pain.* Pain 10:199, 1981.

72. Byrne, M, Troy, A, et al: *Cross validation of the factor structure of MPQ.* Pain 13:193, 1982.

73. Reading, AE: *A comparison of MPQ in chronic and acute pain.* Pain 13:185, 1982.

74. Gracely, RH: *Pain measurement in man.* In Ng, LKY and Bonica, JJ (eds): *Pain, Discomfort and Humanitarian Care.* Elsevier/North-Holland, New York, 1980, pp 111–137.

75. Cosentino, AB, Cross, DL, et al: *Ultrasound effects on electroneuromyographic measures in sensory fibers of the median nerve.* Phys Ther 63:1789, 1983.

76. Mense, S: *Effects of temperature on the discharges of muscle spindles and tendon organs.* Pflugers Arch 374:159, 1978.

77. Parsons, CM and Goetzl, FR: *Effect of induced pain on pain threshold.* Proc Soc Exp Bio Med 60:327, 1945.

78. Melzack, R and Wall, P: *The Challenge of Pain.* Penguin Books, New York, 1982.

79. Lehmann, JF and DeLateur, BJ: *Therapeutic heat.* In Lehmann, JF (ed): *Therapeutic Heat and Cold,* ed 3. Williams & Wilkins, Baltimore, 1982, pp 404–562.

80. Travell, J: *Myofascial trigger points: Clinical view.* In Bonica, JJ, Able-Fessard, DG (eds): *Advances in Pain Research and Therapy,* Vol 1. Raven Press, New York, 1976, pp 919–926.

81. Cattell, M and Hoagland, H: *Response of tactile receptors to intermittent stimulation.* J Physiol 72:392, 1931.

82. Gammon, GD and Starr, I: *Studies on the relief of pain by counter-irritation.* J Clin Invest 20:13, 1941.

83. Hensel, H: *Thermoreception and Temperature Regulation.* Academic Press, New York, 1981.

84. Buchthal, F and Rosenfalck, A: *Evoked action potentials and conduction velocity in human sensory nerves.* Brain Res 3:1, 1966.

PART 2

INSTRUMENTATION: METHODS AND APPLICATION

INSTRUMENTATION CONSIDERATIONS: OPERATING PRINCIPLES, PURCHASE, MANAGEMENT, AND SAFETY

H. T. M. RITTER, III, B.A., C.B.E.T.

In opening this chapter, it is significant to note that most of the earliest applications of electricity in medicine were intended as physical therapy devices. Experiments with electrotherapy are on record from the 18th century.[1] Diathermy was first described late in the 19th century, and ultrasound was under investigation shortly thereafter.[2] Today, there is a greater variety of instrumentation to be found in hospital physical therapy departments than in any other patient care area.

A basic knowledge of electrical principles is essential for safety in the physical therapy department and for an understanding of devices such as ground fault circuit interrupters, diathermy units, and ultrasound generators. The author assumes that the reader has had previous exposure to these basic principles, including electron flow, Ohm's law, capacitance, and inductance. For a comprehensive review of electrical terminology and theory, the reader may refer either to Cromwell[3] or to Spooner.[4]

The objectives of this chapter are to (1) present the basic principles and physiologic effects of 60 Hz alternating current; (2) discuss the reasons for grounding electrical devices and for installing ground fault circuit interrupters in hydrotherapy areas; (3) offer guidelines for prepurchase evaluation, acquisition, and knowledgeable management of equipment; and (4) review general and device-specific inspection procedures including calibration methods and appropriate standards.

ELECTROMAGNETIC ENERGY

The entire range of radiation, or electromagnetic spectrum, includes heat, radio, and light waves as well as ultraviolet, x, and cosmic rays. It is important to know, however, that *ultrasound energy is not electromagnetic,* but rather a mechanical/pressure waveform that cannot be transmitted by air. Notice from careful study of Figure 3–1 that shortwave (SWD) and microwave (MWD) diathermy are both safely in the non-ionizing section.

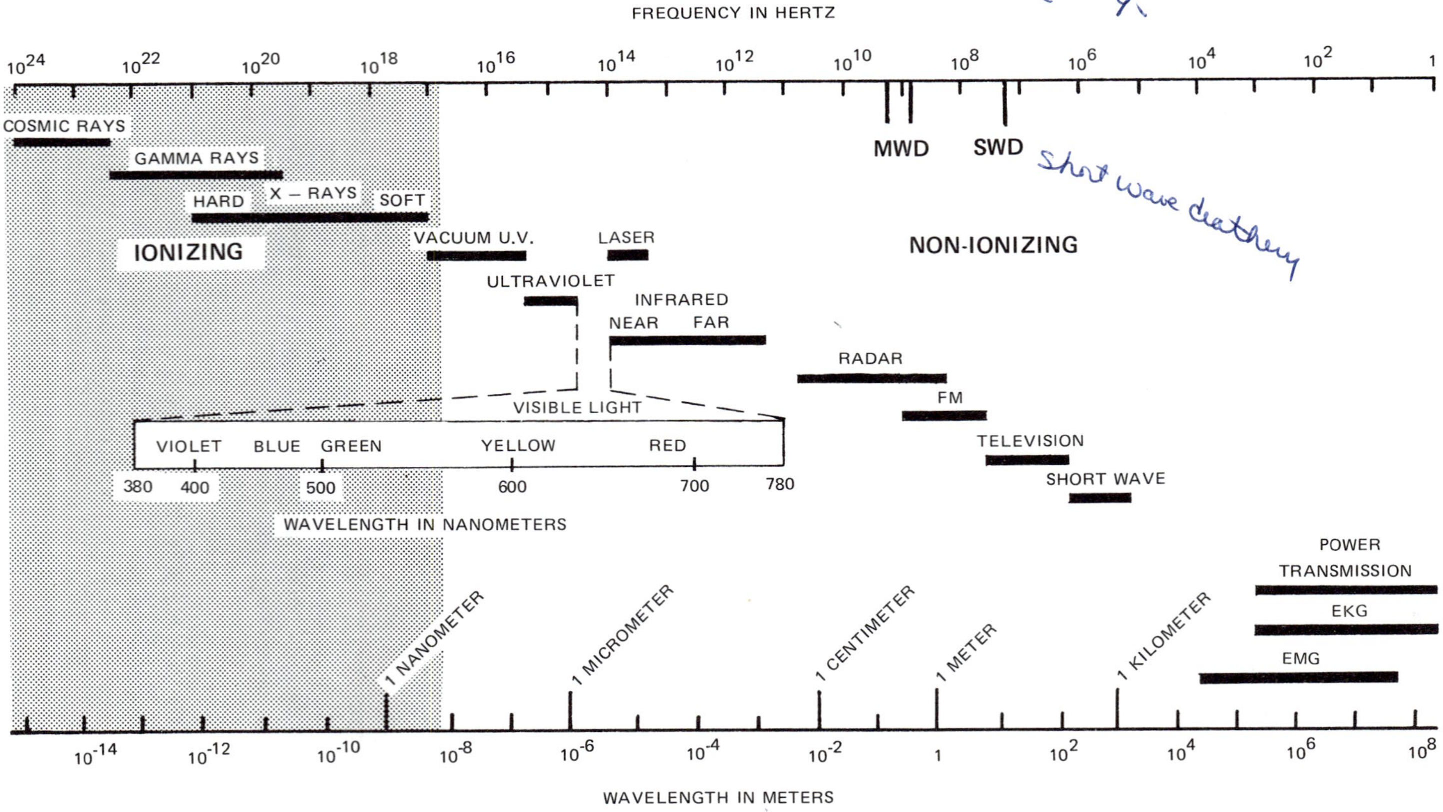

FIGURE 3–1

A graphic representation of the electromagnetic spectrum. (Adapted from *IES Lighting Handbook,* ed 5, 1972.)

This means their radiation effects are thought to be purely thermal. These energies are not capable of stripping electrons from atoms.

The electromagnetic spectrum also reveals that each form of radiation can be described by a frequency (f) and a wavelength (λ). All forms of radiant energy are self-propagating and travel in a vacuum at the speed of light (c), which is 300 million meters per second. The reader should be aware of the formula that interrelates these three quantities: $c = f\lambda$. Since c is a constant, frequency or wavelength can be derived even when just one of them is known. For instance, given that the wavelength of shortwave diathermy is 11.062 meters, calculate its frequency.

$$f = c/\lambda = \frac{3 \times 10^8 \text{ m/sec}}{11.062 \text{ m}} = 27.12 \times 10^6 \text{ cycles/sec} = 27.12 \text{ mHz}$$

Radiation energy is directly proportional to frequency. Therefore, cosmic rays are far more penetrating than is infrared radiation. Within the infrared spectrum, the higher-frequency radiation, near visible light, is more penetrating than "far" infrared. The biologic effects of electromagnetic radiation depend on frequency, exposure duration, tissue characteristics, and power density.

In dealing with instrumentation for thermal therapy, there is no need to be concerned with direct current (DC). The domain of relevant alternating current (AC) frequencies ranges from the 60 Hz power line supply through the megahertz region for diathermy up to infrared radiation.

POWER SUPPLY: "115 VAC – 60 Hz"

Conventional power line voltage in North America alternates at the very regulated frequency of 60 hertz (abbreviated Hz and denoting cycles per second). The accuracy of electric clocks, for instance, depends on this constant, since "line" voltage frequently varies between 110 and 125 volts. Every electrical device intended for operation on line voltage will bear a label that typically lists 110, 115, 117, or 120 volts—alternating current (VAC), as distinguished from direct-current voltage (VDC). (Some heavy-duty devices, such as treadmills, may require a 230 volt source.) The label will also indicate the line frequency (60 Hz) and either a current or a power rating. For instance, a new solid state ultrasound unit specifies "120 VAC 60 Hz, 0.5 amp maximum." The same information could have been conveyed by indicating 60 watts instead of listing current: Power = Voltage (E) × Current (I) = 120 × 0.5.

Voltages and their frequencies can be seen and measured with an oscilloscope. A comparison of symbols and waveforms for DC and AC is illustrated in Figure 3–2.

TRANSFORMERS

Electricity is transmitted from generating stations over long distances at very high voltages (e.g., 230,000 volts). Prior to commercial distribution, it must

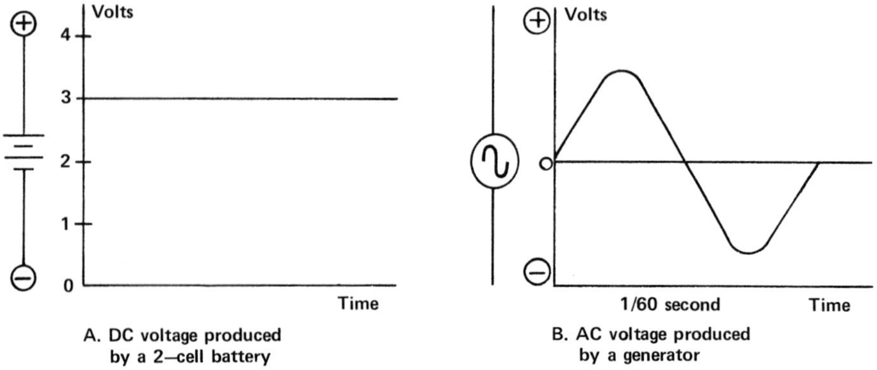

FIGURE 3–2

Symbols and waveforms for direct current (DC) and alternating current (AC).

be dropped to the 115 volt range. While whirlpool motors, paraffin baths, and infrared lamps operate directly off this line voltage, some instruments have power supplies that require a lower AC voltage. Others may require a boosting of voltage at some point.

Transformers accomplish these necessary voltage manipulations. Typically they are composed of two adjacent coils on an iron core and operate on the principle of electrical induction. When alternating current flows through the input or primary winding of a transformer, it creates a surrounding magnetic field. This field, in turn, cuts through the secondary winding and induces an output current. Note that there is no electron flow between primary and secondary windings. Output voltage and current are determined by the ratio of primary to secondary winding turns. When transformer windings have approximately the *same* number of turns, output voltage will equal input voltage, and the unit is referred to as an isolation transformer. This type of transformer, which can be used as a safety device, will be discussed in another section.

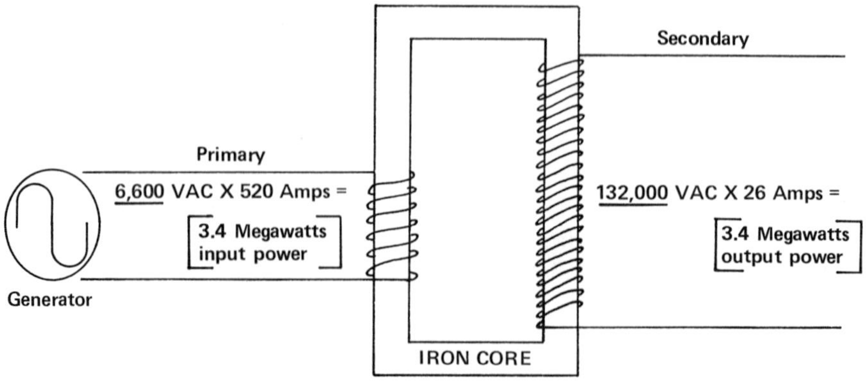

FIGURE 3–3

A step-up transformer used for electrical power transmission. Lowered secondary current greatly reduces losses due to heating of the power distribution wires. (Note: "Step-up" or "step-down" refers to secondary *voltage*.)

The concept of input power equaling output power (assuming no coupling losses) is fundamental to understanding step-up and step-down transformers. Again reviewing the power formula $P = E \times I$, it can be seen that for a given input power to the primary, a stepped-up *voltage* is associated with a proportional reduction in secondary current (Fig. 3–3).

If a transformer secondary has *fewer* turns than its primary winding, output voltage will be reduced. For example, an ultrasound generator has a step-down transformer that drops line voltage to approximately 24 volts, which is then fed to the unit's power supply.

POWER DISTRIBUTION AT THE USER'S END

Figure 3–4 illustrates the terminology and mechanism of power distribution to the familiar point of an electrical receptacle. It also depicts a simplified current flow to, from, and within a representative ultrasound unit.

As previously described, electrical power is commercially supplied in a range of 110 to 125 volts, alternating at the frequency of 60 Hz. Although only two conductors are actually required for a voltage source, a third conductor can be employed to enhance electrical safety. This line is referred to as "ground" and most often is actually connected to a rod in the earth in or just outside a building. As a rule, the plumbing system of a building is also considered to be "grounded." Ground is a universal electrical reference point that is at a zero-voltage potential.

Current circulates to and from the ultrasound unit through wires designated as hot and neutral. In spite of careful design and proper insulation, minute currents will nevertheless stray (much of it capacitively) from the hot/neutral circuit to adjacent conductive surfaces. Then, if a path exists, these so-called leakage currents will flow to any object that is grounded, completing their return back into the power system. (Note carefully in Figure 3–4 that neutral side of the electrical service is also connected to ground.)

If an electrical device loses its line cord/receptacle grounding, a patient or therapist, or both, can become a substitute path for leakage current from its conductive exterior, for instance, to any grounded surface, as illustrated in Figure 3–5. Most people have experienced leakage current as a mild tingling or buzzing sensation in touching certain electrical devices that are powered by two-wire line cords. Since resistance of the human body is in a range of 100 to 1,000,000 ohms (depending, for instance, on how much tissue is between the contact sites and if they are damp or dry), the normally intact ground wire in three-wire line cords, with resistance less than 1 ohm, will divert any nontherapeutic current before it can cause electrical shock. Such current is simply dumped into the receptacle's ground terminal.

Users of electrical devices must know that *leakage current is a normal phenomenon.* Widely recognized standards[5,6] recommend a maximum of 100 microamperes for exterior surface (chassis) leakage. This amount is approximately one-tenth the current believed necessary to stimulate sensory perception. Leakage from an *applicator* (or electrode) intended for direct patient connection should not exceed 50 microamperes.

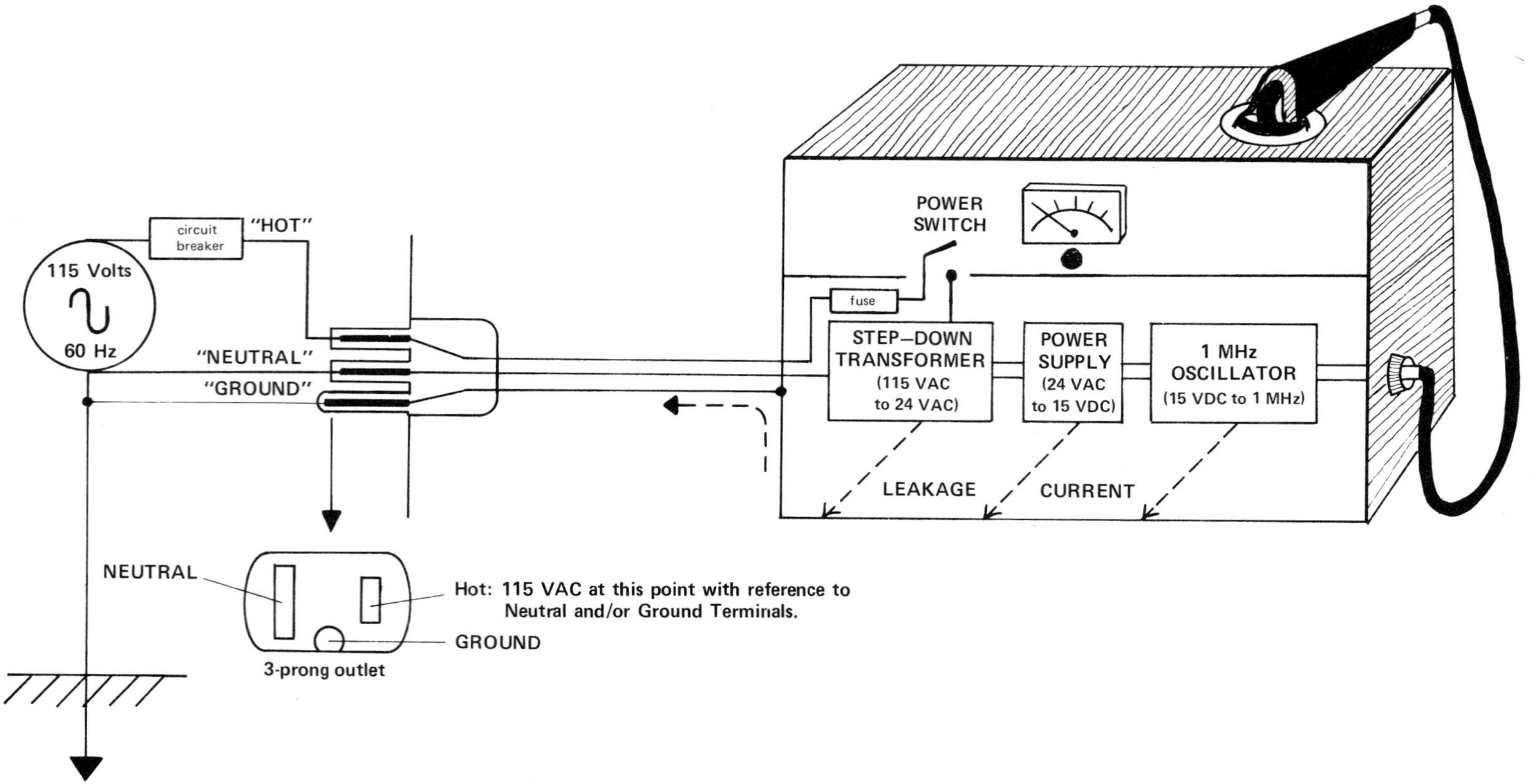

FIGURE 3–4

A device is powered by the voltage between the hot and neutral conductors. Normal leakage current is conducted away from metal housing (chassis) by the ground wire.

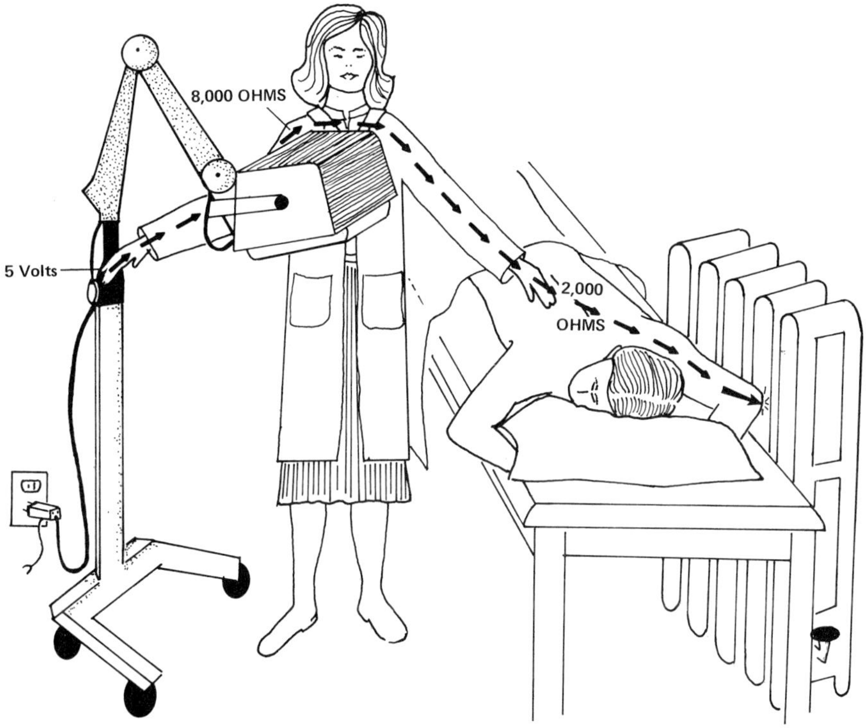

FIGURE 3–5

A realistic leakage current hazard. Three-wire line cord is plugged into a two-blade outlet using a "cheater" plug. Radiator completes circuit to ground.

$$\text{Leakage current} = \frac{\text{Voltage}}{\text{Resistance}} = \frac{5 \text{ volts}}{10{,}000 \text{ ohms}} = 500 \text{ microamperes}$$

In the event of a *major* degradation of electrical insulation (for example, water seepage into the unit's electronic circuits), an unintended path to ground or "ground fault" is likely to result. This would produce excessive leakage current, commonly termed *fault* current. As before, with normal leakage current, the fault current would be conducted away from the unit by its ground wire. The fuse, with a typical current rating of 1 to 2 amperes should then melt open when fault current exceeds that limit.

At this point, visualize the hazard that would exist in the absence of a low-resistance grounding connection: the 1 to 2 amperes could end up flowing to ground through someone's body, with possibly fatal consequences. Ground wire integrity, therefore, must be inspected routinely to verify low resistance between conductive chassis surfaces and the grounding pin of the power plug.

Double insulation is a design technique that introduces a second layer of insulation between the "live" internal components of a device and the operator. Many manufacturers are turning to plastic and other nonconductive materials for chassis fabrication as an alternative method of minimizing risks from stray currents. This usually makes chassis grounding unnecessary and a two-wire line cord would therefore be acceptable. The device should be labeled, preferably on its nameplate, as being double-insulated. Hydrotherapy devices, however, are an exception; these always require grounding

GROUND FAULT CIRCUIT INTERRUPTERS

Equipment used in hydrotherapy areas presents a major potential for electrical hazards arising from ground faults. Installation of ground fault circuit

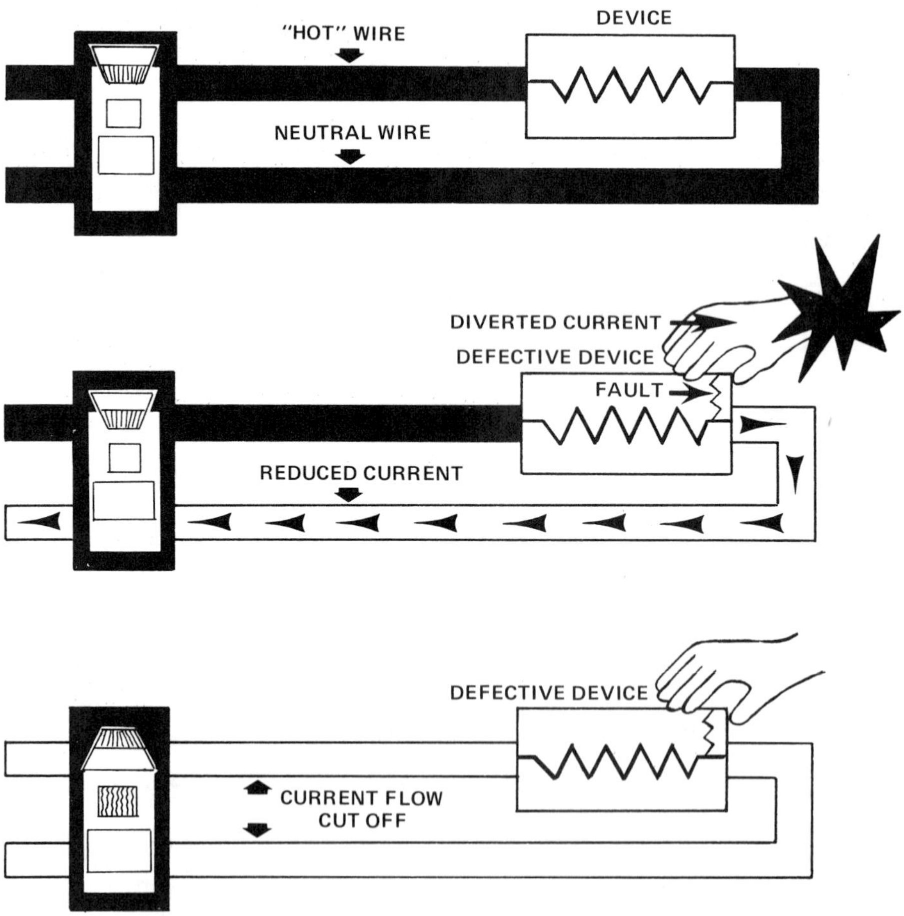

FIGURE 3–6

Operation of a ground fault circuit interrupter (GFCI). (Adapted from Square D Company product information literature.)

interrupter (GFCI) protection for all receptacles that serve these locations can effectively eliminate such hazards. In general, GFCIs are required for all receptacles within 1.52 m of therapeutic tubs.[7]

Note that the name for this device is nearly descriptive: the (power) circuit is interrupted when a ground fault is sensed. The same device is frequently referred to as a ground fault interrupter or GFI. This terminology is misleading, because it suggests that the fault itself is eliminated.

A sensor within the GFCI constantly monitors the currents in the *hot* and *neutral* lines that feed a given receptacle. The assumption is that input current from the hot line *to* a device should very nearly equal current *from* the device back to the neutral line. A substantial difference of 5 milliamperes between hot and neutral suggests that a ground fault exists and is diverting current return from neutral to ground (Fig. 3–6). Since the maximum safe transthoracic current (through intact skin) is deemed to be 5 milliamperes, GFCI activation is set to occur at this level.

Tripping time is almost instantaneous; a button labeled RESET extends out of its channel when the circuit is interrupted. Once the ground fault is identified and eliminated, this same button is depressed to reactivate the GFCI. Depressing the TEST button generates a low-level internal ground fault causing the unit to trip. This test should be exercised monthly to verify operation. Annual inspection of ground fault circuit interrupters using a calibrated external test device is also advocated.[6]

A GFCI can be integrated within a power receptacle or as part of the circuit breaker for that receptacle. Figure 3–7 illustrates both configurations.

ISOLATION TRANSFORMERS

External isolation transformers are fading into history, as older equipment is being replaced. They are used to lower the leakage current of some older devices that generate chassis leakage far in excess of 100 microamperes but that are otherwise safe and functional.

As previously discussed, output voltage of an isolation transformer is of the same magnitude as line voltage. The difference is that the secondary voltage is not referenced to ground. Therefore, the leakage current from a device plugged into the transformer will not seek or flow to ground.

ONE TO SIX THOUSAND MILLIAMPERES

The effects of 1-second exposures to *60 Hz* currents are summarized in Table 3–1. The current levels listed are *average* figures; actual effects would vary as a function of many factors, including body size, physical condition, and age. Wet skin, also, would greatly increase resultant risk current. For perspective in reviewing Table 3–1, it is helpful to know that the current that flows through a 100 watt bulb is almost 1 ampere.

As current frequency increases, its physiologic "shock" hazards diminish. At frequencies greater than 10 kHz, current of sufficient intensity produces tissue heating with no other apparent effect on the neuromuscular

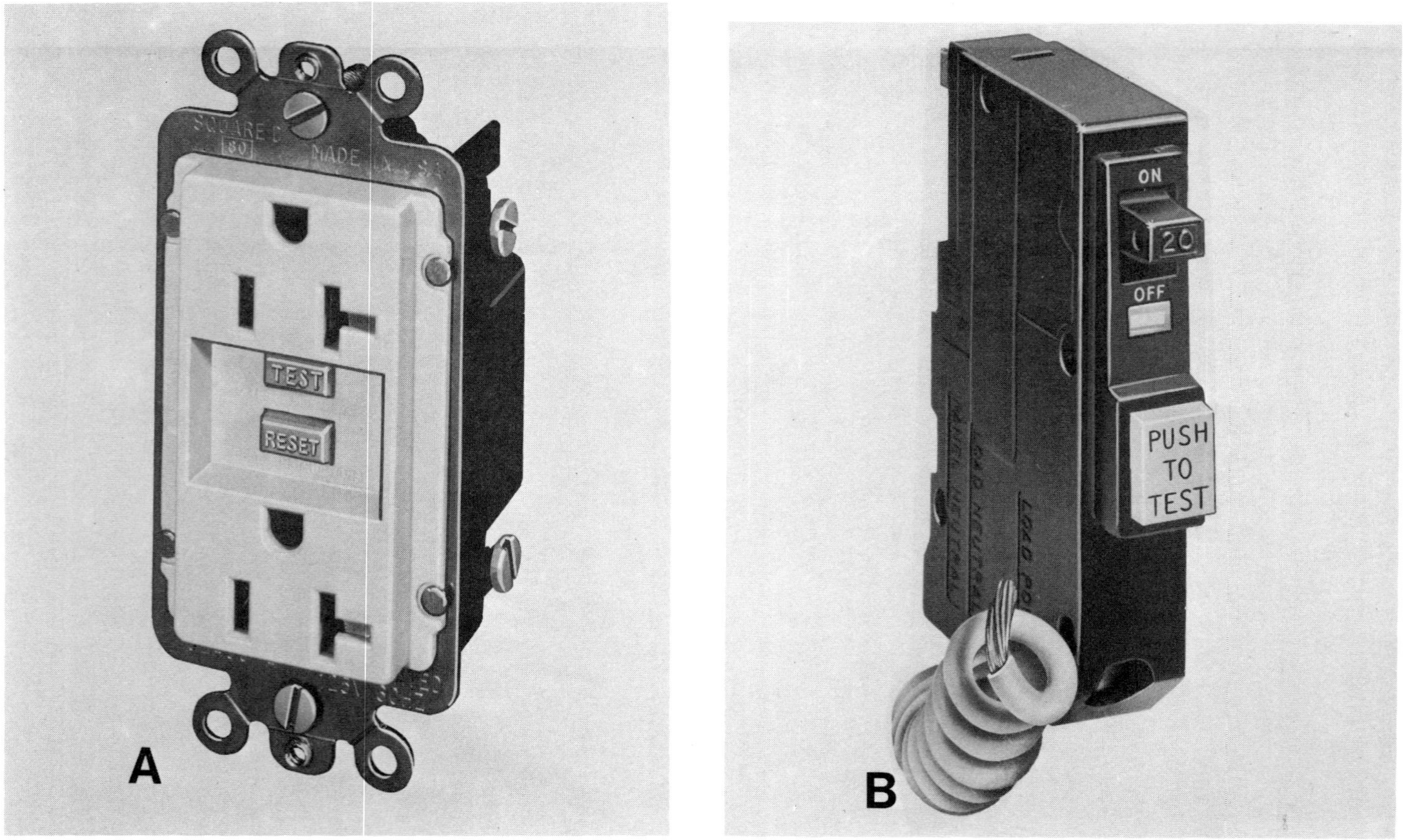

FIGURE 3–7
Ground fault circuit interrupters. *A*, Receptacle style; *B*, Circuit breaker style. (From Square D Company, Lexington, KY, with permission.)

TABLE 3–1
Effects of 60 Hz AC Current Flowing Arm to Arm Through the Chest*

Current in Milliamperes	Physiologic Effect
1	Threshold of perception; tingling.
5	Maximum current considered to be harmless. (Typical GFCI tripping level is 4–6 mA.)
10–20	Sustained muscular contractions.
50	Pain, exhaustion; possible fainting.
100–300	Ventricular fibrillation.
1000–6000 (1–6 amps)	Body muscle system contracts violently; probable respiratory paralysis and burns.

* Adapted from Bruner, JMR: *Hazards of electrical apparatus.* Anesthesiology 28:400, 1967.

system. High-frequency electromagnetic current is the active mechanism of shortwave diathermy delivered with air-gap or pad (capacitive) applicators.

OSCILLATORS

As is commonly known, AC signals in radio frequency range can be directed and transmitted through air. A shortwave diathermy unit, for instance, with a frequency of 27.12 MHz is just a step removed from a citizens' band (CB) radio transmitter. Each device contains an electronic circuit known as an oscillator that develops an alternating or oscillating output from a DC source. *Any* specific (resonant) frequency can be obtained as a function of the associated timing circuit's capacitance and inductance. Waveforms produced can be sinusoidal, square, saw-toothed, or unidirectional pulses, as illustrated in Figure 3–8.

In physical therapy instrumentation, oscillators are integral to ultrasound, shortwave diathermy, and electric stimulator units. For patient treatment, the waveform can be either continuous or cyclically interrupted (pulsed).

PREPURCHASE EVALUATION AND ACQUISITION OF EQUIPMENT

Considering equipment cost and the fact that most devices have a reasonable life expectancy of 8 to 10 years, it is vital that a thorough prepurchase investigation be conducted. Information should be sought and assembled from every possible source. ECRI (formerly, Emergency Care Research Institute) is a nonprofit agency dedicated to health care technology, facilities, and procedures. It offers three publications with associated membership services that should be consulted in the preliminary stage of equipment acquisition. *Health Devices* is a monthly journal which features brand-name evaluations and ratings based on ECRI's testing. *Hospital Product Comparison System,* jointly produced with McGraw-Hill, presents background informa-

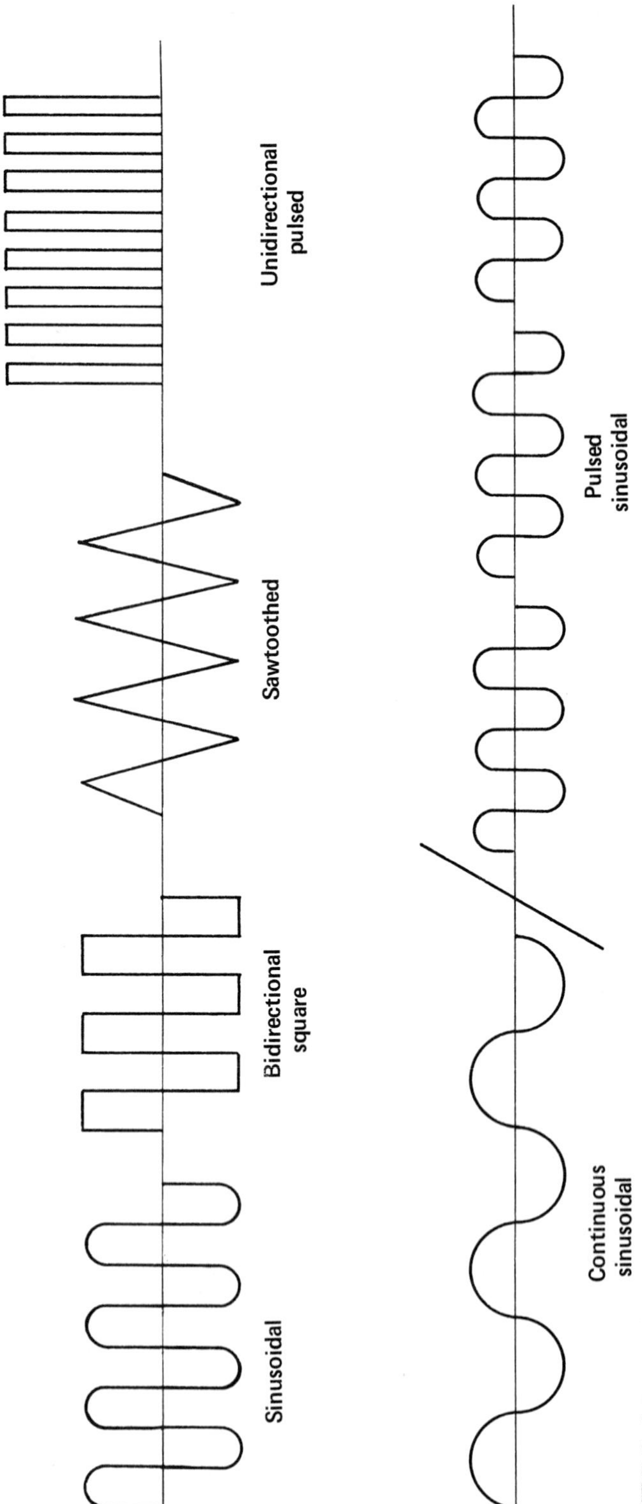

FIGURE 3–8
Oscillator waveforms.

tion on an increasing number of device categories coupled with a listing of manufacturers and a tabulation of specifications and features by model number. The *Health Devices Sourcebook* is a directory of medical devices, trade names, and manufacturers that is updated annually.

It would be additionally advisable to solicit the experiences of therapist colleagues who have used specific devices in various clinics and departments. Review the following questions:

1. Have there been any major defects or failures? (If so, was warranty service readily available?)
2. Have there been any problems in obtaining accessories or product support?
3. Does the device have any operational difficulties?
4. Can clinical effectiveness be assessed?

After limiting the field to perhaps three models, the next step is to arrange for a minimum 1-week trial period for each unit under a normal patient load. The salesperson or a technical representative should perform an in-service for all staff members who will be evaluating the equipment.

During the test period, difficulties are likely to arise under the varying circumstances of patient treatment. A log should be maintained to record all such problems and relevant patient comments so that they can be reviewed with the representative. Careful documentation will help to distinguish genuine deficiencies in the equipment or accessories from operator error.

When available, consult with the biomedical instrumentation* department, a biomedical equipment technician (BMET), or whoever is responsible for maintaining existing equipment. They should be asked to perform an electrical safety inspection on the loaned equipment and to examine its service manual. Review their experience with the product and manufacturer, and establish whether any specialized test equipment would be required for inspection, repair, or calibration. Consider together whether there would be any unusual assembly or installation requirements and estimate associated costs. If accessories are needed for routine operation of the device, their annual cost should be estimated.

Finally, analyze the terms of the warranty; most are for 1 year. Verify that warranty will not start until the equipment is installed and functional. Ascertain how this service would be performed: is it available locally or must the user package and ship the defective unit back to the manufacturer?

The end result of the decision process will be a purchase order (P.O.) for the selected device. In addition to quantity, description, and shipping address, a P.O. should specify:

1. Operator and service manuals (two each: one for the physical therapy department and one for the biomedical instrumentation department).
2. All applicators/accessories agreed upon.
3. An introductory in-service presentation.

---

* May also be referred to as biomedical or clinical engineering.

4. How/where warranty service will be performed and possibly a maximum "down" time limit.
5. Payment will be made after successful completion of an acceptance inspection.

It may bc desirable to notify the sales representative upon delivery of the equipment so that this person can do the unpacking and assembly. If shipping damage has occurred, the representative can handle any necessary adjustments. Otherwise, an in-service orientation can be performed for the entire staff.

In an institution with a biomedical instrumentation department, the new equipment generally will be tagged with a control number to facilitate documentation of inspection and repair. Manufacturer performance specifications should be selectively verified. (For instance, ultrasound and diathermy output frequencies would not normally be checked.) When the unit passes its acceptance inspection, final authorization for payment can be made.

OPERATOR MANUALS

Under ideal circumstances, a therapist should be very familiar with a newly acquired device by the time it is put into service. Many manufacturers provide a checklist for troubleshooting anticipated problems in their operator and/or service manuals (Table 3–2).

In addition, operator manuals typically include the following information: indications, contraindications, and precautions for using the device; function and location of controls; and serial procedures for treatment. Accessories and methods of application are generally illustrated and described. The stocking of certain spare items may also be recommended. A

TABLE 3–2
A Checklist for Troubleshooting for a Hot Pack Unit (Hydrocollator M-2)*

Problem	Cause	Remedy
Unit plugged in, water does not get hot with switch on.	Breaker for electric circuit off.	Turn breaker on.
	Thermostat not functioning.	Replace thermostat.
	Heating element burned out.	Replace element.
	On-off switch broken.	Replace switch.
Cloudiness of water	Seepage from packs (worn out).	Replace packs.
	Too long a period between cleanings.	Drain and clean.
Packs too hot	Thermostat set too high.	Adjust thermostat.
	Thermostat failure.	Replace thermostat.
Unit boils	Thermostat failure.	Replace thermostat.
Packs too cool	Thermostat set too low.	Adjust thermostat.
	Power failure.	Check electric circuit.

* From Chattanooga Corporation, Chattanooga, TN, with permission.

careful review of all operator manuals, therefore, should be a definite part of orientation for employees new to a department.

EQUIPMENT CARE AND SERVICE

Instrumentation service personnel generally estimate that 30 to 60 percent of reported equipment problems turn out to be attributable to operator error of some sort. Before initiating a request for service, therefore, recheck the entire set-up and, if necessary, review the operator manual.

In the absence of a pilot light or output power, first test the electrical receptacle with another device. When either the circuit breaker for the receptacle or the breaker on the instrument is tripped (and the institution does not have a policy requiring an electrician or equipment technician to reset breakers), the therapist can attempt the reset. Circuit breakers *do* occasionally trip for no apparent reason. If, however, a reset breaker immediately trips again, do not attempt to reset it a second time. Remember also to check for a tripped GFCI in situations of interrupted power.

There are three cases of equipment malfunction that should cause a device to be instantly removed from operation. In all situations when anyone experiences an electrical shock, smells an unusual odor (chemical or burning), or actually sees smoke, the device in question should be unplugged and prominently labeled "DEFECTIVE—DO NOT USE." Request an *immediate* investigation by the biomedical instrumentation department. Decide whether an incident report is necessary. Communicate the experience to ECRI directly, by phone, or with a copy of the User Experience Network problem reporting form (Fig. 3–9).

Accidental damage *will* occur: transducers are inevitably bumped and dropped, and fluids have a way of finding chassis ventilation openings. Repeated operator abuse, on the other hand, is inexcusable. Never roll a device over its line cord or pull a power plug by yanking the cord. Avoid wrapping cables and cords over-tightly; it is likely to make them intermittent or degrade their insulation. Do not force controls that are stuck or connectors improperly mated. Significantly, the experience of biomedical instrumentation personnel indicates that the majority of legitimate equipment defects are mechanical rather than electrical. Loose knobs and hardware, broken casters, and damaged strain reliefs are very common defects.

Whenever a nonemergency problem cannot be resolved by the user, it should be reported with *ample* detail to the appropriate service group. Unless this happens to be the manufacturer, it may be necessary for the therapist first to explain the function or demonstrate the operation of the equipment to the service individual. In most cases, the training of biomedical equipment technicians and even clinical engineers tends to focus on operating room and intensive care unit instrumentation. As a result, their inspections of physical therapy equipment are frequently limited to electrical safety checks, with little or no attention to actual performance. Be prepared, therefore, to review jointly each device in the department and to develop protocols for functional inspections. The next section of this chapter offers suggestions relevant to this task.

User Experience Network™

Problem Reporting Form

Use this form to report a problem or hazard related to the use of medical devices or equipment.

Telephone or Telex reports are acceptable. Information may also be sent via telecopier with CCITT Group I or Group II capabilities by calling (215) 834-1275.

Your personal and institutional identities will not be revealed in any way without your permission.

Your Name: ______________________ **Date:** __________
Please type or write legibly

Title: ______________________

Department: ______________________

Institution: ______________________

Address: ______________________

____

Phone: (______)______________ **Ext.** ________

May we identify you to the manufacturer and/or supplier of the device(s) involved? **Yes** ☐ **No** ☐

DEVICE IDENTIFICATION

Please be as specific as possible in identifying the devices involved. Please add any other information that might be helpful, and omit any items that are not known or that appear irrelevant to this particular problem.

Type of Device(s) Involved: ______________________

____

Manufacturer: ______________ Model: ______________

Serial / Lot No.: ______________ Expiration / Use Before Date: ______________

How Long in Use? ______________ Condition: ______________

Date Last Inspected or Serviced: ______________ Date Problem Occurred: ______________

Will You Send the Affected Device to **ECRI** for Examination, if Requested? **Yes** ☐ **No** ☐

Were Other Devices Involved? **Yes** ☐ **No** ☐ If yes, please identify all other units on the reverse side, including the information listed above.

PROBLEM DESCRIPTION

Could (or did) the described problem result in injury? **Yes** ☐ **No** ☐

Please use the **reverse side of this form or separate sheets** to describe the problem or hazard in detail. Include any action you took, and the response of any vendors or manufacturers. Attach copies of any related correspondence, where possible. Sketches, photographs, or copies of portions of operating manuals are often helpful in describing the problem, especially if the affected device is not available for examination at ECRI. Retain all disposable accessories possibly involved in an incident, but do not send them to ECRI until requested.

SIGNATURE: ______________________

Please mail completed form to ECRI, 5200 Butler Pike, Plymouth Meeting, PA 19462
(215) 825-6000 • TWX 510-660-8023

This form may be reproduced without prior permission.

ECRI 5200 BUTLER PIKE
PLYMOUTH MEETING, PENNSYLVANIA 19462

ECRI-02-883

FIGURE 3–9

ECRI User Experience Network Problem Reporting Form.

DEVICE-SPECIFIC INSPECTIONS

Superficial Heat and Cold

Most devices employed to deliver superficial heat or cold therapy incorporate thermostats to maintain defined temperature ranges. For instance, paraffin bath temperatures are usually maintained between 51°C and 54°C.

Thermostats are mechanical switches that may actually turn on and off many times an hour to achieve temperature regulation. They do fail periodically and require replacement. More commonly, however, control settings are tampered with, both inadvertently and intentionally. Calibration, therefore, may be required at any time. The internal thermometers of therapy appliances must also be monitored during inspections.

Some units may have integral timers for terminating treatment after a prescribed interval. Timer accuracy and actual power deactivation and/or alarm functions must be verified on such devices.

Hydrotherapy

Again, with whirlpool baths and Hubbard tanks, thermometer precision must be routinely checked. In fact, it is probably advisable that a therapy department or clinic have its own calibrated electronic thermometer with both air and submersible sensors. This will prove useful for occasional spot-checking of any of its device thermometers.

A whirlpool turbine must never be operated without water fully covering its impeller. Impellers should be checked to ensure free rotation: they are often partially wrapped with bandage material that restricts flow and turbulence.

Experience of some therapists suggests the wisdom of securing a turbine to its bath tank with an additional set screw or bolt.[8] This precaution eliminates the hazard of an energized motor falling into a filled tank during adjustment of turbine ejector height.

Inspections of hydrotherapy locations should additionally test the secureness of hand rails, stools, and overhead patient lifts. If a tank is mobile, the condition of its casters and drain hose should be assessed.

Ultrasound

To date, of all physical therapy devices, Federal Performance Standards exist only for ultrasonic products.[9] (A 1980 proposed standard for microwave diathermy[10] was withdrawn in 1983.) Specifically, in terms of performance, ultrasound units sold since 1979 are required to:

1. Indicate the magnitudes of ultrasonic power and intensity with an accuracy of ± 20 percent (both for continuous and amplitude-modulated waveform operation).
2. Control treatment time: 0 to 5 minutes, ± 0.5 minute; 5 to 10 minutes, ± 10 percent; >10 minutes, ± 1 minute.

Although many generators manufactured before 1979 are still in use, most, with proper calibration, should be able to meet these specifications.

An ultrasound power meter, pictured in Figure 3–10, should be a standard piece of test equipment in a biomedical instrumentation department. Transducer output power is radiated into distilled, degassed water at

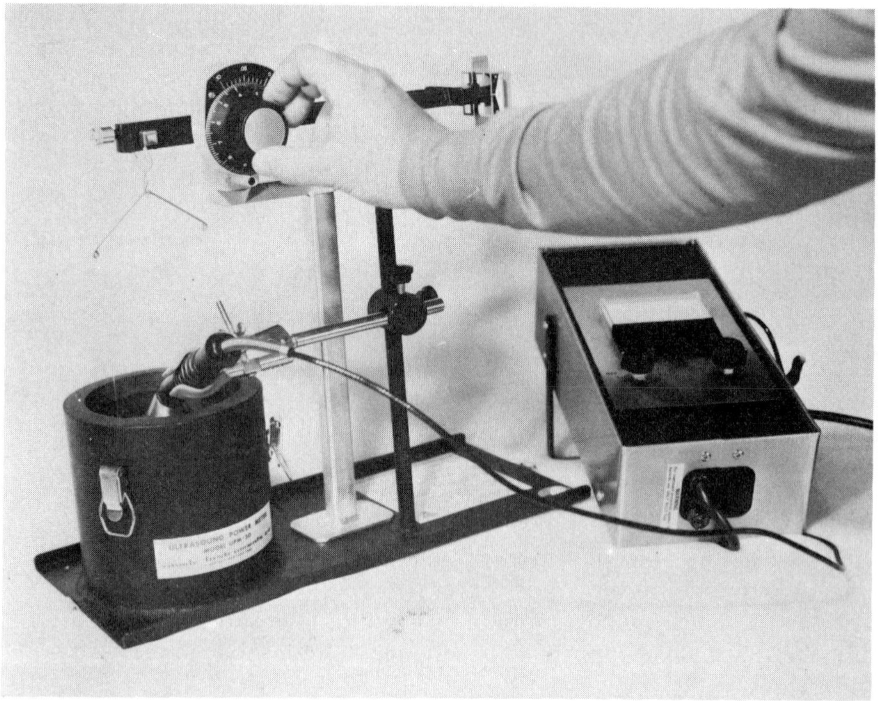

FIGURE 3–10

Testing watt output of ultrasound transducer using a power meter. (From Ohmic Instruments, with permission.)

30°C. Verification of output power accuracy is advisable on an annual basis and recalibration is always necessary when a transducer is replaced.

For more detailed information about transducer beam patterns and intensities, a device known as a hydrophone would be required. Principles of hydrophone operation are illustrated in Figure 3–11. The use of this test instrument is generally limited to ultrasound research applications.

Most problems with ultrasound units are traceable to either the transducer itself or the cable assembly. A therapist can quickly check for ultrasonic output by wrapping a ring of 1-inch tape around the front edge of the transducer and pouring a half inch of water into this cavity. At a power setting of 10 to 15 watts, boiling agitation and possibly a cone will be observed.

During this test, the transducer cable should be flexed, especially at the transducer and chassis connector strain reliefs (Fig. 3–12). If an intermittency exists, it will be manifested by a sudden decrease or interruption of output power, causing the water agitation to diminish or disappear. Defective transducer assemblies are usually returned to the manufacturer for rebuilding.

Diathermy

An accurate, standardized method for verifying output power actually delivered to a patient has not been developed for shortwave diathermy.[11] A

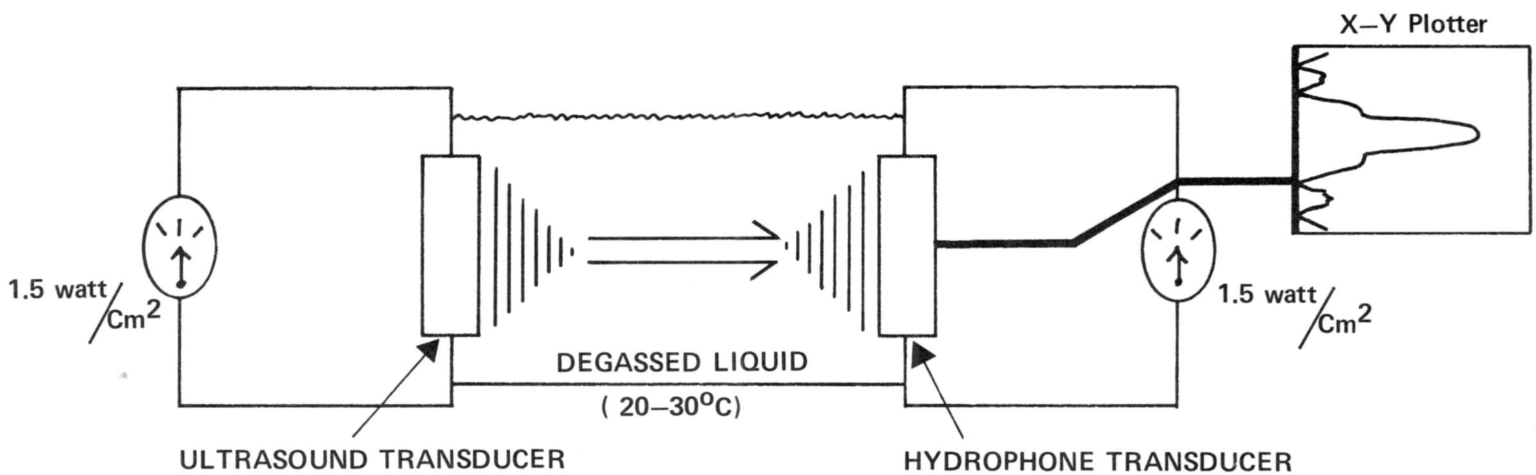

FIGURE 3–11

Piezoelectric materials can convert AC voltage to mechanical vibrations, which can then be converted back to voltage of the original frequency. Using a hydrophone and recorder, a transducer's spatial characteristics can be depicted.

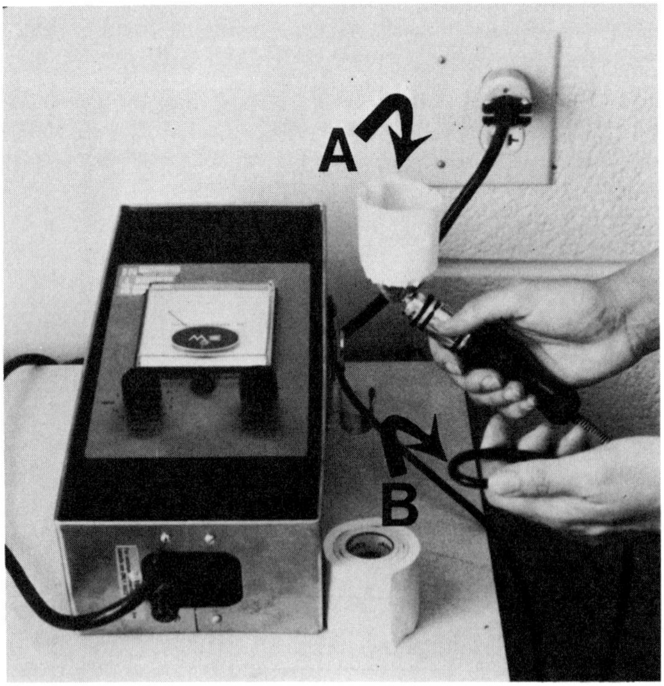

FIGURE 3–12

Therapist checking ultrasonic output (see text for description). *A,* Tape around transducer; *B,* Flexing transducer cable.

new microwave unit (TAG MED Model TDS-2450-2) purports this capability. The electromagnetic energy actually coupled to a patient and the resultant amount of heating produced are functions of operator technique, exposure time, the anatomy, and electrical properties of the treatment location, as well as spatial distribution and temporal characteristics (continuous versus pulsed output) of the radiated energy. At present, commercially available diathermy power meters are of little use other than for gathering baseline data on output, beginning with the acceptance inspection. They merely indicate power delivered to a fixed resistance in a test device.

A simple and inexpensive neon light bulb taped to a tongue blade is generally sufficient to indicate the presence of diathermy output. The bulb will have an orange glow if held near the applicator(s) or next to their cables (unless they are shielded).

Cables should *always* be kept spaced apart and several inches away from anything that is conductive (mattress covers or springs) or that may be grounded (including other energized devices and their line cords and plumbing fixtures). Be additionally cautious of some plastics and synthetics (for example, nylon) which, although nonconductive, may possibly be heated by electromagnetic diathermy.[12]

Timers can be tested against manufacturer specifications. Observe that output power is, in fact, deactivated when a set time expires. Operation of patient emergency cut-off switches and their pull ropes should also be verified.

ELECTRICAL SAFETY

As discussed earlier, electrical safety depends greatly on maintaining the integrity of device grounding and periodically verifying that chassis leakage currents do not exceed 100 microamperes. For equipment in general care areas of hospitals, a minimal testing interval of 12 months is stipulated by the National Fire Protection Association (NFPA). The NFPA along with organizations such as AAMI, ANSI, ECRI, and JCAH (Table 3–3) have developed a variety of guidelines, protocols, and standards for an extensive range of medical instrumentation and facilities.[5,6,13,14] In some cases, legislative bodies have adopted certain standards and made them binding regulations. Hospitals, however, generally comply to reduce potential equipment-related liabilities and to obtain institutional accreditations.

Appropriate documentation for every inspection (and repair) must be generated and kept for each piece of equipment. An inspection interval of less than 12 months may be indicated if a device has an extensive repair history or if utilization is especially heavy.

Equipment that is either portable or mobile tends to be repeatedly plugged in and out of receptacles. For this reason, all AC power receptacles and plugs should be hospital-grade quality (usually signified by a green dot). Annual testing of receptacles is also recommended.[6] Such inspections verify physical integrity of the outlet, as well as grounding continuity, correct polarity of hot and neutral, and grounding blade retention force (≥4 oz).

Documented inspection of devices, receptacles, and ground fault circuit interrupters is generally performed by the hospital's biomedical instru-

TABLE 3–3

Organizations Dealing with Medical Device Information, Standards, and Regulations

AAMI	Association for the Advancement of Medical Instrumentation 1901 North Fort Myer Drive, Suite 602 Arlington, VA 22209 (703) 525-4890
ANSI	American National Standards Institute 1430 Broadway New York, NY 10018 (212) 354-3300
ECRI	5200 Butler Pike Plymouth Meeting, PA 19462 (215) 825-6000
FDA	Center for Devices and Radiological Health Food and Drug Administration 8757 Georgia Avenue Silver Spring, MD 20910 (301) 427-8200 or (800) 638-6725
JCAH	Joint Commission on Accreditation of Hospitals 875 North Michigan Avenue Chicago, IL 60611 (312) 642-6061
NFPA	National Fire Protection Association Batterymarch Park Quincy, MA 02269 (617) 770-3000

mentation department or an outside service contractor. Although standards do not specifically apply to private clinics or offices, these locations should nevertheless have grounded power receptacles throughout and ground fault circuit interrupters in hydrotherapy areas. So-called cheater plugs, which adapt three-blade power plugs to two-blade receptacles (thus defeating grounding), and extension cords are never to be used.

SUMMARY

Effective and safe use of thermal instrumentation requires a thorough familiarity with each device, as well as a general understanding of electrical principles. A therapy department or clinic should establish and maintain a file of clinical and technical information for every piece of equipment in use.

Therapists should develop a close-working relationship with biomedical instrumentation personnel, using their resources to assist with evaluation of new devices and regular inspection and preventive maintenance of existing equipment. Inspections should verify both electrical safety and performance. Appropriate documentation of all inspection and repair activities must be kept for each device. Electrical receptacles and ground fault circuit interrupters require annual testing.

REFERENCES

1. Licht, SH: *History of electrotherapy.* In Stillwell, GK (ed): *Therapeutic Electricity and Ultraviolet Radiation,* ed 3. Williams & Wilkins, Baltimore, 1983.
2. Licht, SH: *History of therapeutic heat.* In Lehmann, JF (ed): *Therapeutic Heat and Cold,* ed 3. Williams & Wilkins, Baltimore, 1982.
3. Cromwell, L, et al: *Medical Instrumentation for Health Care.* Prentice-Hall, Englewood Cliffs, NJ, 1976.
4. Spooner, RB: *Hospital Electrical Safety Simplified.* Instrument Society of America/Prentice-Hall, Englewood Cliffs, NJ, 1983.
5. *Safe Current Limits for Electromedical Apparatus.* ANSI/AAMI **ESI, 1985.**
6. *Safe use of electricity in patient care areas of hospitals.* In *Standard for Health Care Facilities.* National Fire Protection Association 99, Quincy, MA, 1984.
7. *Therapeutic pools and tubs in health care facilities.* In *National Electrical Code.* National Fire Protection Association 70, Quincy, MA, 1984.
8. Gieck, JH: *Precautions for hydrotherapeutic devices.* Clinical Management 3:44, 1983.
9. *Performance Standards for Sonic, Infrasonic, and Ultrasonic Radiation Emitting Products.* 21 CFR 1050:10. Federal Register 43:7166, 1978.
10. *Microwave Diathermy Products: Performance Standard.* 21 CFR 1030. Federal Register 45:50359, 1980.
11. *Evaluation: Shortwave diathermy units.* Health Devices 8:175, 1979.
12. *Shortwave or microwave diathermy: A fire hazard?* Health Devices 12:197, 1983.
13. *Health Devices Inspection and Preventive Maintenance System.* ECRI, Plymouth Meeting, PA, 1984.
14. *Accreditation Manual for Hospitals.* Joint Commission or Accreditation of Hospitals, Chicago, 1985.

CHAPTER 4

CRYOTHERAPY: THE USE OF COLD AS A THERAPEUTIC AGENT

SUSAN L. MICHLOVITZ, M.S., P.T.

Cold agents are used as first aid measures after trauma and as adjunctive tools in rehabilitation of musculoskeletal and neuromuscular dysfunctions. Cryotherapy is an age-old remedy for pain relief, fever reduction, and control of bleeding, and more recently has been applied to prevent or reduce edema of traumatic origin, reduce inflammation, decrease muscle-guarding spasms, and temporarily diminish spasticity.

A number of agents are available to achieve the common goal of reducing tissue temperature. These agents include cold/ice packs, ice cubes for ice massage, ice-soaked towels, vapocoolant sprays, cold baths, and cold units with thermal controls.

The objectives of this chapter are to (1) discuss the physical principles underlying energy transfer with cooling agents; (2) explain the biophysical effects resulting from cold application; (3) discuss the clinical conditions for which cold can be of benefit; (4) discuss the techniques utilized for the administration of cryotherapy; and (5) discuss precautions to be taken to ensure safety of the patient during cryotherapy.

PHYSICAL PRINCIPLES

When heat is removed or lost from an object, this is referred to as heat abstraction or cooling. Therefore, when cold is applied, it lowers the temperature of the skin and underlying tissues by abstracting or removing heat from the body. The two modes of energy transfer used for therapeutic cooling include conduction and evaporation.

Conduction

The most common methods of cooling are placing ice/cold packs over an area or immersing a distal extremity in cool/cold water. The body part comes in direct contact with the cold agent. Energy transfer in these cases is by conduction. *Conduction* is the transfer of heat by the direct interaction of the molecules in the hot area with those in the cooler area. Internal energy is gained by the slower moving cooler particles from the more rapidly moving hotter particles.[1]

The magnitude of the temperature change and secondary biophysical alterations will depend on several factors, including (1) the temperature difference between the cold object and the tissue; (2) the time of exposure; (3) the thermal conductivity of the area being cooled; and (4) the type of cooling agent (for example, ice versus water).

The rate of heat transfer by conduction can be summarized by the following equation:

$$D = \frac{\text{area} \cdot k \cdot (T_1 - T_2)}{\text{thickness of tissue}}$$

where D equals rate of heat loss (calories/second); area equals amount of body surface area cooled or heated (cm^2); k equals thermal conductivity of tissues ($cal/sec/cm^2 \times c/cm^2$) (Table 4–1); and T_1 and T_2 equals temperature of warm and cool surfaces (°C).

The greater the temperature gradient between the skin and the cooling source, the greater will be the resulting tissue temperature change. For example, following a 15-minute immersion of the forearm in a water bath of 1°C, subcutaneous tissue temperature dropped by 24°C.[2] With the same duration and area of exposure at 17°C, the decrease in temperature in the subcutaneous tissue was only 6°C.[3]

When considering the ability of cold to lower the temperature of subcutaneous tissues, muscles, and joints, the time of exposure is important. The deeper the tissue, the longer the time required to lower the temperature (Fig. 4–1). Changes in skin temperature will occur very rapidly (within a minute or less) on exposure to cold. Subcutaneous tissue and muscle temperature can also be reduced by topical cold application, but additional

TABLE 4–1
Thermal Conductivities ($cal/sec)/(cm^2 \times °C/cm$)

Material/tissue	Thermal Conductivity (k)
Silver	1.01
Aluminum	0.50
Ice	0.005
Water at 20°C	0.0014
Bone	0.0011
Muscle	0.0011
Fat	0.0005
Air at 0°C	0.000057

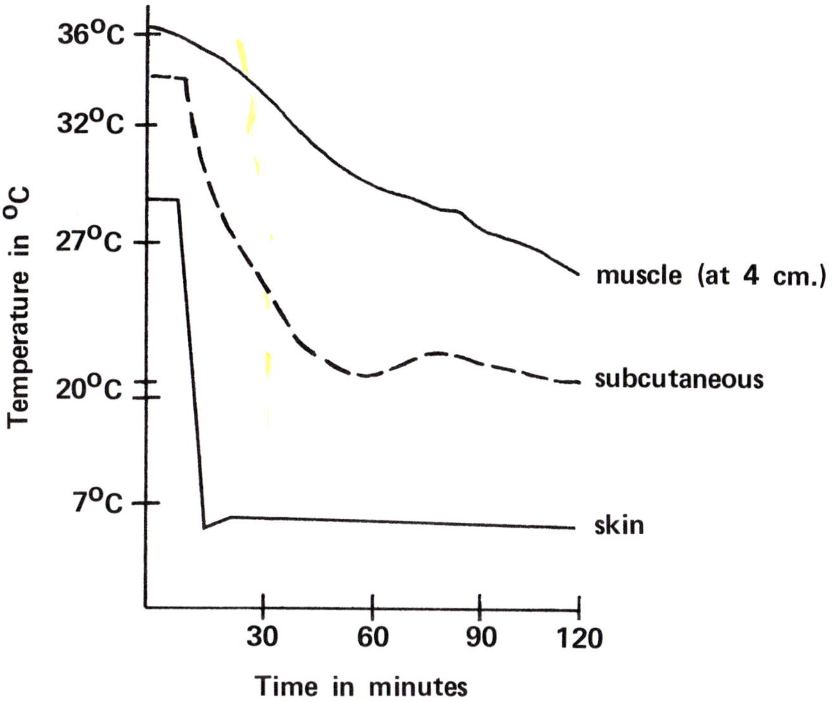

FIGURE 4–1

Temperature changes during ice pack application to the calf. (Adapted from Bierman and Friedlander.[5])

time is required to allow for conduction of energy. Muscle temperature at a depth of 4.3 cm can be lowered by an average of 1.2°C when cooled with an agent at 10°C.[4] It can take as long as 30 minutes, though, to lower muscle temperature at a depth of 4 cm by 3.5°C using ice packs.[5]

Thermal conductivity (Table 4–1) is a measure of the efficiency of a material or tissue to conduct heat. For example, metals are better heat conductors than are nonmetals. Tissues with a high water content, such as muscle, have better thermal conductivity than does adipose tissue. Adipose acts as an insulator, providing resistance to heat flow (for example, gain or loss). The amount of fat may influence the degree and rate at which muscle can be cooled[6,7] and conversely returned back to its precooled temperature.

In addition to the consideration of thermal conductivity, the effects of cold on blood flow to the area are important to understand, with respect to discussing why a cooled area can take such a long time to return to the precooled temperature. In fact, it can take a cooled area longer than a heated area to return to resting values. Arterial blood coming from the body core is warmer than the cooler venous blood returning from the periphery. Arteries and veins course through the body in juxtaposition to each other. Normally, as warm blood flows toward the periphery, it passes by the cooler blood in veins, which are in juxtaposition to the arteries. There is a countercurrent heat exchange between the warmer arterial blood and the cooler venous blood. After an area is heated, the vasodilation of arterioles allows cooler blood to rush into the area and carry away the heat. Cold causes a vasoconstriction of arterioles, decreasing the amount of warm blood flowing into the area. Thus, countercurrent heat exchange is reduced and the area may not rewarm very rapidly. When ice packs were applied around the knee of a dog for 1 hour, it took longer than 60 minutes after removal of the cold source before tissue temperature returned to resting values.[8] When hot packs were applied for the same duration, temperature rose to peak within 15 minutes, and then began to decline. The hot packs caused a vasodilation allowing cooler blood to flow into the area, dissipating heat. As long as the heat being added was greater than that being carried away, temperature remained elevated. After the heat source was removed, heat was rapidly lost by convection and radiation.

Intramuscular temperature of the gastrocnemius remained lowered for at least 3 hours following 20 minutes of cold baths at 10°C;[9] for at least 4 hours following a 30-minute cold bath at 10°C;[10] and for at least 1½ hours following 20 minutes of ice packs.[11] The level of activity can also influence the return of temperature to precooling levels. If exercise is done following cooling, this will facilitate an increase of blood flow to the area, thus, a faster rate of rewarming.

The form in which cold therapy is applied (for example, ice or cold water baths) may contribute to the degree of cooling. The magnitude of temperature change would be expected to be greater when ice packs are used, compared with cold water baths or frozen gel packs. Quadriceps muscle temperature in dogs was reduced by 11.3°C following 1 hour of chipped ice, compared with a decrease of 8.4°C when gel packs were applied for the same time.[12] The ice may be more effective in cooling an area because of the amount of internal energy required to melt the ice; that is, to break apart the solid bonding forces of the ice molecules. The internal energy is used first to change the ice to water before raising its temperature.[1]

Evaporation

Vapocoolant sprays utilize evaporation as a means of energy transfer. Vapocoolant sprays, such as Fluori-Methane (Gebauer Chemical Company, Cleveland, OH), are volatile liquids that are bottled under pressure and are emitted in a fine spray when the bottle is inverted. As the liquid comes out of the bottle, it begins to evaporate. When this transition occurs, the steam cools and upon contact with the skin extracts heat. The vapocoolant spray feels colder than room temperature water sprayed on the skin, because, like alcohol, it evaporates more quickly than water. The fluorocarbon mixture has a lower boiling point than water. The spray is applied for only a few sweeps across the skin. Skin temperature can drop to about 15°C with negligible changes in subcutaneous tissue and muscle temperatures.[13]

BIOPHYSICAL EFFECTS

Many of the clinical uses of cold are predicated on the physiologic changes resulting from tissue temperature reduction. Cold is used in the management of acute trauma, because the resulting (1) arteriolar vasoconstriction reduces bleeding; (2) decrease in metabolism and vasoactive agents (e.g., histamine) reduces inflammation and outward fluid filtration; and (3) elevation of pain threshold affords the patient more comfort. A reduction in skeletal muscle spasm can be postulated to be an interplay of factors, including a decrease in pain and a decrease in sensitivity of muscle spindle afferent fibers to discharge. Spasticity can be temporarily diminished owing to a decrease in the sensitivity of the muscle spindle to stretch. Muscle performance may be temporarily enhanced following cold. Pain and perhaps joint inflammation in certain inflammatory rheumatic diseases can be decreased. But some patients may experience an increase in joint stiffness secondary to the effect of cold on increasing tissue viscosity. When tissue viscosity is increased, the resistance to motion increases.

Hemodynamic Effects

When cold is applied, the immediate response is vasoconstriction of cutaneous blood vessels and reduction in blood flow. The amount of blood flow to an area is inversely proportional to the resistance factors impeding flow. Vessel diameter is the most significant factor relating to blood flow. Any influence that will cause vascular smooth muscle to contract will reduce vessel diameter. Conversely, when smooth muscle tone decreases, as happens with heating, vessel diameter increases.

Generally, exposure to cold for a short duration (15 minutes or less) results in vasoconstriction of arterioles and venules. The mechanisms of action causing vasoconstriction involve an interplay of factors including the direct action of cold on smooth muscle[14] and a reflex cutaneous vasoconstriction.[15]

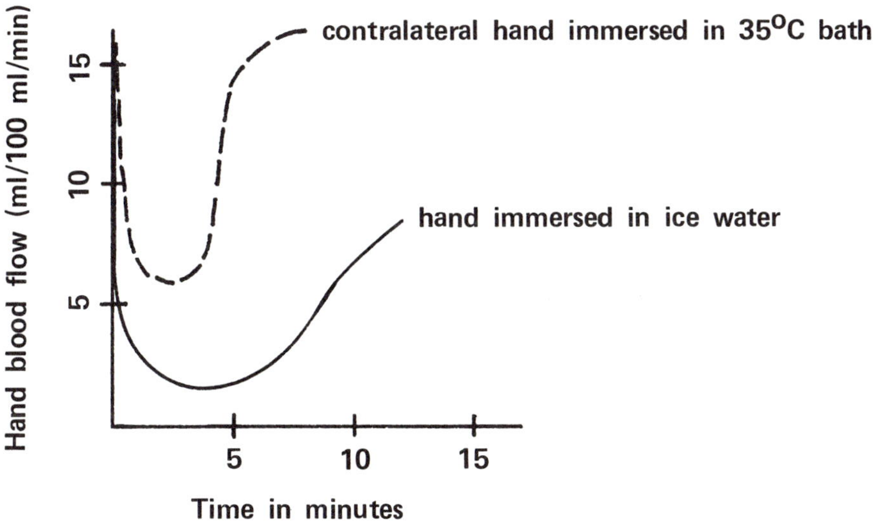

FIGURE 4–2

Blood flow to the hands following ice water immersion of one hand. (Adapted from Folkow et al.[16])

The blood flow to skin is primarily under neural control and plays an important role in thermoregulation.[15] Vasoconstriction of cutaneous vessels occurs as part of the heat retention mechanisms of the body. When skin temperature is lowered, cold thermal sensors (free nerve endings) in the skin are stimulated, causing a reflex excitation of sympathetic adrenergic fibers. Increased activity of these fibers causes vasoconstriction. This reflex vasoconstriction can also result in a generalized cutaneous vasoconstriction. The blood flow decrease is greatest in the area that is directly cooled. For example, blood flow in a hand cooled in ice water changed from a resting value of 16 ml/100 ml/min down to 2 ml/100 ml/min (Fig. 4–2).[16] Contralateral changes resulting from generalized cutaneous vasoconstriction were less pronounced.

As cooled blood returns to the general circulation, it stimulates the heat conservation area in the preoptic region of the anterior hypothalamus. Stimulation of this area will result in further reflex cutaneous vasoconstriction. If a large area of the body is cooled, shivering will occur as a heat retention mechanism.

Decreases in joint blood flow have also been demonstrated.[17] Ten minutes of ice packs at 0°C to the knee joints of dogs resulted in decreases in resting blood flow averaging 56 percent. The flow returned to precooled values approximately 25 minutes after the cold was removed.

The viscosity of blood, in part, determines resistance to blood flow. As viscosity decreases, so does the ease with which blood flows. The increase in blood viscosity resulting from cold exposure contributes to the decrease in blood flow. Figure 4–3 summarizes the mechanisms of action contributing to the reduction in local blood flow caused by cold application.

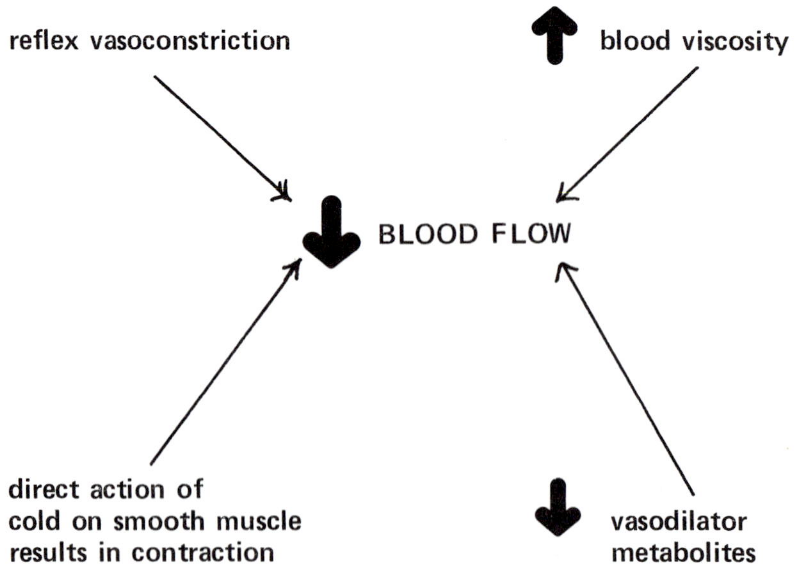

FIGURE 4–3

Action of cold stimulus on local blood flow.

When tissue temperature reduction is maintained for a long time and/or when temperature is reduced below 10°C, a cold-induced vasodilation can follow the initial period of vasoconstriction. This phenomenon was first recognized and reported by Lewis in 1930.[18] He found that when fingers were immersed in an ice bath, skin temperature decreased during the first 15 minutes. This reduction was followed by cyclic periods of increasing and decreasing temperature, which Lewis correlated with vasodilation and vasoconstriction, respectively. During the cycling periods, temperatures never returned to near-preimmersion values. This cycling was termed the "hunting response" and was felt by Lewis to be mediated by activity within an axon reflex. As skin was cooled to less than 10°C, pain would result, causing afferent sensory impulses to be carried antidromically toward skin arterioles. An unidentified neurotransmitter, substance "H," similar in action to histamine, was hypothesized to be released, resulting in arteriolar vasodilation. As warm blood came in and elevated temperature above 10°C, the ice bath was again effective in causing a vasoconstriction.

The "hunting response" appears to occur predominantly in apical areas where arteriovenous (A-V) anastomoses are located in the skin.[18,19]

There has been much speculation and investigation over the ensuing years to clarify the causes of cold vasodilation. In addition to activation of an axon reflex, others feel that cooling to less than 10°C can inhibit myogenic activity of smooth muscle[2,20] or reduce the sensitivity of blood vessels to catecholamines,[15] thus causing vasodilation.

Cold vasodilation can also occur without the "hunting" (cycling) component. Clarke and associates[2] cooled human forearms at a temperature of 1°C. A marked increase in blood flow to three to four times the precooled values occurred after 15 minutes of immersion. Only a slight increase in blood flow was noted with temperatures at 10°C. This cold vasodilation was thought to be a deep response, probably in skeletal muscle. This response was assumed to be local, because no reflex changes were noted in the contralateral extremity.

Post-Traumatic Edema and Inflammation

For the first 24 to 48 hours following injury, cold is usually the thermal agent of choice. The rationale for its use includes (1) less fluid filtration into the interstitium, owing to vasoconstriction; (2) less inflammation and less pain; and (3) a decrease in metabolic rate. The choice of cold has largely been based on empirical evidence. The length of cold exposure and the temperature can have significant effects on tissue swelling. Some animal laboratory studies will be discussed in this section, while clinical reports will be presented subsequently under Clinical Indications for Cryotherapy.

In most of the animal experiments, trauma was induced through some type of crushing force, resulting in soft tissue damage and/or fracture. Cold was then applied for varying lengths of time.

Matsen[21] used ice bags following tibial fractures in rabbits. Those animals treated with ice at temperatures ranging from 5°C to 15°C for 24 hours and at 10°C for 6 hours had more swelling than control animals. The swelling in a group cooled at 20°C to 25°C did not differ from that of the control group.

Jezdinsky and associates[22] also gave prolonged cold for 2, 5, 7, or 10 hours, with a constantly maintained temperature at 11.5°C to 12.5°C for postcrush edema in the rat. They reported a slight tendency for increased edema in the cold-treated animals. In a later group of experiments from the same laboratory,[23] the degree of cooling was less. Cold compresses at an initial temperature of 15°C to 18°C were applied to traumatized rat paws and changed at 30-minute intervals. Tissue cooling was probably not as great as with the first set of experiments,[22] because the compresses increased in temperature during each 30-minute period. There was no apparent "reactive hyperemia" after the compresses, as was reported after constant cold at 11.5°C to 12.5°C. Also, there was less of a trend toward edema formation if cold was applied at 2 hours post-trauma rather than immediately postinjury.

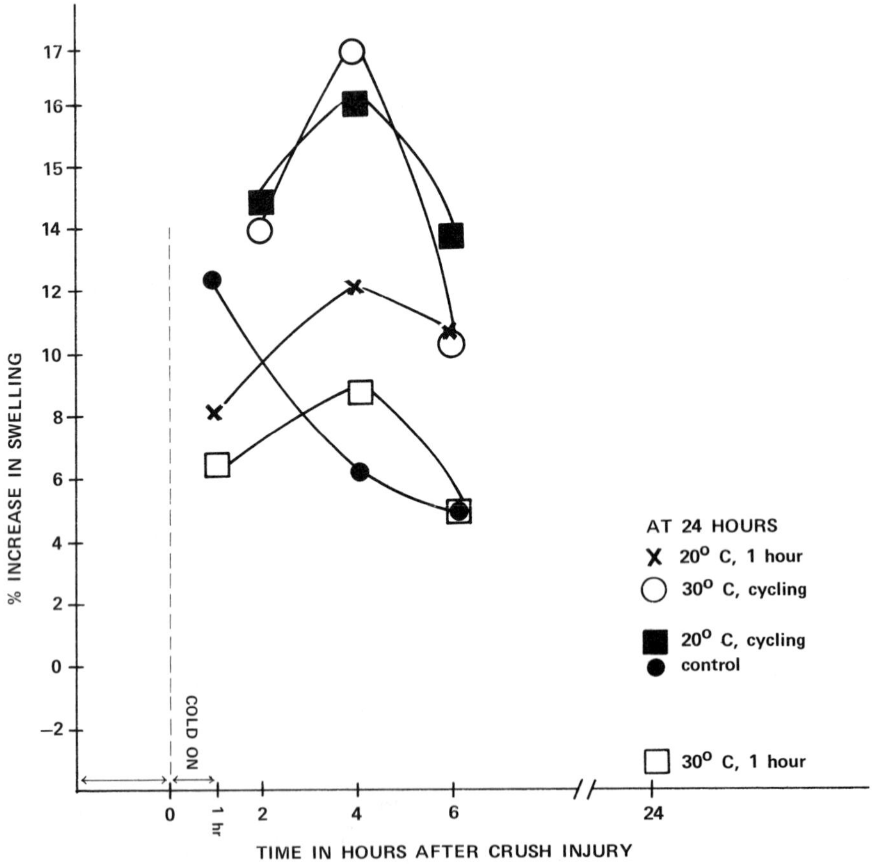

FIGURE 4–4

The effects of cold immersion on post–crush injury swelling in rabbits. Animals treated by "cycling" had three consecutive cycles of 1 hour immersion, 1 hour no immersion. (Adapted from McMaster and Liddle.[24])

Four different protocols were given by McMaster and Liddle[24] to treat crush injuries to rabbit forelimbs. The protocols included limb immersion in (1) 20°C water bath for 1 hour; (2) 30°C for 1 hour; (3) 20°C for 1 hour in, 1 hour out, 1 hour in; and (4) 30°C for 1 hour in, 1 hour out, 1 hour in. Results are detailed in Figure 4–4. It is interesting to note that both groups treated at 20°C had a greater residual edema at 24 hours postinjury than did the control group. It would have been interesting to see the results if compression wraps had been applied after immersion in the baths.

No attempt was made by the investigators described so far to correlate changes in tissue swelling with inflammatory exudates. Farry and Prentice[25] applied crushed-ice packs to treat experimentally induced radiocarpal ligament sprains in pigs. Cold was given for 20 minutes, followed by a 1-hour rest period, followed by another 20 minutes of cold. The protocol was probably more similar to actual clinical practice. Even though the cold produced an increased swelling in subcutaneous tissues, there was histologic evidence of decreased inflammation. Only one out of the 10 treated limbs had signs of a pronounced inflammatory response (that is, numerous polymorphonuclear leukocytes, plasma cells, lymphocytes, and fibrinous exudate). All the others had either no inflammatory cells or occasional to moderate amounts of polymorphs and lymphocytes.

The increases in edema that were observed could have been due to a cold-induced vasodilation or thermal damage secondary to prolonged cold exposures. Most awake humans, in addition, would not tolerate such long exposures. The animal studies reviewed do not seem to support the notion that cold prevents or reduces edema. Certainly, more animal studies using shorter duration cold followed by compression and/or elevation are warranted. These would more closely simulate clinical conditions and perhaps further add to our understanding of the effects of cold on edema.

Effects on Peripheral Nerves

Cold can alter the conduction velocity and synaptic activity of peripheral nerves. If temperature of the nerve is decreased, there will be a corresponding decrease in sensory and motor conduction velocities or even a failure of the nerve to conduct impulses. Synaptic transmission can be impeded or blocked. The quantity of the change elicited depends upon the duration and the degree of the temperature alteration.

Nerve fibers of different diameters and degrees of myelination appear to have different thresholds or sensitivities to the effects of cold.[26] The most "sensitive" fibers (for instance, those that exhibit changes in nerve conduction velocity first) are small-diameter myelinated fibers. The fibers least responsive to decreasing temperature are unmyelinated, small-diameter fibers. A fibers were blocked before C fibers in the saphenous nerve (afferent). Of the A fibers, the smallest diameter—the deltas—were blocked first; the largest fibers—the alphas—were blocked last. In motor fibers of the sciatic nerve, the gammas were blocked before the alphas.

Cold can decrease nerve conduction velocity. Motor conduction velocity of the ulnar nerve after cold application has been investigated by two groups of researchers.[27,28] Following 5 minutes of cold to the elbow, Zankel[27] recorded an average of a 6 percent decrease in motor conduction velocity in 8 out of 10 subjects. In those eight, conduction velocity returned to precooled values within 15 minutes. Zankel postulated that cold can alter the rate of transmembrane ionic flow.

With longer durations of cold, a greater decrease in temperature and conduction velocity is predicted. Ice packs over the ulnar nerve for 20 minutes resulted in an average decrease in motor conduction velocity of 29.4 percent from precooling values.[28] Thirty minutes after the ice packs were removed, the conduction velocity was still 8.3 percent lower than prior to ice application, suggesting a long-lasting effect when ice is given for a longer duration than in the experiments of Zankel. One group of investigators could find no direct correlation between percentage of body fat and velocity or temperature changes.[28]

Li[29] demonstrated in the rat that neuromuscular synaptic transmission was impeded when temperatures dropped as low as 15°C and that it was blocked at 5°C. The peripheral nerve stopped conducting impulses at 4°C.

Cryotherapy resulted in four cases of neurapraxia and one of axonotmesis in young athletes.[30] The ice packs were applied either over a major nerve branch that was superficially located (for example, over peroneal nerve at lateral border of the knee) or around the thigh for up to 2 hours (as in the case of axonotmesis).

Muscle Strength

When designing and implementing exercise programs, the clinician should be aware of the effects of a thermal agent on the ability of a muscle to generate tension. If cold is applied prior to exercise, could this be expected to alter muscle strength? And if it is applied after fatiguing exercise, will this have an effect on the course of postexercise recovery? Both questions have been examined in part. Most of the investigations to date have addressed only isometric strength. There is no evidence to suggest that the effectiveness of cold has been studied as an adjunct to isokinetic, concentric, and eccentric strengthening regimens.

McGown[31] measured isometric strength of the quadriceps before and after 5 minutes of ice massage to the entire anterior thigh of normal subjects. After icing, there was an increase in strength, compared with pretest values and with changes among a control group. There was no further followup reported to see if strength changed over time. Because muscle temperature was not expected to be lowered by such a short duration of ice massage to this large muscle mass, the author felt the increase in strength may have been due to increased muscle blood flow via sympathetic changes. In addition, those who received ice could have been psychologically motivated to perform better on the post-test.

Perhaps the short-duration cold had a facilitatory effect on the alpha motoneuron pool.[32] This notion is also supported by the finding that the facilitation of single motor unit activity is seen after 1 to 2 minutes of icing over the biceps brachii muscle in healthy subjects.[33]

When the duration of cold exposure is lengthened, then muscle temperature can be expected to decrease. Following cold immersion of normal legs for 30 minutes at 10°C to 12°C, Oliver and associates found that muscle temperature and plantarflexion strength decreased. This decrease could have been the result of reduced muscle blood flow at these lowered temperatures or an increase in the viscous properties of the muscle. At 45 minutes postimmersion, plantarflexion strength began to increase over pretreatment values and continued to do so for the next 3 hours (Fig. 4–5).

The findings of Johnson and associates[34] were similar to those of Oliver.[9] Following 30 minutes of immersion of the hand and forearm in a bath of 10°C to 15°C, grip strength was decreased for up to 1 hour, then increased over the pretest values for the next 2 hours.

Neither Johnson nor Oliver carried out post-test measurements past 3 hours. Therefore, time to recovery of the pretest values is not known. Also, both groups only tested one repetition of isometric strength at each interval. This paradigm is not representative of a therapy setting in which

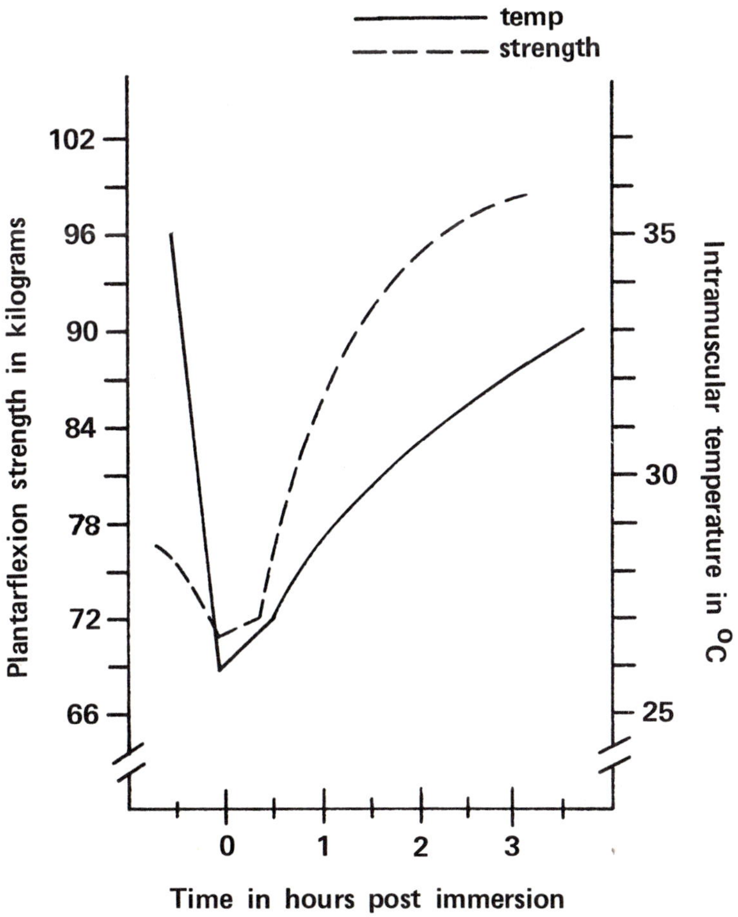

FIGURE 4–5

Plantarflexion strength and intramuscular temperature measurements post–cold immersion at 10°C. (Adapted from Oliver et al.[9])

a patient is often expected to perform multiple repetitions within a few minutes. On the other hand, Clarke[35] reported that cold baths at 10°C following fatiguing isometric exercise did not alter the period of recovery.

The fact that cold can change muscle strength can have important implications when evaluating patients and carrying out treatment plans. Cold could perhaps be used to enhance muscle performance during a therapy program, thus maximizing muscle performance. Because cold can change muscle strength, caution should be taken when performing initial and followup evaluations on patients during a therapy program. The evaluation of strength should be done prior to cold application to that muscle and not for at least a few hours after cooling.

Neuromuscular Effects

The presence of spasticity limits the ability of someone to carry out purposeful movements at the varying speeds required to perform activities of daily living. Spasticity is associated with an increased resistance to passive stretch, increased deep tendon reflexes, and clonus. Many therapeutic agents and regimens are used with the belief that spasticity can be reduced. Cryotherapy can temporarily reduce spasticity. Although the mechanisms responsible for the changes seen have not been fully elucidated, many animal and human studies have been designed to clarify and provide a rationale for these observed responses.

Eldred and associates[36] directly cooled the gastrocnemius muscle in cats and recorded the discharge of muscle spindle primary (Ia) and secondary (II) sensory endings and Golgi tendon organs (GTOs). The muscle spindles were de-efferented in these experiments. As the muscle temperature dropped from 38°C to 28°C, there was a linear decrease in the frequency of discharge of Ia and II afferents. GTO discharge decreased by approximately 50 percent. Between temperatures of 25°C and 20°C, firing became irregular and in some instances ceased altogether.

Newton and Lehmkuhl[37] also directly cooled cat gastrocnemius muscle. Recordings from dorsal root filaments revealed a decrease in action potential firing when muscle was cooled to 25°C. This finding indicates a decrease in muscle spindle afferent discharge secondary to cooling. When isolated muscle is cooled, the axonal discharge in cutaneous sensory afferents may be different than when cold is applied transcutaneously.

Twenty minutes of cold packs were applied to the calves of normal humans by Knuttsson and Mattsson.[32] Skin temperature dropped abruptly (by as much as 25°C) within the first few minutes, and the H response increased in amplitude. This increase in H amplitude would suggest facilitation of alpha motoneuron activity by short-duration cold. The amplitude of the Achilles tendon reflex (ATR) decreased shortly after the cold was started and continued to do so during the 20-minute period. Because ATR amplitude decreased before intramuscular temperature fell, activation of cutaneous afferents could cause reflex changes in muscle activity. The ATR continued to decrease as muscle temperature dropped. Therefore, changes in muscle spindle sensitivity secondary to cooling could also have contributed to the total response. The changes seen probably involve a series of complex mechanisms.

A decrease in monosynaptic reflexes following gastrocnemius cooling in the decerebrate cat was reported by Eldred.[36] Wolf and Letbetter[38] also examined the effects of short-duration cold stimulus on spontaneous electromyogram (EMG) activity of decerebrate cats. Cold was applied to the skin overlying the gastrocnemius muscle. EMG activity and subcutaneous and muscle temperatures were recorded. Rigidity, as measured by integrated EMG activity, decreased within 1 to 5 seconds after the skin was cooled. The decrease in muscle temperature was not as great as that predicted to change muscle spindle afferent activity. Therefore, Wolf and Letbetter concluded that a change in cutaneous afferent firing through reflex mechanisms produced a decrease in skeletal muscle activity.

Ten patients with spasticity were studied by Hartvikksen.[11] Twenty minutes of iced towels over the calf resulted in abolition of ATR and clonus. Decreasing ATR activity was seen before intramuscular temperature dropped; therefore, a reflex decrease in gamma motoneuron activity activated through skin receptors was proposed. These findings were in general agreement of those by Mecomber and Herman,[39] who recorded a decreased tendon jerk response prior to intramuscular temperature drop.

After 10 minutes of cooling muscle temperature, decreases in ATR were recorded by Hartvikksen.[11] This observation may be due to a decrease in muscle spindle firing. The ATR remained depressed for 30 minutes following removal of cold; clonus disappeared for 1½ to 2 hours.

Fifteen minutes of cold whirlpool at 18.3°C to the leg was also successful in decreasing the frequency of clonus or totally abolishing it for 4 to 5 hours.[40] Miglietta[41] studied clonus and muscle contraction time on a large series of patients with spasticity. Cold baths were given for 10, 20, and 30 minutes at 7°C. Muscle twitch time was prolonged before intramuscular temperature decreased, but clonus was not abolished in the majority of the patients until intramuscular temperature dropped. Even though contraction time increased and clonus decreased, the author thought they were not directly related to each other.

Knuttsson[42] used 15 minutes of cold packs to the upper extremity or 20 minutes to the lower extremity of patients with spasticity. Ten out of 15 patients had a decrease in resistance to passive motion, two had no change, and three had an increase. Clonus decreased in frequency, duration, and threshold in all patients who had displayed it initially. Voluntary range of motion improved in two thirds of those who had reduced range of motion.

Urbscheit and associates[43] reported inconsistent findings following cooling of the calf of hemiplegics for 12 to 20 minutes. H responses and ATRs were measured. In addition to having no consistent changes among the patients in H response and ATR, the patients' uninvolved side often responded differently than the involved side.

This points out that the change in spasticity following cold cannot always be accurately predicted. The underlying pathophysiology of the spasticity must be considered in predicting the responses to cold.

In many patients with spasticity, cold application can temporarily decrease the amplitude of deep tendon reflexes and the frequency of clonus, and can improve the patient's ability to participate in therapy programs. Cold facilitates alpha motoneuron activity and decreases gamma motoneuron firing. In order for spasticity to be reduced, the reduction in gamma activity should be proportionally greater than the increase in alpha activity. In summary, spasticity reduction via cold may occur through at least two mechanisms: (1) a reflex decrease in gamma motoneuron activity via stimulation of cutaneous afferents; and (2) a decrease in afferent spindle discharge by direct cooling of the muscle.

CLINICAL INDICATIONS FOR CRYOTHERAPY

Most clinicians will agree that in the acute stages (24 to 48 hours) following trauma, cold would be the thermal agent of choice. Even though cold may be uncomfortable for the patient during the first few minutes, pain will ultimately be reduced, and edema, inflammation, and muscle spasm will most likely occur to a lesser degree. Beyond the acute phase of injury, heat may be the first agent for treatment. But in many cases, cold has been a successful part of a therapeutic regimen to reduce spasticity, facilitate muscle contraction, reduce arthritic joint pain, and lessen muscle spasm.

Musculoskeletal Trauma

One of the most common applications of cryotherapy is for musculoskeletal trauma or postorthopedic surgical swelling and pain. One of the earliest clinical reports supporting cold therapy for edema control and pain management appeared in 1946.[44]

A comparison was made between two groups of patients who had undergone a variety of orthopedic procedures. One group (n = 479) had no ice packs, while the other (n = 345) had ice bags over their soft casts for a 48-hour period. Even though the cooling period was prolonged, the decrease in tissue temperature was probably minimal, owing to the cast interface between the ice pack and the skin.

The group treated with ice packs required less splitting of casts (5.31 percent), compared with that of the non-iced group (42.3 percent). In addition to the benefit of less swelling, the ice-treated group had less inflammation, as evidenced by a lower white blood cell count, and fewer elevated temperatures. None of the experimental group had apparent hematomas or hemarthrosis, compared with 16 of those in the group receiving no ice. Fewer narcotics were taken by those who were ice treated, indicating that their pain was less. Reduction of analgesic intake following cold has been reported by others.[45]

In most acute trauma situations, cold is used in conjunction with compression and elevation. The cold can act to reduce pain and fluid infiltration into the area, but the compression wraps are usually necessary to maintain the decreased tissue swelling. In the animal studies discussed earlier under Biophysical Effects, it was noted that the cold regimens did not incorporate compression as part of the study design. Basur and associates[46] looked at the more common clinical practice of cold and compression compared with compression only in patients following ankle sprain. One group of patients received cold packs once every 4 hours, followed by a compression wrap using a crepe bandage. Those patients treated with cold had a mean period of disability of 9.7 days, compared with 14.8 days for patients receiving only crepe bandaging. Swelling was better controlled in the group treated with ice.

The use of ice in combination with intermittent compression pumps is becoming increasingly popular in sports medicine facilities. These techniques are discussed in Chapter 11.

The duration of cold and the extent of temperature drop are important to the final outcome. To lessen the risk of thermal damage and an increase in limb volume during the acute post-trauma or postoperative phases, cold given for 20 to 30 minutes, a few times a day, in combination with compression and elevation would seem to be a logical treatment.

Even though intuition might lead us to believe that cold rather than heat during the early phases postinjury would lead to a faster recovery, this comparison was not reported until 1982 by Hocutt and associates.[47] One group of patients with ankle sprains was treated with superficial heating agents one to three times a day for 15 minutes and wore Ace wraps within the first 36 hours postinjury. Other ankle sprain patients had cold whirlpools 7°C to 10°C or ice packs for the same duration and frequency as the heat-treated group. A third group of patients was seen after 36 hours and treated with cold. Treatment was continued for a minimum of 3 days among all patients. The patients treated with "early cold" (within the first 36 hours) returned to full activity (running and jumping without pain) an average of 8 days before the other two groups. Therefore, the time at which thermotherapy is initiated following trauma can be expected to influence the time course for functional outcome.

As sequelae to trauma, skeletal muscle spasm and pain limit mobility and function. Many therapeutic techniques, including thermal agents, electrical stimulation and massage are given with the common goals of reducing pain and muscle spasm, thus facilitating a more expedient recovery to normal function. In addition, many of these agents could be given in lieu of pain medication.

Cooling the skin can elevate pain threshold[48] and reduce pain by acting as a counterirritant,[49] thus making motion more comfortable. During an acute episode of tendinitis or bursitis, severe pain can limit motion and could ultimately lead to joint stiffness. To avoid this scenario, a therapeutic regimen should be aimed at reducing pain and inflammation and maintaining range of motion. Lane[50] reported on a patient with bicipital tendinitis who regained full, pain-free range of motion after four treatments with ice massage.

Cryokinetics (cold and exercise) was a technique popularized in the 1960s by Hayden[51] and Grant.[52] Hayden reported on a group of 1000 military patients who sustained sprains, strains, and contusions during training. Ice massage or ice water immersion was used to provide analgesia prior to range-of-motion exercises. All but three of the patients returned to active duty within 2 days; most of them required only one physical therapy treatment. Of the 7000 patients reported on by Grant, 80 percent had no more than three formal treatments with ice massage. Both Grant and Hayden cite that ice massage and exercise have an additional advantage of allowing patients to be more easily instructed in self-treatment.

Cold in combination with static stretch or contract relax techniques has been recommended for reducing muscle spasm or decreasing exercise-induced muscle soreness, thus increasing range of motion. Cold is applied over the painful muscle using ice massage, ice packs, or iced towels. Either during or immediately following the cold application, the exercise is carried out with the idea of returning the muscle to its normal resting length.

Prentice[53] induced muscle soreness in normal subjects through fatiguing concentric and eccentric contraction of the hamstrings. The following day, EMG activity of the exercised muscle was increased from the pre-exercise measurement. EMG activity was measured as an indicator of muscle pain and spasm.[54] Following 20 minutes of cold packs and static stretch to the hamstrings, EMG activity was reduced, suggesting a decrease in muscle soreness and spasm. Cold application, followed by a proprioceptive neuromuscular facilitation (PNF) technique, slow-reversal-hold, was done with another group. This technique was also successful in reducing EMG activity. These techniques were compared with an untreated control group and two groups who were given hot packs and static stretch or PNF. Those who received cold had less measured EMG activity.

With 15 minutes of ice massage only, pain and range of motion did not improve in subjects with exercise-induced soreness in the biceps.[55] No stretching or other form of exercise was given. The combination of ice in conjunction with exercise may successfully decrease muscle soreness. The cold may be used to reduce the pain, thus permitting stretching to be carried out. In addition, cooling of 10 or more minutes may reduce muscle temperature and decrease the sensitivity of the muscle spindle to stretch.

Vapocoolant sprays can also be utilized as a counterirritant to decrease pain thus allowing an increase of range of motion. In a study on normal subjects, Fluori-Methane was sprayed along the length of the hamstrings as a static passive stretch was applied. Passive hip flexion measurements were increased more significantly in the group receiving spray and stretch versus a control group who received only passive stretch.[56]

A series of patients with low back pain was studied by Landen.[57] Patients with chronic pain (an onset of greater than 2 weeks pretreatment) received ice massage or hot packs followed by flexion exercises. Those patients who were treated with ice had a significantly shorter hospitalization period than did those treated with heat—an average of 6.27 days compared with 9.29 days, respectively. Interestingly enough, however, those patients classified as acute had a shorter hospitalization when given hot packs instead of ice massage, an average of 4.08 days compared with 5.53 days, respectively.

Myofascial Pain Syndrome

Myofascial pain syndrome is defined as "pain and/or autonomic phenomena referred from active myofascial trigger points with associated dysfunction."[13] The dysfunction can be manifested as decreased range of motion in the area of the myofascial trigger point or area of referred pain. A trigger point in muscle may result from muscular strain and be associated with sensitized nerves, increased metabolism, and decreased circulation. Trigger points are also thought to be present in skin, ligaments, and nonmuscular fascia.

The pioneering work in trigger point localization and therapy was done by Dr. Janet Travell. She has designated active and latent trigger points. Active points are associated with a decrease in motion and moderate to severe pain. With latent trigger points, the person may have restricted range

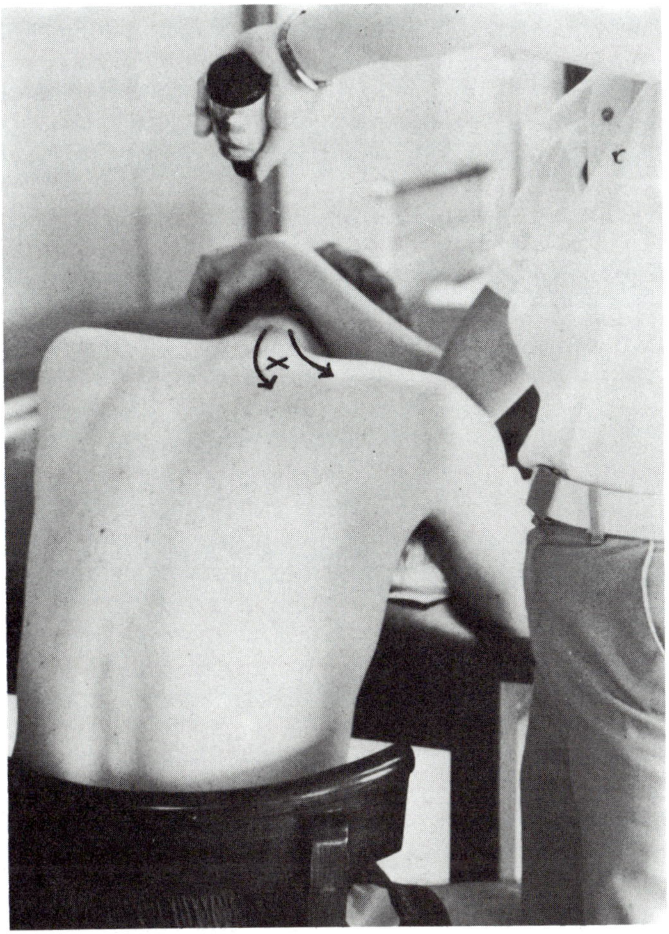

FIGURE 4–6

Stretch and spray with Fluori-Methane. A trigger point has been identified in the levator scapulae muscle (noted by the X). The muscle is put on passive stretch and then sprayed.

of motion but pain is only present on palpation. Trigger points can be located by digital pressure, electronic point locators such as the Neuroprobe (Physio Technology, Inc., Topeka, KS), and thermography.

Trigger points can be treated using a variety of techniques including "stretch and spray," ice massage, deep pressure, ultrasound, and electrical stimulation. The choice of treatment seems to be based upon empiricism.

"Stretch and spray" is a method taught by Travell that involves putting the affected muscle on passive stretch, then spraying over the area with a vapocoolant while maintaining the stretch (Fig. 4–6). The skin is then rewarmed by the therapist's hand or a moist hot pack and the stretch and spray is repeated if necessary. Spraying over the trigger point and area of referred pain is thought to stimulate cutaneous afferents, producing a reflex decrease in gamma motoneuron firing and thus permitting more passive stretch of the muscle.

Common areas of trigger points can be around the cervical spine, shoulder girdle, and low back. Poor body mechanics and faulty posture are probably contributing factors. Therefore, in addition to stretch and spray techniques, a complete therapeutic program should include postural exercises and instruction in proper body mechanics.

Reduction of Spasticity

Spasticity associated with upper motoneuron lesions often interferes with the performance of activities of daily living and gait. Cryotherapy can be used as an adjunct in the total treatment plan of the patient with spasticity to reduce temporarily the hypertonicity, thus permitting instruction in purposeful movements and activities.

Levine and associates[58] suggested cryotherapy as part of the treatment regimen. Cold is applied over the hypertonic muscle for 10 to 30 minutes. The method of application (for example, iced towels and cold packs) depends on accessibility, size, and contour of the body area to be treated. Once the area has been cooled and the spasticity reduced, an exercise program is carried out. The effects of the cold can be expected to last about 1 to 1½ hours.

As discussed earlier in the chapter, many researchers have documented decreases in ATR and clonus following cold. These measures, though, do not directly relate to an ability to perform skillful and purposeful activities. Hedenberg[59] reported on a series of hemiplegic patients with onset of their disability from 3 months to 10 years. All patients had hypertonia and hyperreflexia in the involved arm. The study was designed to measure upper extremity function, using a standardized test to evaluate if cryotherapy contributed to improvement of function. The hemiplegic upper extremities of the patients were immersed in a 12°C water bath for 15 minutes. Following immersion, all patients improved on test scores. Seventeen of the 24 had significant improvements. The greatest improvements in skill were with precision movements involving the thumb and the index and middle fingers.

Certainly more clinical documentation and information sharing on the use of cryotherapy for patients with spasticity should be encouraged. In fact, this technique could be appropriate for patients, caretakers, and family members to apply in the home prior to exercise and selected ADL.

GENERAL GUIDELINES FOR METHODS OF CRYOTHERAPY

Cold is administered by a variety of means. The methods that will be discussed include cold packs, ice massage, iced towels, cold baths, vapocoolant sprays, and controlled cold units. The choice of which agent to use depends on accessibility, body part to be treated, and size of the area to be cooled. For example, the foot may be best covered by a cold immersion bath, the knee by a cold pack wrapped circumferentially. Treating the ankle and leg can be done more efficiently with cold packs than with ice massage.

When considering cryotherapy, the therapist must be familiar with the patient's medical status. (Precautions for cryotherapy are discussed in the next section.) Prior to actual treatment, particularly before ice massage or cold immersion bath, a small area of skin should be tested for hypersensitivity.[60] If hypersensitivity is apparent, this should be documented and the cold discontinued. Generally speaking, conductive cooling is administered for 10 to 30 minutes, with the longer time periods being recommended for obese patients.[6]

Oftentimes, the skin underlying the cooling agent will redden. This can occur for one of two reasons. First, oxygen does not dissociate as freely from hemoglobin at lowered temperatures; therefore, the blood passing through the venous system is highly oxygenated, giving a red color to the skin. Second, after a 10- to 15-minute period of chilling or upon removal of the cold stimulus, a reactive hyperemia may occur, bringing a greater amount of blood in the area.[15]

For an hour or two after cryotherapy, the patient should avoid stresses that could potentially reinjure or aggravate the pathology for which they were treated. The analgesia produced by the cold could mask exercise-induced pain, thus giving the patient a false sense of security. Lowering of joint temperature can increase stiffness,[61] thereby decreasing reaction time and velocity of motion.[62] This fact, in combination with analgesia, predisposes the patient to further injury.

Cold Packs

Cold packs can be purchased or easily made. The commercial brands usually contain a silica gel or sand slurry mixture encased in vinyl and are available in a variety of sizes and shapes to contour the area to be treated. The packs can be stored in a special refrigeration unit or in a household freezer. Storage temperature should be approximately −5°C for at least 2 hours prior to use. For hygienic reasons, a layer of towel should be placed between the pack and the skin surface. Air is a poor thermal conductor; therefore, a moist towel will facilitate energy transfer by eliminating as much air interface as possible. If the towel is wet with room temperature or lukewarm water, the initial contact will be more comfortable for the patient. The packs can be secured by a strap, with the patient positioned so that the area is well supported.

There are a number of cold packs chemically activated by squeezing or hitting them against a hard surface. These packs are usually marketed for first aid and designed for one-time use only. The chemical reaction inside some of the packs is at an alkaline pH and can cause skin burns if the package splits open and the contents spill out.

An economic method of making cold packs is to fill a self-sealing plastic bag with crushed ice and isopropyl alcohol at a 2:1 ratio. These packs will remain cold in the freezer but will not totally solidify; therefore, the packs can easily contour an extremity. Either commercial gel packs or "homemade" packs are suitable for home use. Cold packs will remain at a sufficiently low temperature for 15 to 20 minutes. If longer treatment time is desired, then the pack should be replaced.

Ice Massage

Ice massage is usually done over a small area—for instance, over a muscle belly, tendon, or bursa, or over trigger points prior to deep pressure massage. The technique is simple and can be taught to reliable patients for home use.

Water is frozen in Styrofoam or paper cups to make handling of the ice by the therapist easier. The cup is pealed back as the ice melts. As an alternative, ice "lollipops" can be made by putting a wooden tongue depressor in the cup with the water. The ice pop can be taken out of the cup and held by the tongue depressor for application. An area 10 cm by 15 cm can be covered in 5 to 10 minutes.[63] The ice is rubbed over the skin using small overlapping circles.

During ice massage, the patient will most likely experience four distinct sensations, including intense cold, burning, aching, then analgesia. The stages of burning and aching should pass rapidly within about 1 to 2 minutes. It has been the author's experience that a prolonged phase of aching or burning resulted either if the area covered was too large or if a hypersensitive response was imminent (see under Precautions for Cryotherapy). Skin temperature will usually not drop below 15°C when this technique is employed; therefore, the risk of damaging tissue is minimal.

Ice Towels

If a terrycloth towel is put in a bucket of crushed ice and then removed and lightly shaken, ice particles will adhere to the towel. Alternatively, towels can be soaked in a slush mixture, then wrung out. The towel can be wrapped around a joint or over a muscle from origin to insertion, providing good contact. The towels can be held on by the therapist or strapped on while exercises are performed. This approach allows the clinician easily to do contract-relax procedures for increasing range of motion. The towel must be changed after 4 to 5 minutes, because it will warm fairly rapidly.

Cold Baths

When cooling is indicated for the distal extremities, immersion of that part in a cold bath is most practical. This approach ensures circumferential contact of the cooling agent. Water temperatures for immersion vary from 13°C to 18°C. The lower the temperature range, the shorter the duration of immersion. In fact, immersion at 13°C will often be very uncomfortable. A basin of water or a small whirlpool filled with water and crushed ice can be used.

Vapocoolant Sprays

Fluori-Methane is a nonflammable and nontoxic vapocoolant spray. It is bottled under pressure and emitted as a fine spray when the bottle is inverted. Ethyl chloride spray, a topical anesthetic, was originally used for trigger point treatment, but is no longer recommended because it is volatile, inflammable, and can freeze the skin.

After locating the treatment area, the patient is comfortably positioned and the muscle is maintained on passive stretch. The bottle of vapocoolant spray is inverted and held at an acute angle (30 degrees) approximately 45 cm from the skin. Further stretch is applied as tolerated.

When treating trigger points, spraying is done in unidirectional parallel sweeps along the muscle over the trigger area, then over the area of referred pain. If muscle is sprayed to increase range of motion when no specific trigger areas have been identified, then the entire length of muscle from proximal attachment to distal attachment should be covered (Fig. 4–7). The skin should be covered two to three times at a rate of about 10 cm per second. Further treatment, whenever necessary, should be undertaken after rewarming, to avoid frosting of the skin. If spraying is done around the face, the eyes should be covered and precautions should be taken to avoid inhalation of the vapors.

Controlled Cold-Compression Units

Controlled cold-compression units like the Cryotemp (Jobst Corporation, Toledo, OH) can be adjusted to selected temperatures (ranging from approximately 10°C to 25°C) and maintained during the time the unit is turned on. Cooled water is circulated through a sleeve that is applied over

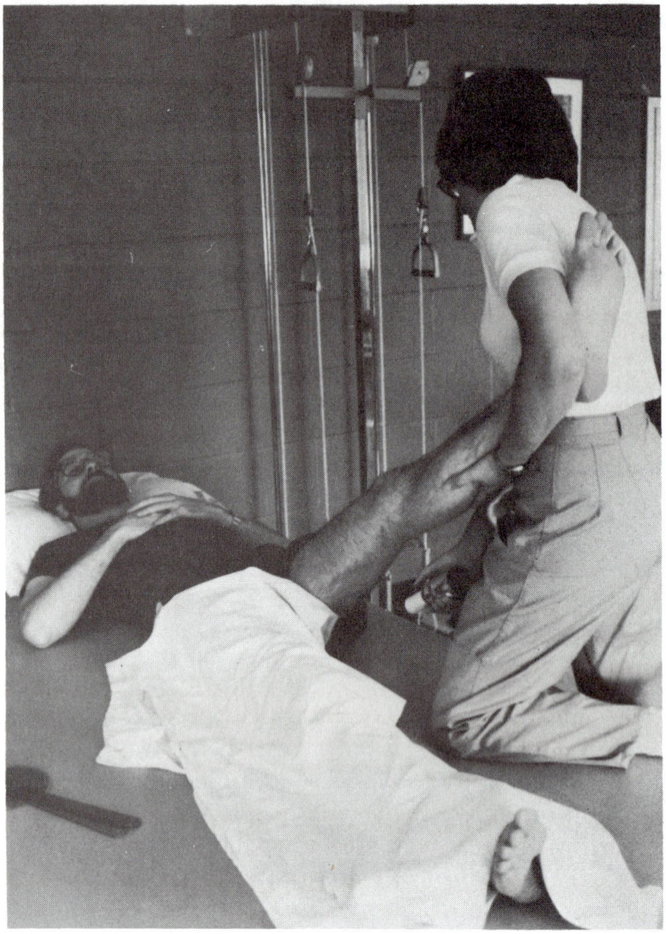

FIGURE 4–7

Stretch and spray with Fluori-Methane spray for hamstring tightness. The skin over the hamstrings is sprayed from proximal muscle attachment toward distal muscle attachment, while the therapist holds the leg with the muscle in a stretched position.

an extremity. The sleeve is inflated intermittently to "pump edema fluid" from the extremity.

These units are probably most commonly seen in centers that treat a multitude of musculoskeletal injuries.

PRECAUTIONS FOR CRYOTHERAPY

Cryotherapy should be avoided in patients with cold sensitivity symptoms. These symptoms include, but are not limited to, cold urticaria, cryoglobinemia, cold intolerance, Raynaud's phenomenon, and paroxysmal cold hemoglobinurias.[64]

Cold urticaria or hypersensitivity can include both local and systemic reactions. In patients experiencing local reactions, wheals occur, having erythematous raised borders with blanched centers.[65,66] Mast cell degranulation causes histamine release into the area, thus markedly increasing capillary permeability.[67] This phenomenon can lead to local redness and swelling in addition to the wheals. Systemic reactions can include flushing of the face, a sharp drop in blood pressure, increased pulse rate, and syncope.[68]

Cryoglobinemia is a disorder characterized by an abnormal blood protein that forms a precipitate or gel at low temperatures. Precipitate or gel formation can lead to ischemia or gangrene. This condition can be found in association with multiple myeloma, leukemia, systemic lupus erythematosus, rheumatoid arthritis, and some other disorders.[64]

Cold intolerance can occur in some types of rheumatic diseases, following crush injuries, and following digital or partial extremity replantation surgery. It can manifest itself by severe pain, numbness, and color changes including redness, cyanosis, and mottling.

Raynaud's phenomenon, a vasospastic disorder, can be idiopathic or associated with some rheumatic diseases, particularly scleroderma and systemic lupus erythematosus. In addition, about 50 percent of patients with thromboangiitis obliterans (Buerger's disease) have cold sensitivity of Raynaud's type.[69] Attacks of cyanosis, blanching, or rubor and numbness of distal parts of extremities can be precipitated by cold exposure or emotional stress.[65]

Paroxysmal cold hemoglobinuria can occur following local or general exposure to cold. Hemoglobin, which is normally found within red blood cells (RBC), is released from lysed RBC and appears in the urine.

Cold should not be applied over circulatory compromised areas. In particular, in patients with peripheral vascular disease affecting the arterial system, the vasoconstrictive effects of cold could further compromise an already nutritionally deprived area.

Because cold can cause a transient increase in systolic and diastolic blood pressure,[70,71] care should be taken when considering cryotherapy for the hypertensive patient. If the decision is made to use cold, the patient's blood pressure should be monitored throughout treatment. Treatment should be discontinued if an elevation of blood pressure is noted.

Wound healing may be impaired by cold temperatures. Lundgren and associates[72] demonstrated a 20 percent reduction in wound tensile strength in rabbits kept at environmental temperatures of 12°C compared with those kept at 20°C. The decreased healing might be caused by a decreased blood supply to the area. Only innervated animals showed this impaired healing response, suggesting a reflex cutaneous vasoconstriction. Until demonstrated otherwise, it is probably a prudent decision to avoid vigorous cold application directly over a wound during the initial 2- to 3-week period of healing.

As mentioned earlier in this chapter, prolonged cold application, from 1 to more than 2 hours, over an area containing a superficial peripheral nerve (for example, around the medial epicondyle of the elbow or fibular head) can lead to neuropraxia or axonotmesis.[30]

In addition to certain physiologic reasons contraindicating use of cryotherapy, the psychologic response of the patient to this form of treatment should be taken into account. There are some people who have an aversion toward cold, and thus would not tolerate this thermal agent. This consideration is particularly important if cold is being used to decrease pain and promote skeletal muscle relaxation.

SUMMARY

The use of cryotherapy is based on the physiologic responses to a decrease in tissue temperature. Cold decreases blood flow and tissue metabolism, thus decreasing bleeding and acute inflammation. Spasticity and muscle guarding spasms can be diminished, allowing for a greater ease of motion. Pain threshold is elevated, thus allowing exercises to be carried out with increased comfort.

Cold can be easily applied through a variety of means including cold packs, ice massage, ice soaked towels, cool baths, vapocoolant sprays, or controlled cold devices. Caution should be taken, though, to avoid undue exposure to cold in persons with cold hypersensitivity syndromes, impaired circulation, and hypertension.

REFERENCES

1. Nave, CR and Nave, BC: *Physics for the Health Sciences,* ed 2. WB Saunders, Philadelphia, 1980, p 178.
2. Clarke, RSJ, Hellon, RF, and Lind, AR: *Vascular reactions of the human forearm to cold.* Clin Sci 17:165, 1958.
3. Abramson, DI: *Physiologic basis for the use of physical agents in peripheral vascular disorders.* Arch Phys Med Rehabil 46:216, 1965.
4. Wolf, SL and Basmajian, JV: *Intramuscular temperature changes deep to localized cutaneous cold stimulation.* Phys Ther 53:1284, 1973.
5. Bierman, W and Friedlander, M: *The penetrative effect of cold.* Arch Phys Ther 21:585, 1940.
6. DeLateur, BJ and Lehmann, JF: *Cryotherapy.* In Lehmann, JF (ed): *Therapeutic Heat and Cold,* ed 3. Williams & Wilkins, Baltimore, 1982.
7. Lowdon, BJ and Moore, RJ: *Determinants and nature of intramuscular temperature changes during cold therapy.* Am J Phys Med 54:223, 1975.
8. Wakim, KG, Porter, AN, and Krusen, KH: *Influence of physical agents and of certain drugs on intra-articular temperature.* Arch Phys Med 32:714, 1951.
9. Oliver, RA, et al: *Isometric muscle contraction response during recovery from reduced intramuscular temperature.* Arch Phys Med Rehabil 60:126, 1979.
10. Johnson, DJ, et al: *Effect of cold submersion on intramuscular temperature of the gastrocnemius muscle.* Phys Ther 59:1238, 1979.
11. Hartvikksen, K: *Ice therapy in spasticity.* Acta Neurol Scand 38:79, 1962.
12. McMaster, WC, Liddle, S, and Waugh, TR: *Laboratory evaluation of various cold therapy modalities.* Am J Sports Med 6:291, 1978.
13. Travell, JG, and Simons, DG: *Myofascial Pain and Dysfunction. The Trigger Point Manual.* Williams & Wilkins, Baltimore, 1983.
14. Perkins, J, et al: *Cooling and contraction of smooth muscle.* Am J Physiol 163:14, 1950.
15. Berne, R, and Levy, MN: *Cardiovascular Physiology,* ed 4. CV Mosby, St Louis, 1981.
16. Folkow, B, et al: *Studies on the reactions of the cutaneous vessels to cold exposure.* Acta Physiol Scand 58:342, 1963.
17. Cobbold, AF and Lewis, OJ: *Blood flow to the knee joint of the dog: Effect of heating, cooling and adrenaline.* J Physiol 132:379, 1956.

18. Lewis, T: *Observations upon the reactions of the vessels of the human skin to cold.* Heart 15:177, 1930.

19. Fox, RH and Wyatt, HT: *Cold-induced vasodilatation in various areas of the body surface in man.* J Physiol 162:289, 1962.

20. Major, TC, Schwinghamer, JM, and Winston, S: *Cutaneous and skeletal muscle vascular responses to hypothermia.* Am J Physiol 240 (Heart Circ Physiol 9):H868, 1981.

21. Matsen, FA, Questad, K, and Matsen, AL: *The effect of local cooling on post fracture swelling.* Clin Orthop 109:201, 1975.

22. Jezdinsky, J, Marek, J, and Ochonsky, P: *Effects of local cold and heat therapy on traumatic oedema of the rat hind paw. I. Effects of cooling on the course of traumatic oedema.* Acta Universitatis Palackianae Olomucensis Facultatis Medicae 66:185, 1973.

23. Marek, J, Jezdinsky, J, and Ochonsky, P: *Effects of local cold and heat therapy on traumatic oedema of the rat hind paw. II. Effects of various kinds of compresses on the course of traumatic oedema.* Acta Universitatis Palackianae Olomucensis Facultatis Medicae 66:203, 1973.

24. McMaster, WC and Liddle, S: *Cryotherapy influence on post traumatic limb edema.* Clin Orthop 150:283, 1980.

25. Farry, PJ and Prentice, NG: *Ice treatment of injured ligaments: an experimental model.* NZ Med J 9:12, 1980.

26. Douglas, WW and Malcolm, JL: *The effect of localized cooling on conduction in cat nerves.* J Physiol 130:53, 1955.

27. Zankel, HT: *Effect of physical agents on motor conduction velocity of the ulnar nerve.* Arch Phys Med Rehabil 47:787, 1966.

28. Lee, JM, Warren, MP, and Mason, SM: *Effects of ice on nerve conduction velocity.* Physiotherapy 64:2, 1978.

29. Li, C-L: *Effect of cooling on neuromuscular transmission in the rat.* Am J Physiol 194:200, 1958.

30. Drez, D, Faust, DC, and Evans, JP: *Cryotherapy and nerve palsy.* Am J Sports Med 9:256, 1981.

31. McGown, HL: *Effects of cold application on maximal isometric contraction.* Phys Ther 47:185, 1967.

32. Knuttsson, E and Mattsson, E: *Effects of local cooling on monosynaptic reflexes in man.* Scand J Rehabil Med 1:126, 1969.

33. Clendenin, MA and Szumski, AJ: *Influence of cutaneous ice application on single motor units in human.* Phys Ther 51:166, 1971.

34. Johnson, J and Leider, FE: *Influence of cold bath on maximum handgrip strength.* Percept Mot Skills 44:323, 1977.

35. Clarke, DH: *Effect of immersion in hot and cold water upon recovery of muscular strength following fatiguing isometric exercise.* Arch Phys Med Rehabil 44:565, 1963.

36. Eldred, E, Lindsley, DF, and Buchwald, JS: *The effect of cooling on mammalian muscle spindles.* Exp Neurol 2:144, 1960.

37. Newton, M and Lehmkuhl, D: *Muscle spindle response to body heating and localized muscle cooling: Implications for relief of spasticity.* J Am Phys Ther Assoc 45:91, 1965.

38. Wolf, SL and Letbetter, WD: *Effect of skin cooling on spontaneous EMG activity in triceps surae of the decerebrate cat.* Brain Res 91:151, 1975.

39. Mecomber, SA and Herman, RM: *Effects of local hypothermia on reflex and voluntary activity.* Phys Ther 51:271, 1971.

40. Miglietta, O: *Electromyographic characteristics of clonus and influence of cold.* Arch Phys Med Rehabil 45:508, 1964.

41. Miglietta, O: *Action of cold on spasticity.* Am J Phys Med 52:198, 1973.

42. Knuttsson, E: *Topical cryotherapy in spasticity.* Scand J Rehabil Med 2:159, 1970.

43. Urbscheit, N, Johnston, R, and Bishop, B: *Effects of cooling on the ankle jerk and H-response in hemiplegic patients.* Phys Ther 51:983, 1971.

44. Schaubel, HH: *Local use of ice after orthopedic procedures.* Am J Surg 72:711, 1946.

45. Conolly, WB, Paltos, N, and Tooth, RM: *Cold therapy—an improved method.* Med J Aust 2:424, 1972.

46. Basur, R, Shephard, E, and Mouzos, G: *A cooling method in the treatment of ankle sprains.* Practitioner 216:708, 1976.

47. Hocutt, JE, et al: *Cryotherapy in ankle sprains.* Am J Sports Med 10:316, 1982.

48. Benson, TB and Copp, EP: *The effects of therapeutic forms of heat and ice on the pain threshold of the normal shoulder.* Rheumatol Rehabil 13:101, 1974.

49. Gammon, GD and Starr, I: *Studies on the relief of pain by counterirritation.* J Clin Invest 20:13, 1941.

50. Lane, LE: *Localized hypothermia for the relief of pain in musculoskeletal injuries.* Phys Ther 51:182, 1971.

51. Hayden, CA: *Cryokinetics in an early treatment program.* J Am Phys Ther Assoc 44:990, 1964.

52. Grant, AE: *Massage with ice (cryokinetics) in the treatment of painful conditions of the musculoskeletal system.* Arch Phys Med Rehabil 45:233, 1964.

53. Prentice, WE: *An electromyographic analysis of the effectiveness of heat or cold and stretching for inducing relaxation in injured muscle.* J Orthop Sports Phys Ther 3:133, 1982.

54. Cobb, CR, et al: *Electrical activity in muscle pain.* Am J Phys Med 54:80, 1975.

55. Yackzan, L, Adams, C, and Francis, KT: *The effects of ice massage on delayed muscle soreness.* Am J Sports Med 12:159, 1984.

56. Halkovich, LR, et al: *Effect of Fluori-Methane[R] spray on passive hip flexion.* Phys Ther 61:185, 1981.

57. Landen, BR: *Heat or cold for the relief of low back pain?* Phys Ther 47:1126, 1967.

58. Levine, MG, et al: *Relaxation of spasticity by physiological techniques.* Arch Phys Med Rehabil 35:214, 154.

59. Hedenberg, L: *Functional improvement of the spastic hemiplegic arm after cooling.* Scand J Rehabil Med 2:154, 1970.

60. Olson, JE and Stravino, VD: *A review of cryotherapy.* Phys Ther 52:840, 1972.

61. Wright, V and Johns, RJ: *Physical factors concerned with the stiffness of normal and diseased joints.* Bull Johns Hopkins Hosp 106:215, 1960.

62. Fox, RH: *Local cooling in man.* Br Med Bull 17:14, 1961.

63. Waylonis, GW: *The physiologic effect of ice massage.* Arch Phys Med Rehabil 48:37, 1967.

64. Ritzmann, SE and Levin, WC: *Cryopathies: A review.* Arch Intern Med 107:186, 1961.

65. Austin, KF: *Diseases of immediate type hypersensitivity.* In Isselbacher, KJ, et al (eds): *Harrison's Principles of Internal Medicine,* ed 9. McGraw-Hill, New York, 1980.

66. Day, MJ: *Hypersensitive response to ice massage: Report of a case.* Phys Ther 54:592, 1974.

67. Shelley, WB and Caro, WA: *Cold erythema: A new hypersensitivity syndrome.* JAMA 180:639, 1962.

68. Horton, BT, Brown, GE, and Roth, GM: *Hypersensitiveness to cold with local and systemic manifestations of a histamine-like character: Its amenability to treatment.* JAMA 107:1263, 1936.

69. Strandness, DE: *Vascular diseases of the extremities.* In Isselbacher, KJ, et al (eds): *Harrison's Principles of Internal Medicine,* ed 9. McGraw-Hill, New York, 1980.

70. Boyer, JT, Fraser, JRE, and Doyle, AE: *The haemodynamic effects of cold immersion.* Clin Sci 19:539, 1980.

71. Claus-Walker, J, et al: *Physiological responses to cold stress in healthy subjects and in subjects with cervical cord injuries.* Arch Phys Med Rehabil 55:485, 1974.

72. Lundgren, C, Muren, A, and Zederfeldt, B: *Effect of cold vasoconstriction on wound healing in the rabbit.* Acta Chir Scand 118:1, 1959.

CHAPTER 5

BIOPHYSICAL PRINCIPLES OF HEATING AND SUPERFICIAL HEAT AGENTS

SUSAN L. MICHLOVITZ, M.S., P.T.

Warmth is associated with tranquillity and relaxation. Heating tissue has been used for centuries as an antidote for pain relief and reduction of muscle spasm. In physical rehabilitation, locally applied heat agents are used not only to promote relaxation and pain relief but also to increase blood flow and facilitate tissue healing and to prepare stiff joints and tight muscles for exercise.[1] The physiologic effects occurring as a result of temperature elevation are considered a rationale for including these agents as part of a therapy protocol. For example, elevation of collagen tissue temperature can alter viscoelastic properties, thus enhancing the effects of passive stretch for increasing range of motion.[2]

There are numerous thermal agents available for tissue heating. These generally fall within one of two broad categories: superficial and deep-heating agents. The former are those agents that primarily increase skin temperature with little change in the temperature of underlying structures. Superficial or surface heat agents, such as hot packs or paraffin, are used (1) to heat joints, such as those of the hand, that have relatively little soft tissue covering; or (2) to cause an effect in deeper structures, such as muscle, through reflex mechanisms. When the goal of treatment is to elevate tissue temperature at a deeper-seated pathology level (for example, the knee joint or the muscle belly of cervical muscles), then a deep-heating agent is logically chosen. Deep-heating agents, including the diathermies and ultrasound, can increase tissue temperature at depths ranging from 3 to 5 cm without overheating skin and subcutaneous tissue. These deep-heating agents will be discussed in Chapters 7 and 8.

The objectives of this chapter are to (1) discuss biophysical responses to local heating; (2) describe the biophysical principles underlying application of superficial heating agents; (3) discuss clinical techniques and rationale for the use of superficial heating agents; (4) discuss safety and precautions to be taken with these agents; and (5) discuss clinical decision-making principles for logical and effective application of thermal agents.

BIOPHYSICAL EFFECTS OF TEMPERATURE ELEVATION

Many sequelae can occur as a result of an increase in temperature of body tissues. The occurrence and magnitude of these physiologic changes will be dependent upon a number of factors, including (1) the extent of the temperature rise; (2) the rate at which energy is being added to the tissue; and (3) the volume of tissue exposed. In order to meet therapeutic levels of vigorous heating, Lehmann states that temperature must be elevated to between 40°C and 45°C. Within these temperatures, hyperemia, which is indicative of increased blood flow, will occur. Above this range, there is potential for tissue damage. Below 40°C heating is considered to be only mild.[1,2]

The rate of rise in temperature in response to the addition of thermal energy can influence physiologic responses. Temperature elevation increases local blood flow;[3–9] thus, cooler blood comes into the area and acts to remove some of the heat produced. If the rate of temperature increase is very slow, then the amount of heat added could be balanced out by the convective effect of cooler blood. Therefore, therapeutically effective levels may not be obtained. On the other hand, if temperature rises faster than excess heat can be dissipated, then heat may build up to the point that stimulation of pain receptors will occur.

Physiologic alterations can occur at the site of local temperature rise and can also occur in areas remote from the area of heat absorption. Usually, the larger the tissue volume affected by the addition of thermal energy, the greater the likelihood for reflex or consensual changes in other areas and for systemic alterations. An increase in forearm temperature as a result of hot pack application could be expected to cause an increase in local blood flow, with no or minimal alterations in overall peripheral vascular resistance. On the other hand, immersion of a person in a water bath of 40°C could result in systemic changes such as a decrease in mean blood pressure, increase in heart rate, and increase in pulmonary minute ventilation.[1]

A number of physiologic responses to temperature elevation are important to discuss and understand when considering a heat agent for therapeutic intervention. The most relevant changes to address include alterations in metabolic activity, hemodynamic function, neural response, skeletal muscle activity, and collagen tissue physical properties. These changes, in part, serve as a foundation for the use of heat as an effective therapeutic agent. An understanding of adverse reactions to the addition of thermal energy is imperative for the execution of a safe treatment.

Metabolic Reactions

Chemical reactions in cells of the body are influenced by temperature. Generally speaking, chemical activity in cells and metabolic rate will increase two- to threefold for each 10°C rise in temperature.[6,10] Therefore, energy expenditure will increase with increasing temperature. As temperature rises past a certain point, usually 45°C to 50°C, human tissues will burn because the metabolic activity required to repair tissue is not capable of keeping up with thermally induced protein denaturation.

An increase in chemical reaction rate can also have positive effects on human function. Oxygen uptake by tissues will increase.[3] Therefore, theoretically, more nutrients will be available to promote tissue healing.

Vascular Effects

Increasing tissue temperature is usually associated with vasodilation and, thus, with an increase in blood flow to the area.[3–9] This blanket statement, however, can be misleading. The question can be raised about which regions have an increased blood flow. The control mechanisms for flow to different structures—for example, skin versus skeletal muscle—are different. Therefore, their responses to temperature change will not always be the same; or if the response is in the same direction, it still may not be of the same magnitude.

Skin blood flow has an important role in the maintenance of constant body core temperature and is primarily under the control of sympathetic adrenergic nerves.[11] Vasodilation of resistance vessels of the skin will occur as a means of losing heat through local or reflex mechanisms. The skin is unique in that it has specialized vessels, arteriovenous (A-V) anastomoses, which have an important role in heat loss.[11] These shunt vessels go from arterioles to venules and venous plexuses, thus bypassing the capillary bed. The blood flow through these anastomoses is under neural control. Activation occurs in response to reflex activation of temperature receptors or stimulation of heat loss mechanisms triggered in part by the circulation of warmed blood through the preoptic region of the anterior hypothalamus. These A-V shunt vessels are found in the hands (palms and fingertips), feet (toes and soles), and face (ears, nose, and lips).

Blood flow changes in the skin, as mentioned earlier, can be due to local[5,12] or reflex mechanisms. Vasodilation of the heat-exposed skin can be proposed to occur owing to three factors: (1) an axon reflex; (2) release of chemical mediators secondary to temperature elevation; and (3) local spinal cord reflexes. Heat applied to the skin stimulates cutaneous thermoreceptors. These sensory afferents carry impulses to the spinal cord. Some of these afferent impulses are carried through branches antidromically toward skin blood vessels, and a vasoactive mediator is released. This results in a vasodilation through an axon reflex (Fig. 5–1).

Heat produces a mild inflammatory reaction. Chemical mediators of inflammation including histamine and prostaglandin are released in the area and act on resistance vessels to cause vasodilation. In addition, temperature elevation causes sweat secretion; the enzyme kallikrein is released from sweat glands. This acts on a globulin, kininogen, to release bradykinin.[13] Vasodilation of resistance vessels and an increase in capillary and postcapillary venule permeability occur owing to the action of these chemical mediators on smooth muscle tone and endothelial cell contractility,

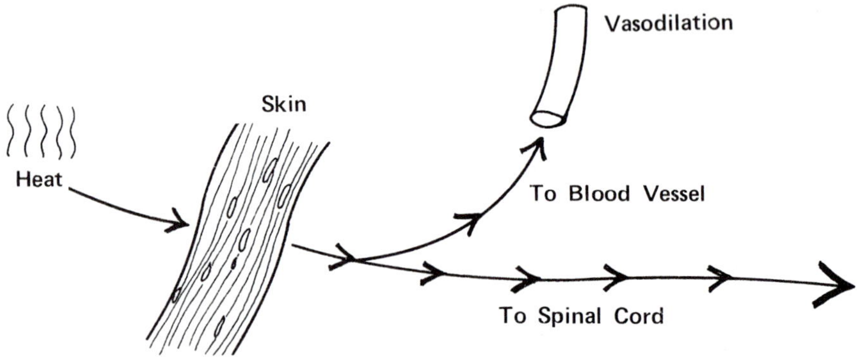

FIGURE 5–1
Schematic diagram of an axon reflex.

respectively. Because of an increase in capillary hydrostatic pressure and permeability, outward fluid filtration from vascular to extravascular space is favored. Therefore, heat within the therapeutic range can potentially increase interstitial fluid and cause a mild edema.

A local spinal cord reflex is elicited through heat-activated cutaneous afferent stimulation. This reflex results in a decrease in postganglionic sympathetic adrenergic nerve activity to the smooth muscles of blood vessels.[14] A schematic of the reflex is diagrammed in Figure 5–2.

Vasodilatory effects of this reflex response are not only limited to the area heated, but there will be a consensual response in areas remote from the site of application. When one area of the body (for instance, hand or low back) is heated, increases in skin blood flow occur in distal extremities at areas of the body that are not directly heated.[15–17] This principle of reflex vasodilation is felt to be safe to use with patients with peripheral vascular disease.[15] For example, cutaneous blood flow to the feet could be increased by heat application to the low back.

Skeletal muscle blood flow is primarily under metabolic regulation and demonstrates the greatest response to increases or decreases in levels of exercise. When surface heat agents are given, minimal to no change in skeletal muscle, blood flow is expected. This notion is supported by two reports on infrared application. Crockford and Hellon[4] measured venous oxygen content following 20- to 30-minute exposures of the forearm. Superficial venous oxygen content increased, but there was no change in deep vein oxygen content. This would suggest there was no change in muscle blood flow. Wyper and McNiven[18] reported no change in muscle blood flow following infrared treatment.

Cobbold and Lewis[19] measured blood flow to the knee joint of the dog following exposure to radiant heat. The magnitude of temperature change was not as great, though, as when ice packs were applied to the animals. Their work does not support the earlier suggestion of Horvath and Hollander[20] that heat will cause a reflex decrease in joint temperature and blood flow, and cold will cause the opposite response.

Heat is often used prior to exercise. Both modalities will increase local blood flow. Hot packs alone, exercise alone, and hot packs plus exercise

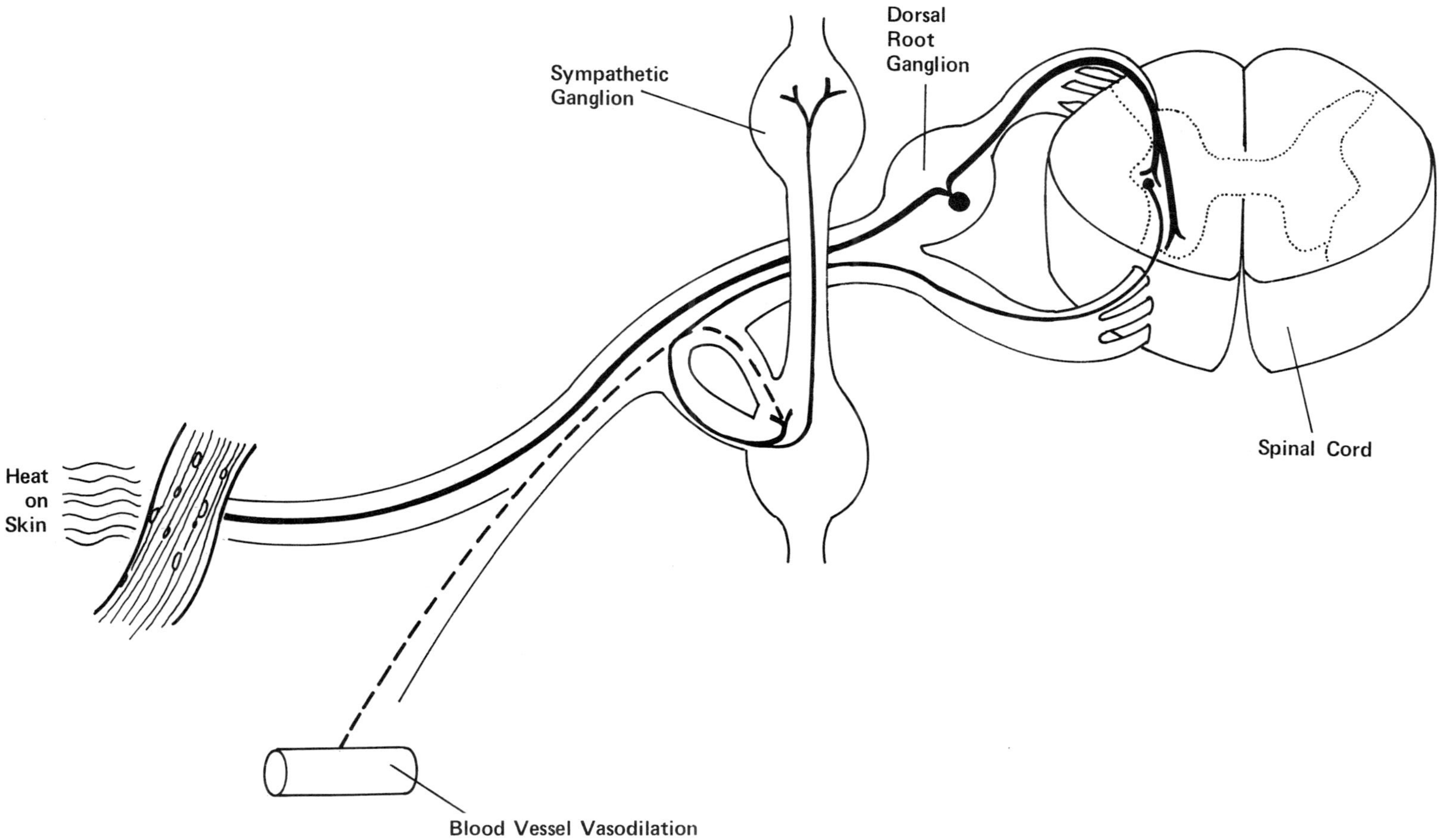

FIGURE 5–2

Heat applied to the skin leads to vasodilation. The change in activity of postganglionic sympathetic adrenergics secondary to local heating is diagrammed.

were compared by Greenberg.[7] Heat application was for 20 minutes; exercise consisted of squeezing a rubber ball once per second for 1 minute. The increase in blood flow from exercise was greater than that with heat; but the effects of hot packs and exercise in combination were additive and greater than either modality used alone.

Neuromuscular Effects

Heat is used therapeutically to provide analgesia and assist in the resolution of muscle-guarding spasms. Although the mechanisms of action are not totally understood, the underlying basis for use may relate to the ability of heat to elevate pain threshold,[21] alter nerve conduction velocity,[22–24] and change muscle spindle firing rates.[25] In addition, temperature elevation of skeletal muscle can temporarily change the ability to build tension and sustain prolonged activity.[26,27]

Raising subcutaneous tissue temperature by 1.2°C[24] to 4.23°C[23] using infrared radiation has been reported to increase sensory nerve conduction velocity. The most pronounced changes appear to occur during the first 1.5°C to 2.0°C temperature increase.[23] The relevance of these findings, however, to the therapeutic use of heat is not readily apparent.

Heating over the area of a peripheral nerve can elevate pain threshold. Fifteen minutes of high-intensity infrared radiation was administered over the medial aspect of the elbow—that is, over the ulnar nerve. Pain threshold measurements distal to the side of application, over the tip of the little finger, revealed analgesia.[21] Direct heating over the area of pain measurement also produced analgesia. Therefore, heat can be a useful adjunct to reduce pain prior to exercise or positioning.

Muscle spasms can result from overuse of a muscle during exercise or from activation of a protective mechanism to guard against movement of painful joints. Pain can be the event triggering a reflex, tonic muscle contraction, thus beginning the pain-spasm-pain cycle.[28] The muscle spindle afferents, which alter their rate of firing primarily in response to tonic or static stretch, are the II afferents. Elevation of muscle temperature to about 42°C will decrease firing rate of the II afferents and increase firing of the Ib fibers from Golgi tendon organs (GTOs).[25] Therefore, with decreased firing of II afferents and increased GTO activity, we could predict a decreased firing of the alpha motoneuron, thus reducing tonic extrafusal fiber activity.

Surface heating agents most likely will not elevate muscle temperature to the degree necessary to alter II or Ib afferent activity. Therefore, another mechanism must be postulated to account for the reduction in muscle spasm when the skin overlying the muscle is heated. Heating the skin has been demonstrated to produce a decrease in gamma (γ) efferent activity.[6] With a decrease in γ activity, the stretch on the muscle spindle would be less, thus reducing afferent firing from the spindle. This indirect method, then ultimately results in decreased alpha motoneuron firing.

Elevating muscle temperature can also alter strength and endurance. In a study of normal volunteers, Chastain[26] used a deep-heating agent, shortwave diathermy, over the quadriceps. During the first 30 minutes following discontinuance of the heat, isometric strength was decreased, followed by an increase for the next 2 hours of measurement. Strength and endurance decreases have also been reported in other studies on humans.[27,29]

Immediately after immersion in whirlpools ranging from 40°C to 43°C, quadriceps strength and endurance were reduced. Edwards and associates[27] found similar results following immersion of the lower extremity in a water bath of 44°C for 45 minutes. The muscle temperature following the 45-minute immersion had reached a value of 38.6°C from a normal mean of 35.1°C.

The physical therapist should be aware of the changes in muscle performance following heat application, particularly when planning strengthening programs or doing valid evaluations of performance.

Connective Tissue Effects

Temperature elevation in combination with a stretch can alter the viscoelastic properties of connective tissues.[30] The viscous properties of connective tissue permit a residual elongation of connective tissue after stretch is applied, then released. This is referred to as plastic deformation or elongation. An elastic structure will stretch under tension but will return to its original length when the load is removed. The elastic properties of connective tissue result in recoverable deformation.[31]

Connective tissue will progressively shorten and joint contractures develop following injury if full range of motion exercises are not performed.[32] Immobilization of structures will result in connective tissue shortening. Adhesions, or the loss of ability for tissue layers to glide past one another, will develop, further limiting mobility. Lacerations and crush and burn injuries will result in scar tissue, further limiting mobility.

Heat and stretch of connective tissue will result in plastic elongation. Two factors must be considered in determining effective treatment strategies, including (1) temperature elevation—site, time, and amount; and (2) stretch—duration, amount, and velocity.

Greater residual length changes with less damage will occur when a stretch is applied during the time tissue temperature is elevated at therapeutic levels; that is, between 40°C and 45°C.[2] For in vivo experiments on rat tail tendon, temperature was elevated in a water bath of 45°C for 10 minutes, then elongation was performed and maintained until cooling to resting values occurred.[33] This was compared with stretch in a water bath of 25°C. Length increases were greater in the 45°C bath, with less evidence of tissue damage.[34]

There are three techniques for obtaining permanent elongation of collagen tissue: (1) constant load of enough magnitude to overcome tissue elasticity, (2) rapid stretch followed by a period of holding in that position, and (3) constant rate of stretch using a slow, low, steady stretch.[2] Lower loads of longer duration result in less tissue damage[34] and greater increases in range of motion.[32,34,35]

Joint stiffness is a common complaint among patients with rheumatoid arthritis and osteoarthritis. Joint stiffness has the physical components of elasticity, viscosity, inertia, plasticity, and friction. Joint stiffness in normal subjects and in patients with rheumatoid arthritis is mainly attributable to the elastic properties of joint capsular structures.[36] Following immersion of the hands into a water bath of 43°C for 10 minutes, there was a slight decrease in finger joint stiffness.[37] Surface heating of the hand to 45°C with infrared resulted in a 20 percent reduction in metacarpophalangeal stiffness, when compared with heating to a temperature of 33°C.[36] Clearly, heating can result in decreased joint stiffness and increased tissue extensibility, thus facilitating ease of motion and gains in motion.

BIOPHYSICAL PRINCIPLES AND TECHNIQUES OF SUPERFICIAL HEATING

Changes in surface tissue temperatures from superficial heat agents depend on the intensity of the heat applied, the time of heat exposure, and the thermal media (product of thermal conductivity, density, and specific heat) for surface heat.[38] Superficial heating agents elevate skin temperature and tissues within 0.5 cm from the surface to the greatest degree. In areas of adequate blood supply, temperature will increase to a maximum within 6 to 8 minutes of exposure.[3,7,39] Muscle temperature at depths of 1 to 2 centimeters will increase to a lesser degree and will require longer durations of exposure, 15 to 30 minutes, to reach peak values.[3,39] At a depth of 3 cm, using clinically tolerable intensities, muscle temperature elevation can be expected to be 1°C or less.[3,40] Fat provides an insulation against heat; it has a low thermal conductivity (see Table 4–1). Therefore, tissues below adipose may be minimally affected by surface heating agents. In order to elevate deep temperatures to therapeutically desirable levels without burning skin and subcutaneous tissue, a deep heat agent should be chosen.

In joints of the hand/foot *or* hand and foot with relatively little soft tissue covering, superficial heat agents can raise intra-articular temperature.[41–43] In fact, a 20-minute exposure of the foot to dry heat at 47.8°C was shown to increase joint capsule temperature in the foot by as much as 9°C.[41] Even though there can be a reflex vasodilatory response on the unheated opposite extremity, no reflex temperature changes would be expected to occur.[43]

After the peak temperature is obtained there is a plateauing effect or slight decrease in skin temperature over the remainder of the heat exposure.[3,7,39] Typical temperature responses of areas with intact circulation are diagrammed in Figure 5–3.

Conductive Heat Agents: Hot Packs and Paraffin

The most commonly used superficial heat agents are hot packs and paraffin. These both transfer their heat energy to the body by conduction. The hot

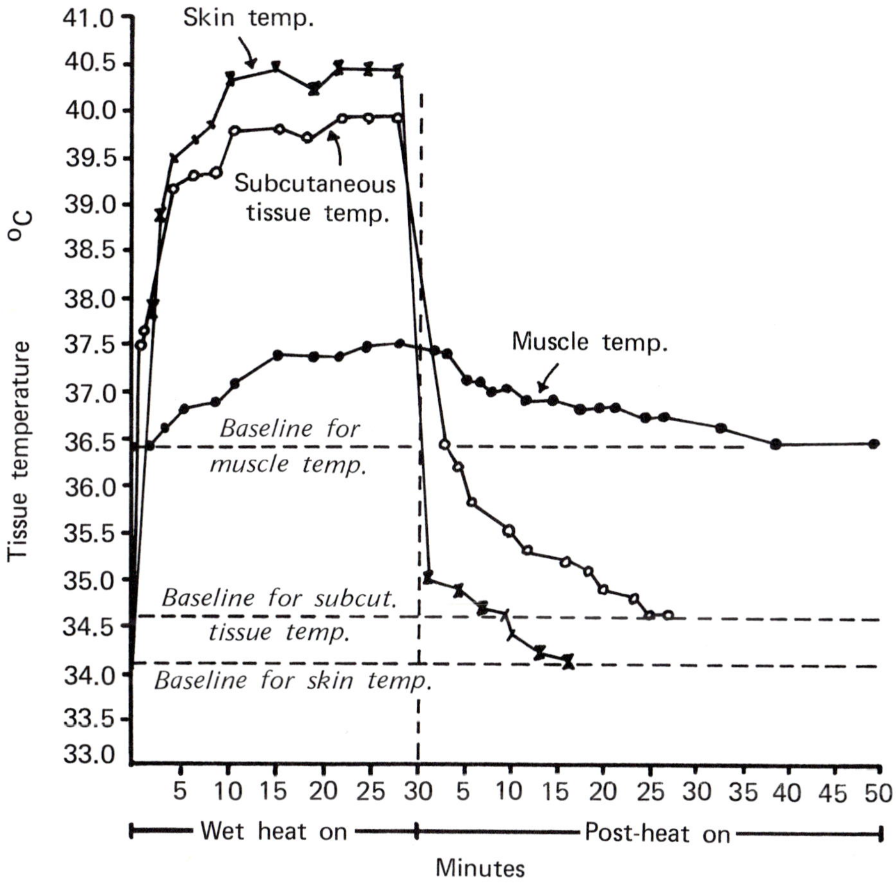

FIGURE 5–3

Curves representing changes in skin, subcutaneous tissue, and muscle temperatures, obtained during and after 30 minutes of wet heat topically applied to the forearm. (From Abramson et al,[3] with permission.)

pack or paraffin is at a much higher temperature than the skin surface to which it is applied. Thermal energy is lost from the agent and gained by the tissues. The quantity of heat gained and the subsequent physiologic responses to that heat gain are dependent on several factors including but not limited to (1) thermal conductivity of tissues, (2) body volume exposed, and (3) time of exposure (see previous discussion of conduction in Chapter 4).

HOT PACKS. Hot packs provide a superficial, moist heat. Commercial packs consist of a canvas case usually filled with bentonite, a hydrophilic silicate, or some other hydrophilic substance. The packs are stored in a thermostatically controlled cabinet in water at a temperature of 71.1°C to 79.4°C.[1] The packs are wrapped in toweling prior to application. Towel layers typically range from six to eight, depending on individual towel thickness, storage temperature of the pack, and patient tolerance. (As with all the superficial heats, the patient should only experience a mild to moderate sensation of heat during application; following the old adage "the hotter the better" could result in skin burns). Between treatments, the packs should be completely immersed in water in the heating unit. Reheating usually takes about 30 minutes. Old, worn packs will leak bentonite; they should be discarded when this occurs.

Hot packs come in a number of sizes and shapes and should be chosen on the basis of the size and contour of the surface to be covered. The packs should totally cover the intended area and then should be secured in place by a wrap. Five minutes after initiating heating, the therapist should remove the pack and check the patient's skin for any blotching—mottled erythema. An uneven, blotchy red and white in Caucasians or darker and lighter areas in blacks could be a sign of overheating. If the heat is too intense, more toweling can be added.

Patients should not lie on top of the hot packs, particularly when the intended area of treatment is on the trunk. Body weight will squeeze water from the pack and accelerate the rate of heat transfer. In addition, local circulation could be reduced, thus reducing convective cooling. Both of these factors could cause overheating of the skin.

PARAFFIN. Paraffin wax, with a melting point of 54.5°C, will stay liquid at temperatures above 47.8°C when mixed with mineral oil. The mineral oil acts to lower the paraffin melting point; this combination has low specific heat. Therefore, the ability for someone to tolerate paraffin at these temperatures ranging from 47.8°C to 54.4°C is better than it would be to water within the same temperature range.[44] The lower end of the temperature range is used for newly healed skin such as skin after a burn.[45] The paraffin mixture comes commercially available and is melted and stored until use in a thermostatically controlled stainless steel container.

Paraffin is most commonly used for heat application to the distal extremities. There are two techniques of application: (1) dip and wrap, and (2) dip and reimmerse. For both methods, the hands or feet to be treated should have jewelry removed, then should be washed and dried. If treating the hand, the fingers are spread apart gently; then the hand and wrist are quickly dipped into and out of the tank. This dipping is repeated for a total of eight to 10 times, until a solid "glove" is formed. Wrap the hand in a plastic bag, then a towel to help retain heat. If there is a potential for edema to increase secondary to the heat, the part should be elevated above heart level until treatment time is over. With the dip and reimmerse technique, after the "glove" is formed, the area covered by the "glove" is put back into the wax bath and kept there for the duration of the heat treatment. The most vigorous responses with respect to temperature elevation and blood flow changes will occur with the dip and reimmerse technique.[46] This technique will not be well suited for most patients, particularly if they have any predisposing factors that could encourage edema or if they cannot sit comfortably in the position required for treatment.

Paraffin should not be applied over open wounds, owing to the risk of burning the area, nor should it be applied over infected skin lesions, since it could exacerbate these lesions.

RADIANT HEATING: INFRARED LAMPS. Radiant energy is emitted from a substance with a temperature greater than absolute zero. Unlike conductive heating, which requires an intervening medium, this form of energy can flow without a medium for support at an approximate velocity of 3×10^8 m/sec. Radiant energy can be absorbed 100 percent by "block bodies" but can also be reflected off reflecting surfaces. The net transfer of heat by thermal radiation is the difference between the radiation emitted by a surface and that which it receives.[10] Human skin acts as a "block body," as a nonreflecting surface for the infrared spectrum. Infrared lamps provide a superficial, dry heat.

The energy for clinical use falls within both the near and far infrared spectrum Fig. 3–1, on the electromagnetic spectrum). Near infrared lamps, also called "luminous" because they have some visible light in their design, are within the wavelength range of 770 to 1500 nanometers. The generators usually consist of a tungsten or carbon filament that heats up very rapidly when a current is introduced across the element. Owing to the visible light emitted, some of the energy is reflected at the skin surface.

Far infrared, also called "nonluminous," is within the 1500 to 12,500 nanometer range on the electromagnetic spectrum. The depth of penetration is slightly less (2 mm compared with 5 to 10 mm) than with near infrared; therefore, the skin may feel warmer during treatment.

Because tissue temperature rises and physiologic responses are very similar with either far or near infrared, the choice of lamp should really depend on accessibility of equipment and staff preference.

With infrared heating, only one body surface at a time can be heated, unlike hot packs, which can easily heat all sides of an extremity. But there is no discomfort from the weight of an object when infrared is used, compared with that of hot packs.

The output of infrared lamps is determined by the wattage. Intensity is controlled by varying the wattage and the distance of the lamp from the surface to be heated. Distance is typically 45 to 60 cm (Fig. 5–4). Using the inverse square relationship, we could predict that the intensity varies inversely to the square of the distance. So, for example, if the distance of the point source of radiation is decreased by one half, the intensity increases fourfold. This relationship cannot be taken as an exact measure of intensity, because the metal reflectors surrounding the infrared source must be taken into account. The angle at which the light beam is incident to the skin will also change the intensity. A larger area of skin will be covered by an infrared beam of perpendicular incidence. If the beam is at an acute angle to the skin, it will reduce the intensity by the cosine of the angle (Cosine Law).[1]

FLUIDOTHERAPY. Fluidotherapy is a dry heat agent that transfers energy by forced convection. Warm air is circulated through a container holding fine cellulose particles (Fig. 5–5). The solid particles become suspended when air is forced through them, thus the properties of fluidotherapy are similar to those of liquids. The viscosity of the air-fluidized system is low, permitting exercise with relative ease.[47]

Fluidotherapy units come in varying sizes. Whereas the smaller units have the capability of treating only distal extremities, a larger model is

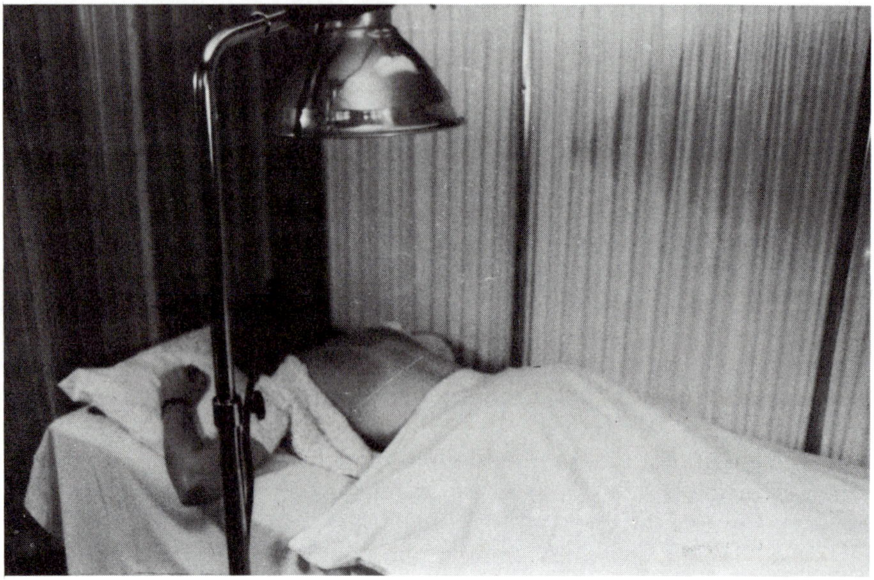

FIGURE 5–4
Infrared lamp is being utilized to apply superficial heat to the thoracic area.

available on which a patient can lie. A netting covers the area that the patient lies on, and the warm air and particles heat up against the netting.

Both temperature and amount of particle agitation can be varied. Temperature ranges for treatment are typically from 37.8°C to 45°C. The lower ranges are recommended for patients who have a greater predisposition for edema formation. Agitation can be controlled for patient comfort. In addition, varying degrees of agitation can be used in a program of desensitization for hypersensitive areas.

Patients can carry out exercises while their hand and wrist or foot and ankle are within the cabinet. If heat and stretch are desired, dynamic splinting can be used during the time of heat treatment, to provide a gentle stretch.

If areas with open wounds are placed in the cabinet, the wounds should be protected by a plastic bag to prevent particles from becoming imbedded in the wound and to minimize the risk of cross-contamination.

CLINICAL APPLICATION: PRINCIPLES AND INDICATIONS

Surface heat agents are used in therapeutic programs to assist in reduction of pain and stiffness, alleviate muscle spasm, increase range of motion, and improve tissue healing by increasing blood flow and nutrients to an area. When superficial heat is applied to the trunk, face, shoulders, hips, or knees, it is considered a mild heat. The site of dysfunction often is well below the

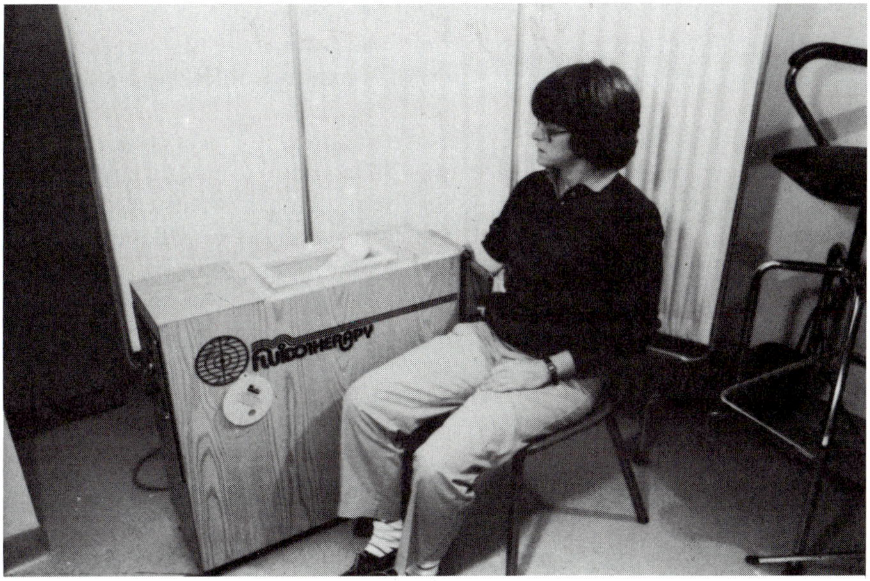

FIGURE 5–5
Hand and wrist are heated with a Fluidotherapy unit.

surface, and the heat will produce desired responses through reflex mechanisms by stimulation of cutaneous afferents. Mild heating usually elevates temperature at the site of pathology to less than 40°C and may be thought of as having a soothing counterirritant effect.[2]

When a higher temperature, between 40°C and 45°C, is desired at the involved structure, then the appropriate agent for "the job" must be chosen. Paraffin, for example, may be a vigorous heater of the finger joints but only a mild heater of the shoulder. The principles of mild versus vigorous heating are summarized in Table 5–1.

TABLE 5–1
A Comparison of Mild and Vigorous Heating[1]

	Mild	Vigorous
Temperature Elevation at Site of Pathology	Low	High
Degree of Temperature Increase	Comfortable sensation of warmth—up to 40°C	Near tolerance levels up to 45°C
Rate of Rise of Temperature	Slow	Rapid
Duration of Peak Temperature Elevation	Relatively short period	Relatively long period
Clinical Examples	Hot packs to cervical area for reducing muscle spasm in upper trapezius	Fluidotherapy at 45°C to the hand for increasing tissue extensibility

Treatment time with all superficial heating agents varies from 20 to 30 minutes. After this time, no further significant increases in blood flow occur.[3] This duration will allow time for maximum tolerable increases in tissue temperatures and blood flow.

Despite the widespread clinical use of surface heat agents, there is a dearth of well-designed clinical studies that address the efficacy to these modalities in a therapeutic regimen. In the remainder of this chapter, some of those studies will be discussed, but most of the text will serve just as treatment suggestions based on suspected physiologic rationale and on the author's clinical experience.

REDUCTION OF PAIN AND MUSCLE SPASM

Symptomatic resolution of pain or elevation of pain threshold can be justification for giving a superficial heat agent prior to exercise, posture, or gait training. Muscle spasm can perpetuate pain and limit motion. Alleviation of the spasm can be accomplished by using a heat agent.

Heat may be used prior to stretching exercises to reduce pain. A comparison was made among normal subjects of the effects of heat alone, stretch alone, and heat plus stretch.[48] In one group, an electric heating pad at a temperature of 43°C was used for 20 minutes over the back and sides of each subject's thigh. Then range-of-motion measurements were taken and compared to pretest values. The second group had exercise only, including contract-relax followed by passive stretch of the hamstrings. The third group had heat and exercise as described for the first two groups. No changes in range of motion were measured with the heat only group; the greatest change was measured in hip flexion in the "heat and stretch" group, compared with the stretch-only group. The technique of heat application would not be expected to alter the viscous properties of underlying muscle due to minimal or no temperature elevation of those structures. Therefore range of motion increases could probably be attributed to the analgesic effect of heat, thus allowing the person to tolerate the stretch better.

A comparison between hot packs and shortwave diathermy (SWD) was made for trigger point therapy.[49] Hot packs or shortwave diathermy were administered for 20 minutes over trigger points in the thoracic, lumbar, or gluteal region. Heat was adjusted to patient tolerance. Pain was measured at the trigger points by tolerable grams of pressure from a pressure algometer. Both hot packs and SWD were effective in reducing pain in the most sensitive trigger points. SWD was more effective in treating less-sensitive trigger points. (An interesting comparison would be between cold versus heat for trigger point therapy.)

Cervical pain of varying origins (injury, arthritis, or "tension") was treated with hot packs, deep massage, and exercise.[50] About one half of all patients were reported to have "good improvement," but the criteria for improvement were not defined by the investigators.

Hot packs reduced muscle spasms in patients with cervical osteoarthritis and neck or hamstring spasms secondary to poliomyelitis.[51] A decrease in spasm was correlated with a decrease in resistance to passive stretch. A static force balance, which measures the force required to initiate movement about a joint, was the measurement tool utilized. No comparisons were made to non–heat-treated patients.

When treating a patient with pain, muscle spasms, or both, the patient's position for treatment must be carefully selected. The patient should be in the most comfortable position possible. If muscle spasm is present, the muscle should not be in a position of "undue stretch" until some analgesia has occurred. If the patient has joint pain, the joint should be positioned in an open-packed position[52] with the ligaments and joint capsule in a slackened position. In this position, intra-articular pressure[53] and stress on joint structures will be lessened.

IMPROVING RANGE OF MOTION

In addition to heat decreasing the pain associated with stretching, if the temperature of tightened structures is elevated to high but tolerable levels, then tissue is stretched, so that range of motion can improve. The stretch should begin after temperature levels reach their maximum, and a slow, prolonged stretch should be held throughout the period necessary for the tissues to cool back to preheat values.

Range of motion during one treatment session could be expected to increase up to 5 degrees.[2] If increases are more dramatic, one could predict that either tissue was overzealously stretched (thus, damaged) or that the cause of limited motion was not due to alterations in connective tissue.

Even though "heat and stretch" has been well tested in the laboratory on normal tissue, little clinical evidence on contracted tissue has appeared in the literature. There was, however, a clinical report on techniques for stretching burn contractures. Paraffin and sustained stretch reduced contractures in freshly healed burns.[45] Owing to the decreased viability of newly healed skin, more mineral oil than usual was added to the paraffin mixture to lower the temperature to 38°C. Certainly more studies or reports on the efficacy of "heat and stretch" would be a welcome addition to our current body of knowledge.

CONTRAINDICATIONS AND PRECAUTIONS IN SUPERFICIAL HEATING

Prior to the decision to use heat in a therapeutic regimen, sensitivity to temperature and to pain, as well as the status of circulation, should be made known to the therapist. An area of skin overlying the intended treatment surface can be tested for sensation using warm and cool objects and a pinprick for pain. This information is necessary, because determining the safe level of heat requires that the patient be able to perceive when pain threshold has been reached.

Patients with circulatory impairment, particularly arterial disease, should be treated by heating with caution or not at all over areas of arterial insufficiency.[54] Dangerous levels of heat could accumulate in the area. Metabolic demands will increase and not be satisfied, owing to impaired arterial inflow. Therefore, there is a high risk of tissue burns.

A mottled erythema may be an indication of overheating but is not always a reliable sign. Persons who have had prolonged repeated use of superficial heat may have a mild erythema ab igne, which mimics a mottled erythema.

Areas that are prone to increased bleeding or hemorrhage should not be treated with heat because of the ability of heat to increase blood flow. Conditions that are included in this category are hemophilia, post–acute trauma (when bleeding may not be controlled), and patients on long-term steroid therapy who have capillary fragility.

Elevating tissue temperature at the site of malignancy may increase the rate of growth of the cancer.

CLINICAL DECISION MAKING

The decision to use a thermal agent as part of a treatment program should be based on a combination of factors, including the patient's diagnosis and medical status, and the objective findings on physical therapy evaluation. It is not until this information is gathered that treatment goals are established. The plan of treatment to obtain these goals can include a thermal agent when indicated. Treatment is executed and followup done. The procedures for clinical decision making and carrying out the treatment are outlined in Table 5–2.

Heat Versus Cold

There are clinical situations when either heat or cold may be selected to meet treatment objectives or when one is clearly preferred over the other. Often the choice between heat and cold is empirical, but before the decision is made, certain factors should be considered: (1) stage of injury or disease, (2) area of body treated, (3) medical status, (4) patient preference, which may be determined by cold or heat hypersensitivity, and (5) decision to use thermal agent as part of a home program. Cold is the preferred agent during

TABLE 5–2

Procedure for Clinical Decision Making and Execution of Treatment with a Thermal Agent

1. Evaluate patient.
2. Establish treatment goals.
3. Select treatment plan including thermal agent when applicable to meet these goals.
4. Choose thermal agent.
5. Select position for treatment.
6. Apply thermal agent.
7. Reassess and determine if treatment will continue or be modified or discontinued.
8. Establish home program (which can include a thermal agent).

the acute stages of inflammation; heat at this stage may further aggravate inflammation. In patients who can tolerate cryotherapy, this may be chosen for reduction of muscle spasm (see discussion, Chapter 4). Cold also can reduce pain around joints prior to range-of-motion exercises and may be easier for the patient to apply at home. On the other hand, heat may be better psychologically tolerated by persons with pain or muscle spasm, thus increasing patient compliance with treatment programs. Temperature elevation will decrease joint stiffness and increase connective tissue extensibility; so, clearly, if the treatment goal is either of these, heat is the agent of choice. In addition, heat to distal extremities seems to be tolerated better than cold.

A sample clinical case is described in Figure 5–6, in which either heat or cold can be considered as part of the therapeutic program. The advantages and disadvantages of the thermal agents are listed and the outcome determined from the process.

Superficial Versus Deep Heat

The decision to use superficial versus deep heat primarily depends on the location of the involved structure and the degree of temperature elevation desired. Generally speaking, though, deep heat is usually selected during the chronic phases after an injury or a disease, when tissue contracture persists.

Wet Versus Dry Heat

Many patients say they have heard that moist heat is more penetrating, and thus effective, than dry heat. Clinical studies that examine the efficacy of one versus the other in obtaining treatment goals are not available. However, it has been determined that dry heat can elevate surface temperatures to a greater degree but that moist heat can elevate temperature to a slightly deeper tissue level.[55]

Until otherwise proven, it is probably safe to say that the choice between moist and dry heat depends on patient preference and availability or accessibility of the thermal agent in your clinic.

SUMMARY

The use of heat in a therapeutic program is predicated on the biophysical effects of temperature elevation, including elevation of pain threshold, decrease in muscle spasm, decrease in joint stiffness, increase in blood flow, and increase in collagen tissue extensibility.

Superficial heat agents include hot packs, infrared, Fluidotherapy, and paraffin. Guidelines for their clinical use and safety precautions have been presented.

PATIENT CASE

A 25-year old female is seen in physical therapy 8 weeks following reduction and short-arm casting of a right Colles' fracture. The cast was removed yesterday. There is mild swelling on the dorsum of the hand. Range of motion of the wrist is limited in all planes. Metacarpophalangeal (MCP) flexion is reduced in all digits. Pain is present on active and passive motion but not at rest.

Goals

1. Reduce and maintain reduction of edema.
2. Reduce pain.
3. Increase range of motion of wrist and MCPs.

TREATMENT CHOICE: HEAT VS COLD

Heat		Cold	
Advantages: ↓ pain ↑ tissue extensibility ↓ stiffness	*Disadvantages:* May ↑ swelling	*Advantages:* May prevent further swelling ↓ pain	*Disadvantages:* ↑ stiffness ↓ tissue extensibility

DECISION

Heat agent—paraffin.

Raise above heart ↓ paraffin

RATIONALE

Owing to the period of immobilization, one would expect that decreased range of motion is due to capsular shortening and adhesions. Heat followed by exercise can increase tissue extensibility. Paraffin application can be expected to increase temperature of the involved structures. With paraffin on, the hand can be elevated during treatment to help prevent further edema. Passive and active exercises can be performed in elevation following the removal of the paraffin glove.

FIGURE 5–6

Clinical decision making: heat versus cold. A patient case is presented, goals are defined, and advantages and disadvantages of heat and cold for this case are then outlined. The treatment decision and rationale for the choice is given. (*Note:* The reader should first cover over the decision and rationale, then uncover them after having had time to formulate a decision.)

REFERENCES

1. Lehmann, JF and deLateur, BJ: *Therapeutic heat.* In Lehmann, JF (ed): *Therapeutic Heat and Cold,* ed 3. Williams & Wilkins, Baltimore, 1982.
2. Warren, CG: *The use of heat and cold in the treatment of common musculoskeletal disorders.* In Kessler, RM and Hertling, D: *Management of Common Musculoskeletal Disorders.* Harper & Row, Philadelphia, 1983.
3. Abramson, DI, et al: *Changes in blood flow, oxygen uptake and tissue temperatures produced by the topical application of wet heat.* Arch Phys Med Rehabil 42:305, 1961.
4. Crockford, GW and Hellon, RF: *Vascular responses of human skin to infra-red radiation.* J Physiol 149:424, 1959.
5. Crockford, GW, Hellon, RF, and Parkhouse, J: *Thermal vasomotor response in human skin mediated by local mechanism.* J Physiol 161:10, 1962.
6. Fischer, E and Solomon, S: *Physiological responses to heat and cold.* In Licht, S (ed); *Therapeutic Heat and Cold,* ed 2. Waverly Press, Baltimore, 1965.
7. Greenberg, RS: *The effects of hot packs and exercise on local blood flow.* Phys Ther 52:273, 1972.
8. Krusen, EM, et al: *Effects of hot packs on peripheral circulation.* Arch Phys Med 31:145, 1950.
9. Randall, BF, Imig, CJ, and Hines, HM: *Effects of some physical therapies on blood flow.* Arch Phys Med 33:73, 1952.
10. Hardy, JD and Bard, P: *Body temperature regulation.* In Mountcastle, VB (ed): *Medical Physiology* (Vol 2), ed 13. CV Mosby, St Louis, 1974.
11. Berne, R and Levy, MN: *Cardiovascular physiology,* ed 4. CV Mosby, St Louis, 1981.
12. Fox, HH and Hilton, SM: *Bradykinin formation in human skin as a factor in heat vasodilatation.* J Physiol 142:219, 1958.
13. Milnor, WR: *Autonomic and peripheral control mechanisms.* In Mountcastle, VB (ed): *Medical Physiology* (Vol 2), ed 13. CV Mosby, St Louis, 1974.
14. Guyton, AC: *Textbook of Medical Physiology,* ed 6. WB Saunders, Philadelphia, 1981.
15. Abramson, DI, et al: *Changes in blood flow, 0_2 uptake and tissue temperatures produced by therapeutic physical agents, III. Effect of indirect or reflex vasodilation.* Am J Phys Med 405:5, 1961.
16. Abramson, DI, et al: *Indirect vasodilation in thermotherapy.* Arch Phys Med Rehabil 46:412, 1965.
17. Wessman, MS and Kottke, FJ: *The effect of indirect heating on peripheral blood flow, pulse rate, blood pressure and temperature.* Arch Phys Med Rehabil 48:567, 1967.
18. Wyper, DJ and McNiven, DR: *Effects of some physiotherapeutic agents on skeletal muscle blood flow.* Physiotherapy 62:83, 1976.
19. Cobbold, AF and Lewis, OJ: *Blood flow to the knee joint of the dog: Effect of heating, cooling and adrenaline.* J Physiol 132:379, 1956.
20. Horvath, SM and Hollander, JL: *Intra-articular temperature as a measure of joint reaction.* J Clin Invest 28:469, 1949.
21. Lehmann, JD, Brunner, GD, and Stow, RW: *Pain threshold measurements after therapeutic application of ultrasound, microwaves and infrared.* Arch Phys Med Rehabil 39:560, 1958.
22. Abramson, DL, et al: *Effect of tissue temperatures and blood flow on motor nerve conduction velocity.* JAMA 198:1082, 1966.
23. Currier, DP and Kramer, JF: *Sensory nerve conduction: Heating effects of ultrasound and infrared.* Physiother Can 34:241, 1982.
24. Halle, JS, Scoville, CR, and Greathouse, DG: *Ultrasound's effect on the conduction latency of the superficial radial nerve in man.* Phys Ther 61:345, 1981.
25. Mense, S: *Effects of temperature on the discharges of muscle spindles and tendon organs.* Pflugers Arch 374:159, 1978.
26. Chastain, PB: *The effect of deep heat on isometric strength.* Phys Ther 58:543, 1978.
27. Edwards, HT, et al: *Effect of temperature on muscle energy metabolism and endurance during successive isometric contractions, sustained to fatigue, of the quadriceps muscle in man.* J Physiol 220:335, 1972.
28. DeVries, H: *Quantitative electromyographic investigation of the spasms theory of muscle pain.* Am J Phys Med 45:119, 1966.

29. Wickstrom, R and Polk, C: *Effect of whirlpool on the strength endurance of the quadriceps muscle in trained male adolescents.* Am J Phys Med 40:91, 1961.

30. LeBan, MM: *Collagen tissue: Implications of its response to stress in vitro.* Arch Phys Med Rehabil 43:461, 1962.

31. Sapega, AA, et al: *Biophysical factors in range-of-motion exercise.* Phys Sports Med 9:57, 1981.

32. Kottke, FJ, Pauley, DL, and Ptak, RA: *The rationale for prolonged stretching for correction of shortening of connective tissue.* Arch Phys Med Rehabil 47:345, 1966.

33. Lehmann, JF: *Effect of therapeutic temperatures on tendon extensibility.* Arch Phys Med Rehabil 51:481, 1970.

34. Warren, GC, Lehmann, JF, and Koblanski, JN: *Heat and stretch procedures: An evaluation using rat tail tendon.* Arch Phys Med Rehabil 57:122, 1976.

35. Light, KE, et al: *Low-load prolonged stretch vs. high-load brief stretch in treating knee contractures.* Phys Ther 64:330, 1984.

36. Wright, V and Johns, RJ: *Physical factors concerned with the stiffness of normal and diseased joints.* Bull Johns Hopkins Hosp 106:215, 1960.

37. Backlund, L and Tiselius, P: *Objective measurement of joint stiffness in rheumatoid arthritis.* Acta Rheum Scand 13:275, 1967.

38. Hendler, E, Crosbie, R, and Hardy, JD: *Measurement of heating of the skin during exposure to infrared radiation.* J Appl Physiol 12:177, 1958.

39. Lehmann, JF, et al: *Temperature distributions in the human thigh produced by infrared, hot pack and microwave applications.* Arch Phys Med Rehabil 47:291, 1966.

40. Whyte, HM and Reader, SR: *Effectiveness of different forms of heating.* Ann Rheum Dis 10:449, 1951.

41. Borrell, RM, et al: *Comparison of in vivo temperatures produced by hydrotherapy, paraffin wax treatment and Fluidotherapy.* Phys Ther 60:1273, 1980.

42. Mainardi, CL, et al: *Rheumatoid arthritis: Failure of daily heat therapy to affect its progression.* Arch Phys Med Rehabil 60:390, 1979.

43. Wakim, KG, Porter, AN, and Krusen, KH: *Influence of physical agents and of certain drugs on intra-articular temperature.* Arch Phys Med Rehabil 32:714, 1951.

44. Zeiter, WJ: *Clinical application of the paraffin bath.* Arch Phys Ther 20:469, 1939.

45. Head, MD and Helms, PA: *Paraffin and sustained stretching in the treatment of burn contractures.* Burns 4:136, 1977.

46. Abramson, DI, et al: *Effect of paraffin bath and hot fomentation on local tissue temperature.* Arch Phys Med Rehabil 45:87, 1965.

47. Borrell, RM, et al: *Fluidotherapy: Evaluation of a new heat and modality.* Arch Phys Med Rehabil 58:69, 1977.

48. Harrison, AS, et al: *The effect of heat and stretching on the range of hip motion.* J Ortho Sports Phys Ther 6:110, 1984

49. McGray, RE and Patton, NJ: *Pain relief at trigger points: A comparison of moist heat and shortwave diathermy.* J Ortho Sports Phys Ther 5:175, 1984.

50. Fountain, FP, Gersten, JW, and Senger, O: *Decrease in muscle spasm produced by ultrasound, hot packs and IR.* Arch Phys Med Rehabil 41:293, 1960.

51. Cordray, YM and Krusen, EM: *Use of hydrocollator packs in the treatment of neck and shoulder pains.* Arch Phys Med Rehabil 39:105, 1959.

52. Kessler, RM and Hertling, D: *Management of Common Musculoskeletal Disorders.* Harper & Row, Philadelphia, 1983.

53. Eyring, EJ and Murray, WR: *The effect of joint position on the pressure of intra-articular effusion.* J Bone Joint Surg 46-A(6):1235, 1964.

54. Abramson, DI: *Physiologic basis for the use of physical agents in peripheral vascular disorders.* Arch Phys Med Rehabil 46:216, 1965.

55. Abramson, DI, et al: *Comparison of wet and dry heat in raising temperature of tissues.* Arch Phys Med Rehabil 48:654, 1967.

CHAPTER 6

HYDROTHERAPY: THE USE OF WATER AS A THERAPEUTIC AGENT

MARK WALSH, M.S., P.T.

Hydrotherapy is one of the oldest therapeutic methods for managing physical dysfunctions.[1] The use of hydrotherapy has been advocated for the treatment of joint stiffness, painful scars, adhesions, and arthritis, and as a warmup to assist with exercise.[2] Water therapy is utilized for its effects on body tissues of heating,[3] cooling, debridement,[4,5] pain relief, and relaxation of muscles. When treatment is not well planned or executed, it can have adverse side effects, primarily on the cardiovascular system.

Hydrotherapy achieves its desired effects through the physical properties of water, temperature, and agitation. The basic understanding of these physical principles, normal physiology, and the pathology involved serve as a foundation for the decision to use hydrotherapy in the treatment of a specific dysfunction. The objectives of this chapter are to (1) provide the reader with a knowledge of the physical principles underlying hydrotherapy (2) discuss the biophysical effects of water immersion, (3) describe equipment preparation and maintenance, (4) discuss specific clinical techniques and pathologies, and (5) discuss safety in hydrotherapy.

PHYSICAL PRINCIPLES

Forces Existing in Water

Water has the inherent forces of buoyancy, pressure, cohesion, and viscosity, which play a role in the effects produced on the body from hydrotherapy. The most important of these is Archimedes' principle of buoyancy. This principle states that a body immersed in a liquid experiences an upward force equal to the weight of the displaced liquid.[6] Thus, the body appears to weigh less in water than it does in air. Buoyancy may be affected by (1) postural alignment, (2) the surface area immersed, (3) weight of the bones in relationship to muscle and fat, and (4) vital capacity. The buoyancy of water can be used to assist with exercise in the extremities and to minimize stress of joints and muscles. Work can be done in the opposite direction against the assist of buoyancy; thus, resistance to motion can be exerted. In addition, by varying the speed of exercise in water, the difficulty of the exercise can be changed or graded.

Specific gravity is the ratio of the weight of a volume of substance to the weight of an equal volume of water. The specific gravity of the body is approximately 0.974. Objects with a specific gravity below 1.0 will float in water. Therefore, the specific gravity of the body can be an advantageous assist to exercise in water.

Water exerts a perpendicular pressure against the surface of the body. This hydrostatic pressure is the ratio of the magnitude of the force exerted by the fluid per body surface area. This pressure is dependent on the depth of the submersed part and the density of the liquid. Hydrostatic pressure increases as depth and density of the liquid increase. Therefore, motion is performed more easily near the surface of the water than at greater depths.

Water molecules are cohesive; they have a tendency to attract each other. This results in an increase in viscosity of the medium, as compared with that of air, and an increase in resistance to motion. Viscosity is internal friction, the property of liquids that resists relative motion within it. The greater the speed of the liquid, the higher the viscosity. Resistance to motion is also dependent on the shape of the body. The more streamlined the body or object, the less force is required to move it through the water. The larger and more spread out the object moving through the water, the greater the resistance to motion.

Methods of Heat Transfer

Hydrotherapy is performed in water tanks of varying sizes and shapes. Tanks used for partial body immersion (that is, immersion of one or two extremities) are termed whirlpools. (Often the terms hydrotherapy and whirlpool are used interchangeably.) Those tanks used for full body immersion are referred to as Hubbard tanks or walking tanks. Thermal energy is exchanged by water in the tank and the body immersed by two methods: conduction and convection.

Conduction is the exchange of thermal energy in which there is physical contact between two surfaces. If water temperature is higher than skin temperature, then heat will be conducted to the skin and temperature will rise. Since fat acts more as an insulator than as a conductor, it has a tendency to hold heat in or to keep it out. This point is important for two reasons: (1) the effect of superficial heating via conduction will be lessened as the body fat composition increases; and (2) the higher the body fat content, the less able the body is to dissipate heat, which may cause an increase in core temperatures to dangerous levels. Therefore, with the obese person, superficial heating with the whirlpool may not achieve the intended effects. Caution must be taken when a large body surface area is immersed; the person may not be able to dissipate internal heat and maintain proper core temperature. This may present a dangerous situation, requiring other methods of heat loss such as evaporation and convection to work overtime causing dehydration and increased cardiac output. A particular patient's medical condition may not tolerate this situation.

Convection is a more rapid process than conduction, which occurs when a portion of the fluid moves from one place to another. Energy transfer by convection occurs when the patient is moving in the water or when the water swirls across the skin surface. Convection plays an important role in heating or cooling tissues as well as dissipating or retaining body heat.

Convection occurs between the core and shell of the body. Surface body heat can be carried by the venous blood toward the core, thus potentially increasing core temperature. Conversely, convection will assist with heat dissipation by carrying heat away from areas of the body that are being heated. This method of heat transfer is compromised when the patient has cardiovascular or peripheral vascular disease. In this circumstance, heating an entire extremity or full body may create a dangerous situation of overheating because the extremity or body is unable to dissipate heat from the treated area in order to maintain tissue temperature at safe levels.

Thus far, the methods of heat transfer discussed were used to transport heat in either direction in the body. Two other methods of heat transfer will be discussed as methods of dissipating heat from the body during or following therapy. Radiation is the exchange of electromagnetic energy and occurs when there is a difference in temperature between the skin and the surrounding environment. As convection and conduction bring the heat from within the body to the level of the skin, *radiation* assists in the transfer of this heat from the skin to the air. This ability to eliminate heat through radiation will be lost in the areas immersed in the whirlpool.

The other heat transfer mechanism used to dissipate heat is *evaporation*. No temperature gradient is necessary. Evaporation occurs via the loss of fluid from sweating and by the pulmonary system during exhaling. Any disturbance with the autonomic nervous or pulmonary systems' functions may interfere with loss of heat by evaporation. Therefore, when administering hydrotherapy, sufficient body surface must be exposed to the air to allow heat loss; otherwise, water temperatures must be kept low.

Heat loss is affected not only by the medical condition of the patient and his or her ability to cope with heat but also by the environmental factors of humidity and temperature. If either humidity or ambient temperature, or both, are too high, the body will have great difficulty with heat loss. On the other hand, should the ambient temperature be too low and the area dry, heat loss may occur to a greater extent than needed, thereby causing a chill. Therefore, muscle and joint stiffness secondary to the reduction in peripheral circulation could occur. Therefore, strong consideration should be given to the design and environment of the hydrotherapy area.

BIOPHYSICAL EFFECTS

Thermal Effects

One of the principal reasons for using hydrotherapy is to gain the therapeutic value of heat or cold. The same physiologic effects of heat and cold apply to hydrotherapy as to other thermal agents, except that usually a larger body surface area is immersed in water than that which is covered by a hot or cold pack. Therefore, exposure of the body to varying temperatures will have not only a local effect (see Chapter 5), but also systemic effects on the cardiovascular and other organ systems. The greater the difference in temperature between the water and skin, the more intense the reaction. Cold application to the whole body decreases heart rate and lengthens diastole. The tone of the cardiac muscle is enhanced and blood pressure is raised as a result of peripheral vasoconstriction. The increase in peripheral resistance requires the heart to work harder to maintain adequate blood flow to the periphery. Other effects of cold immersion can be reviewed from Chapter 4.

The application of heat to the entire body will cause an initial increase in blood pressure, followed by a decrease in blood pressure as a result of vasodilation. The initial rise in blood pressure may be quite marked and prolonged if the temperature of the bath is very high, above 40°C. Respiratory rate will increase owing to application of heat *or* cold, although the increase may be less marked with the application of heat. Dawson and associates[7] studied the effects of hydrotherapy on cardiac output, oxygen consumption, heart rate, and blood pressure, both while in the resting states (positioned supine and sitting) and while exercising (the step test). The subjects were immersed in the whirlpool to hip level for 20 minutes in 40°C water. The mean cardiac output and oxygen consumption increased but not significantly. Pulse rate increased 1.3 to 1.5 times over the sitting or supine resting level, and the mean blood pressure increased 1.1 times over the supine resting values.

In addition, sweating will increase; the amount is dependent on the temperature, size of body surface exposed, and the length of treatment. Whether the use of hydrotherapy bath increases diuresis remains controversial,[8,9] but diuresis seems to be affected by the hydrostatic pressure, which increases with depth of immersion. This influence may have more of an effect on urinary output than does water temperature itself.

Increasing tissue temperature and blood flow are physiologic effects of heat that can have therapeutic value. The depth to which this vasodilation occurs and its relationship to tissue temperature are important. If whirlpool does not increase circulation and temperature to sufficient depths to meet therapeutic goals, it may not be the agent of choice. When one arm was immersed in a water bath 45°C for 20 minutes, there was a 4.17°C rise in subcutaneous tissue temperature, a 1.4°C rise in muscle temperature of the forearm, and an increase in blood flow.[10,11] There is a direct relationship between the increase in superficial blood flow and temperature with the arm immersed in a water bath from 37°C to 42°C.[12] Borrell and co-workers[13] confirmed the penetrating ability of whirlpool in their study in which the thumb joint capsule temperature rose 4°C in a whirlpool bath of 38.9°C when given for a 20-minute period.

Mechanical Effects

WHIRLPOOL AGITATION. Whenever the effects of both cold or superficial heat and water are indicated for a rehabilitation program, the use of whirlpool has been advocated. Physiologically, the whirlpool acts as an analgesic agent, relaxes muscle spasm, relieves joint pain and stiffness, improves mechanical debridement,[14] and facilitates exercise.[15] Based on these facts, its use has been suggested for debriding necrotic tissue and dirt,[3,5,8,14,15] before exercising,[3] and for various musculoskeletal problems.[2] The agitation created by the whirlpool serves as a course of mechanical stimulation to skin receptors, which may explain its sedative and analgesic effect. The agitation may act as a counterirritant or may act as a stimulus to large sensory afferents, thus blocking pain input.

Cohen and associates[16] studied the effects of agitation on blood flow by comparing agitation and nonagitation on diseased and normal extremities. There was no significant effect on blood flow in limbs immersed in whirlpool baths of 38.6°C without agitation and 37.7°C with agitation.[16]

Determining what effects agitation has on body tissues requires some understanding of the pressure and turbulence created in the whirlpool. This has been studied in several types of whirlpools. In general, pressure was significantly influenced by the amount of air allowed to enter into the agitation, and there was more turbulence toward the surface than deeper in the water.[17] The importance of these concepts will be clarified further on in this chapter, especially regarding exercise and open wound care.

GENERAL DESCRIPTION AND UNIT OPERATION

Whirlpool Types

There are basically two types of whirlpools, portable and fixed. In most cases, with the exception of full body therapeutic tubs such as the Hubbard tank or walk tank, any size or style of whirlpool can be either fixed or portable. There are basically three styles of whirlpool baths, depicted in Figure 6–1. The "extremity" tank is used for the treatment of arms and legs. These come in varying widths, usually 15 inches; lengths of 28 to 32 inches; and depths of 18 to 25 inches. The deeper models can be used for lower extremities up to the midthigh region. The "low boy" tank also has varying widths, usually of 24 inches; lengths of 52 to 66 inches; and depths usually of 18 inches. The dimensions of the third style, the "high boy" tank (commonly referred to as the leg or hip tank), are widths of 20 to 24 inches; lengths of 36 to 48 inches; and a usual depth of 28 inches. Each of these tank styles have specific applications that will be discussed later.[18] All require

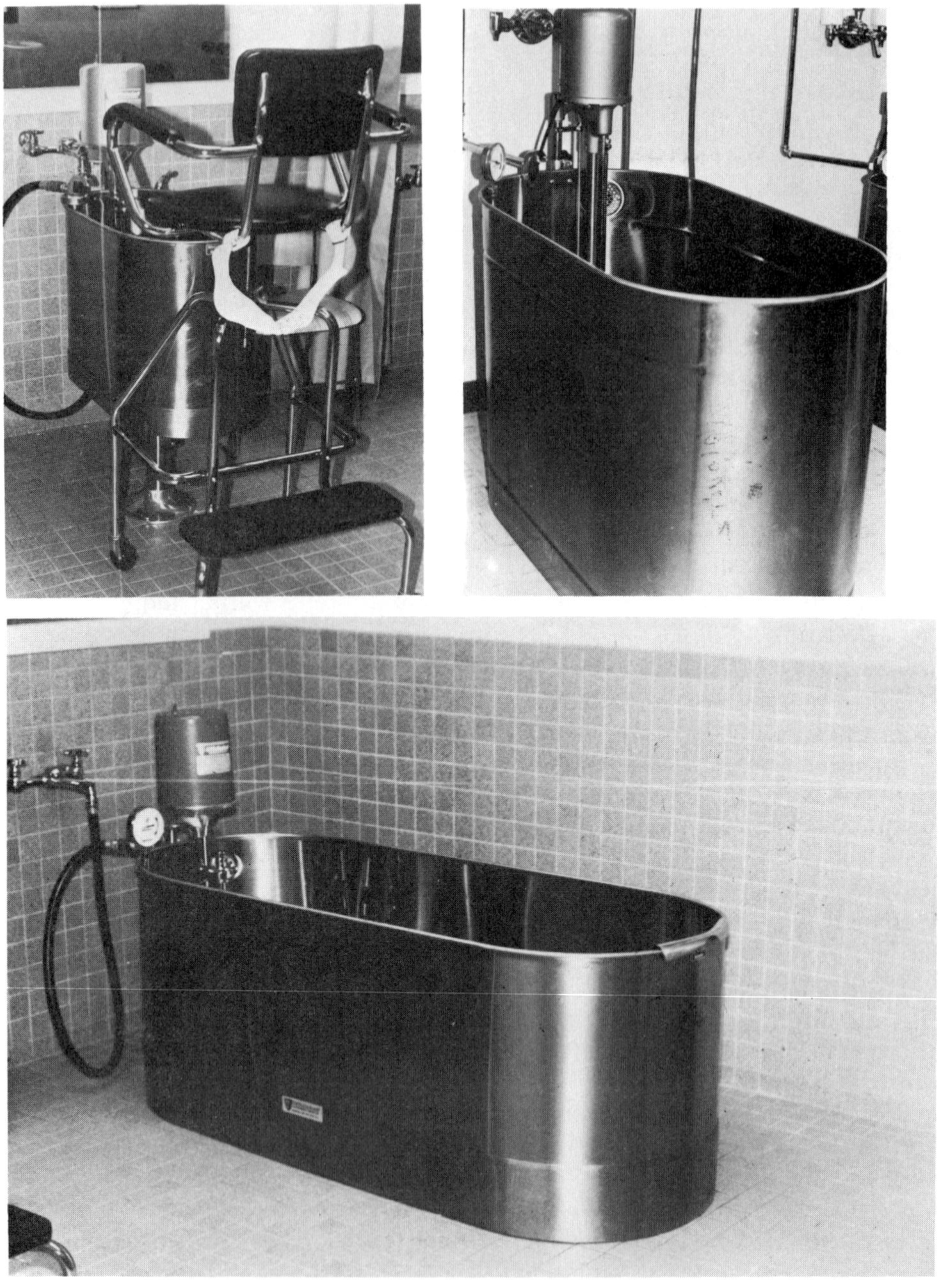

FIGURE 6–1

Styles of whirlpool baths. *Top left,* extremity tank; *top right,* leg or hip tank (high boy); *bottom,* low boy.

an ample supply of hot and cold water and some means of blending them for the desired temperature. The water may be mixed via a thermostatic control valve or manually. Both means of introducing water should include a vacuum breaker on the faucets to prevent the suctioning of water from the whirlpool into the water system.

Hydrotherapy Area

The room temperature in the hydrotherapy area should be higher than in other treatment areas in the physical therapy department. The area should be adequately ventilated to prevent the condensation of moisture on the walls, floors, and equipment. The area for hydrotherapy is best when it is kept separate from other treatment areas and when it contains adequate storage for bandages and other supplies. It should also contain a sink for hand and equipment washing and an area for dressing wounds. The room should be of adequate size to allow for maneuvering of wheelchairs and stretchers.

Turbine

The movement of water and air is regulated by the water pump, or turbine. The whirlpool operates by mixing water and air to control turbulence. Turbulence is created and controlled by combining aeration (the amount of air mixed with the water) and agitation (the movement of the water). In general, the more aeration, the greater the turbulence. Agitational patterns are not uniform from one piece of equipment to another. In any piece of equipment the turbulence is greater toward the surface of the water.[17]

The turbine is mounted on a tubular column, which is a spring-loaded circular vice attached to the whirlpool. The circular vice functions to assist with raising and lowering the turbine, as well as rotating it horizontally. The turbine assembly consists of an electrical motor pump located above the water to which two tubular shafts are connected. The first tube is the drive shaft, which contains an impellor, housed in a casing at the bottom of the tube. A control valve located near the whirlpool motor regulates the opening at the end of the tube, to control the amount of water introduced into the whirlpool system. At the top of the second tube, which is called the breather tube, is a variable pressure control valve to control the amount of aeration; a water jet is attached at the bottom of this tube. Therefore, by regulating the water and air intake via these controls, the turbulence or pressure can be controlled. The various parts of the whirlpool are shown in Figure 6–2. The agitational pattern may be controlled by rotating the turbine assembly to direct the air/water jetstream to the right or left, creating a circular pattern, or to direct it at various points toward the center of the tub, which decreases the circular motion but increases central turbulence. The agitation can be further controlled by raising or lowering the assembly.

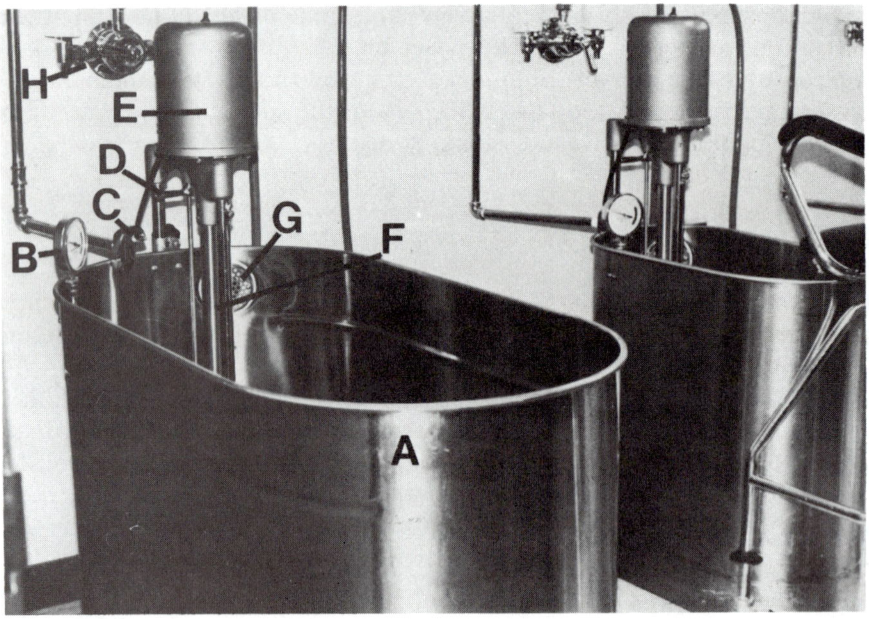

FIGURE 6–2

Whirlpool parts. A, stainless steel tank; B, thermometer; C, inlet spout; D, water control valve; E, turbine motor; F, impellor and breather tubes; G, overflow drain; H, mixing valve.

Whirlpool Care and Safety Precautions

Care of the whirlpool entails cleansing the tank and turbines after each use. The external surface of the tank can be polished with a commercial stainless steel polish. Cleansing the inside can be a problem, especially when patients with contagious or infected open lesions are treated in the tank. For proper cleansing, the tank should be drained immediately after use. The inside of the tank should be scrubbed with a commercial disinfectant, rinsed thoroughly with clean water, and dried. The areas of the tank that should be cleaned most carefully are the tub edges, where the side walls meet the floor; the drain; the tubes of the turbine assembly; and the thermometer. For disinfecting these hard-to-reach places, the use of a glutaraldehyde and a hydrotherapy sterilizing system has been found to be most effective.[19] Exact disinfecting protocol is available from the manufacturers of the glutaraldehyde disinfecting systems. In addition, chlorine and/or povidone iodine have been advocated as a disinfecting or antibacterial agent.[20,21] Routine culturing of the tanks should be done. Guidelines for culturing can be obtained through an appropriate clinical laboratory or hospital infection-control department.

Safety is an important matter to consider when using hydrotherapy equipment. The turbines must be grounded, including both the plug and the motor. The electrical outlet should have a ground fault circuit interrupter installed either at the circuit breaker or in the wall socket itself. This is designed to trip at 5 milliamps, which is below the recommended safety level of 8 milliamps.[22] Finally, if the motor support, which is spring loaded and controlled by the vice grip, is released without the counterblance of the weight of the whirlpool turbine, the assembly spring may catapult the support, creating a hazardous situation. If the support becomes stuck, there should be no attempt to correct this situation while water or a patient is in the tank (see Chapter 3).

CLINICAL TECHNIQUES

Preparatory Considerations

Before initiating a whirlpool treatment, objectives of treatment should be determined, possibly including (1) stimulation of circulation for wound care, (2) promotion of muscle relaxation and pain relief, (3) removal of exudates and necrotic tissue, and (4) facilitation of exercise either as assistance or resistance.

Next, the proper temperature should be selected, based on the patient's medical condition and treatment objectives. Commonly used temperatures and their corresponding generic names are located in Table 6–1. In general, temperatures from 36.5°C to 40.5°C are accepted temperatures when using heat,[2] except in the presence of peripheral vascular disease, sensory loss, or full body immersion. With peripheral vascular disease, the skin temperature of the extremity to be immersed can be a guideline to help determine water temperature. In the presence of cardiovascular or pulmonary disease, the temperature should not exceed 38°C.

The part to be treated should be inspected for its temperature, presence of edema, open lesions, color, muscle spasm, sensation, and those conditions previously noted. The treatment procedure and unit operation should be explained to the patient to reduce anxiety. The patient should be positioned comfortably. The whirlpool may then be activated and the agitation force adjusted initially at a minimal level and increased as desired. Be sure not to direct the agitation specifically toward any body area that could suffer

TABLE 6–1
Whirlpool water temperatures and frequent descriptive terminology

Descriptive Terminology	F°	C°
Very Cold	34–55	1–13
Cold	55–65	13–18
Cool	65–80	18–27
Tepid	80–92	27–33.5
Neutral	92–96	33.5–35.5
Warm	96–98	35.5–36.5
Hot	98–104	36.5–40
Very Hot	104–115	40–46

further damage or not withstand the force of the agitation. The patient should not be left unattended during the treatment session.

Whirlpool Duration

The decision on the length of time for treatment in a whirlpool must be based on sound physiologic judgment and on the objectives the therapist is attempting to achieve through use of the whirlpool. The duration will change, depending on the specific pathologies involved. When used strictly as a heating modality and the patient's medical condition permits, the usual duration is 20 minutes. Borrell and colleagues[13] demonstrated that 20 minutes was a long enough period of time to increase skin, muscle, and joint capsule temperature in the hand and foot. Abramson and associates[11] demonstrated that a 20-minute application of moist heat increased blood flow and that further exposure of up to 2 hours had no real effect on increasing the peak response obtained at the 20-minute mark. When the treatment is concluded, the agitator should be turned off and the patient assisted out of the tub. At no time should the patient operate the agitator controls. Once again, the area treated should be checked for any evidence of adverse effects from the treatment. Occasionally, when full body immersion has been performed, the patient may experience some lightheadedness.

Lower Extremity Technique

Lower extremity immersion, or immersion to the midthoracic level, can be achieved with two of the basic whirlpool types. The high boy tank requires the patient to be able to flex the hip and knee. The length of this tub does not allow for full extension of the average adult lower extremity, and limits the amount of range-of-motion exercise or activity one can perform while in this whirlpool. However, its depth allows a greater body surface area to be submerged safely and comfortably, to as high as the midthoracic region.

The low boy tank is not as deep but has greater length than the high boy, and it affords the patient the ability to fully extend the lower extremities and perform full-motion exercises for the knees. When only the distal portion of the lower extremity has to be immersed, the extremity tank with the use of the whirlpool chair is the appropriate choice. In summary, the high boy and low boy afford greater body surface immersion than the extremity tank does, while the low boy may allow for greater lower extremity extension than the high boy does.

In the event that the patient is unable to negotiate transfer into any of the tubs, they each can be fitted with a hydraulic chair lift or "hoyer lift" to assist the patient in and out of the tub.

Upper Extremity Technique

When treating the upper extremity, the patient should be seated comfortably next to the extremity tank with a towel or other form of padding on the

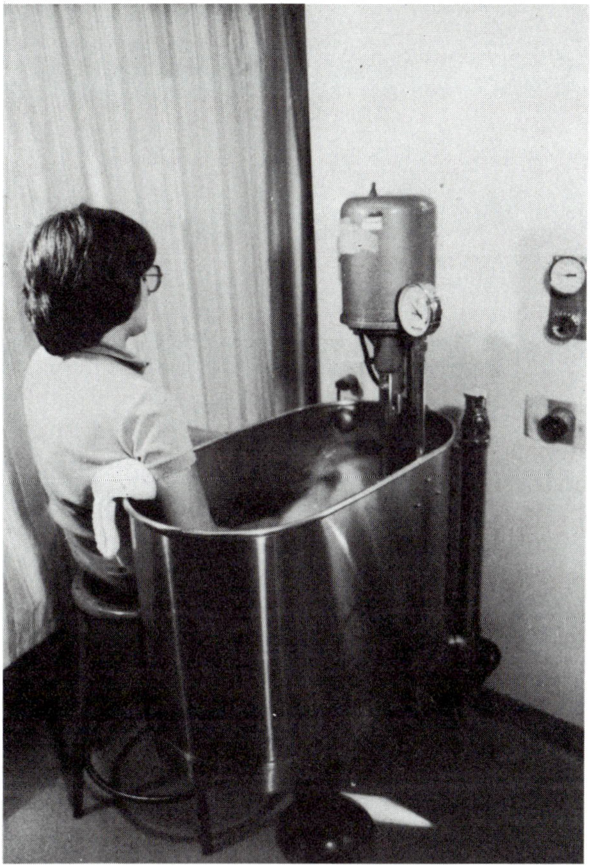

FIGURE 6–3

Whirlpool treatment to the hand and forearm. Caution should be used to avoid a totally dependent position of the hand. If possible, active range-of-motion exercises should be performed during the treatment, to encourage venous and lymphatic return, thus minimizing edema formation.

tank edge to avoid constriction of the circulatory and lymphatic system of the upper extremity (Fig. 6–3). The use of the whirlpool for upper extremity deserves special consideration, because edema can form. It is well accepted that edema of the hand is one of the adverse effects of whirlpool, and the reduction of edema is the primary concern of the treating therapist.[23] Magness and co-workers[24] studied the effect of whirlpool on volume in the upper extremity. They measured upper extremity volume in 20 normal male and female volunteers before and after the immersion of this same extremity in a whirlpool bath at temperatures ranging from 33.5°C to 44.4°C for 20 minutes. In addition, 20 patients with various upper extremity disorders were also treated by whirlpool in the same manner at temperatures from 37.8°C to 40°C for 20 minutes. The results revealed a significant increase in volume for the normal subjects that was directly related to the increase in water temperature. There was also a significant increase in volume of the patient's extremity, and the rise in volume was greater than in the normal subjects at the specific temperatures treated.

Several attempts have been made to determine the causes of this edema and how it could be controlled. Schultz[25] used 20 normal subjects and 20 upper extremity–injured patients to determine the effect of active exercise on edema formation during whirlpool treatment at 37°C. She found no significant difference in edema formation, when comparing active exercise during whirlpool treatment with no exercise during whirlpool treatment, for both normal subjects and upper extremity–injured patients. Walsh[26] studied the effect of elevation versus nonelevation on the upper extremity during whirlpool on 30 healthy volunteers at temperatures of 37.6°C and 40°C. He also found a significant increase in extremity volume in the 40°C whirlpool group. Although not statistically significant, the data supported the theory of nondependency toward the reduction of edema. Therefore, these studies suggest exercising discrimination when choosing whirlpool for the treatment of upper extremity disorders in patients for whom edema is a primary concern.

Hubbard Tank

A tank available for full body immersion is the Hubbard tank, as shown in Figure 6–4. The tank is usually used in conjunction with an overhead lift and/or stretcher to place the patient into the water. Examples of uses for the Hubbard tank can include treatment of (1) an arthritic patient who is at present in an exacerbation phase and unable to negotiate transfer into the smaller tank but who requires the use of heat and water to assist with exercising, maintain range of motion, and provide pain relief; (2) a patient with neurologically involved paralysis who is actively able to move his or her extremities in the buoyancy of water but unable to do so in air; (3) a burn patient; or (4) an elderly patient with an open wound. The major advantage of the Hubbard tank is that its design allows for motion of all the extremities and accessibility of patient by the therapist.

The Hubbard tank (figure 8) is shaped with 15-inch insets, which permits the therapist access to the patient. Its dimensions are a length of 7 feet 2 inches; upper width 6 feet, middle width 35 inches, and lower width 4 feet 2 inches; and a usual depth of 22 inches. It has approximately a 425-gallon capacity, unless the tank has a walking trough, which requires approximately 700 gallons of water. It is equipped with two whirlpool turbines that can be moved around the perimeter of the tank to direct and control the agitation pattern. Other accessories include an optional walking trough with parallel bars for gait training.

For treating open wounds, the Hubbard tank should be drained and cleaned, as previously discussed, and the same preparatory techniques observed. The walking tank, because of its greater gallonage, frequently is hooked to its own filtration system, so open wounds should not be immersed in this tank.

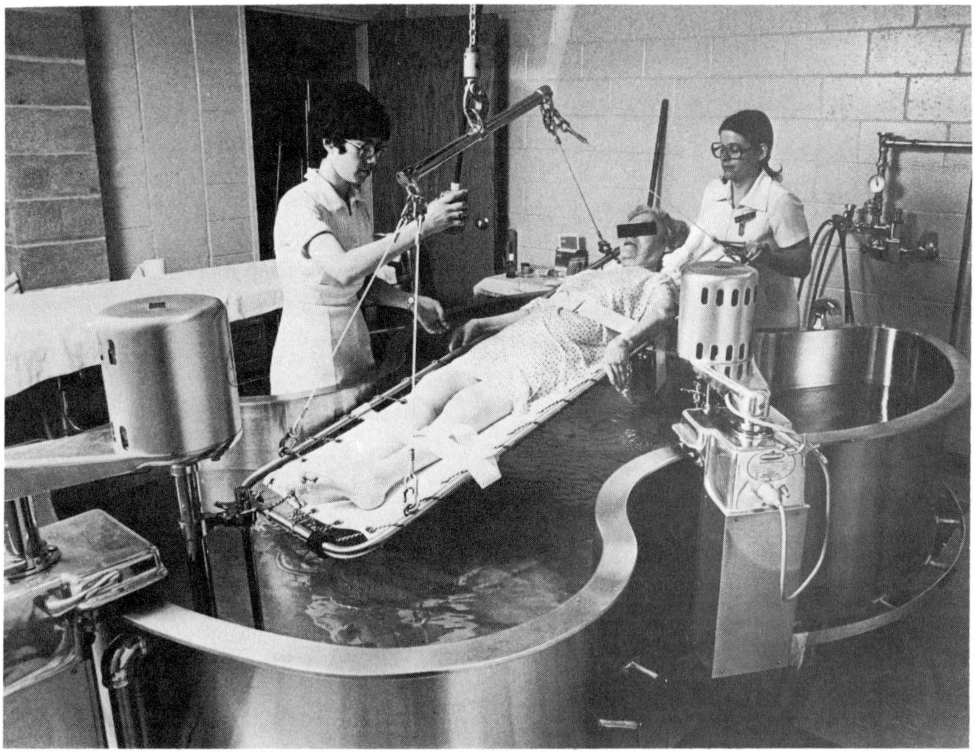

FIGURE 6–4

Hubbard tank with overhead lift. (From Lower Bucks Hospital, Bristol, PA, with permission.)

Contrast Bath

One special technique in the treatment of distal extremities for which the whirlpool can be used is the contrast bath. This requires the use of whirlpool kept at a temperature from 38°C to 44°C and an additional basin containing water kept at a temperature from 10°C to 18°C. The basin should be large enough to enable immersion of the extremity to at least the level of the injury. The extremity to be treated is placed into the warm whirlpool for 10 minutes, then immersed in the cold water in the basin for 1 minute, and then returned to the warm whirlpool for 4 minutes. The cycle continues for 30 minutes, with the last immersion in the warm whirlpool. Although these specific times do not have to be followed, the generally accepted hot: cold ratio is 3:1 or 4:1. The theory, although not well researched, involves the vasodilation (hot water) and vasoconstriction (cold water) caused by the contrast bath. The net result is hypothesized to stimulate local circulation in the treated extremity and, to a lesser extent, to increase circulation in the contralateral untreated extremity. This last point is important and can be of assistance to the therapist when treating a patient with peripheral vascular disease. If the use of heat or cold is contraindicated for a specific extremity, the contralateral extremity may be treated using the contrast bath, causing an increase in circulation in the affected extremity via this crossover phenomenon.

Contraindications for the use of the contrast bath would be small vessel disease secondary to diabetes or arteriosclerotic endarteritis and Buerger's disease. Caution should be exercised in patients with any peripheral vascular disease if the water temperature is higher than 40°C. Contrast baths have been advocated for arthritis of peripheral joints, joint sprains, muscular tenderness strains, some peripheral vascular diseases (in selected cases), and to toughen amputation stumps. No well-controlled studies, though, discussing the efficacy of contrast baths are available in the literature.

WOUND CARE

The whirlpool is commonly used in the care of open wounds. The whirlpool provides an effective method of debriding a wound to remove necrotic material and of cleansing, through the addition of a bactericidal agent. In addition, the mechanical effects of the whirlpool assist in stimulating formation of granulation tissue and, in conjunction with the appropriate water temperature, can assist in softening tissues and stimulating circulation to the affected area. The increase in local circulation raises the levels of oxygen, antibodies, leukocytes, and nutrition supplied to the tissues, and enhances the removal of metabolites. In addition, the amount of systemic medications, such as antibiotics, available to the wound area is increased by the improved circulation, which assists in diminishing or preventing infection. The whirlpool also creates sedation and analgesic effect, which may aid in reducing pain caused by the open wound or surrounding tissues.

Whirlpool Additives

An antibacterial agent added to the whirlpool water helps prevent or reduce infection. Two common additives are a povidone-iodine solution,[20] especially prepared for whirlpools, and sodium hypochlorite 5.25 percent, household bleach. The sodium hypochlorite has been found to be effective in dilution up to 1:160;[27] however, dilutions of 1:60 or 1:120 are recommended. In my experience, the 1:60 dilution is at times painful or may cause irritation to the surrounding tissues and therefore, the 1:120 dilution is recommended. The proper dilutions for common whirlpool types for povidone-iodine and sodium hypochlorite in a 1:120 ratio are listed in Table 6–2. Povidone-iodine in 4 parts per million added to the whirlpool bath has been found to reduce the colony count in bacterial cultures by more than 90 percent.[20] Therapists should be aware that addition of an antibacterial agent in the stronger concentrations or simultaneous use of more than one whirlpool with additives can produce vapors that have the potential to cause lightheadedness, dizziness, and even syncope.

TABLE 6–2
Betadine and chlorine bleach concentrations in standard whirlpools at therapeutic levels

Whirlpool Type	Betadine (oz)	Chlorine Bleach (oz)
Foot/Hand	4	26
Leg/Hip	13.5	102
Low Boy	10	96

Wound Type and Condition

SKIN GRAFTS

The second consideration in determining the proper use of whirlpool for wound care is the wound itself. We must consider what effects temperature, agitation, and duration will have on the wound. In the case of a skin graft, at 3 to 5 days postgraft, the skin's viability is still delicate, as it may not be well adherent to the granular bed of the wound nor be sufficiently invaded with capillaries to provide nutritional support to the graft. The graft will not tolerate the high shearing forces and turbulence that can be created in the whirlpool; therefore, whirlpool aeration is adjusted to minimal levels, or it is absent and is only administered for a short duration of 5 minutes. This would allow for softening of the tissues and cleansing with the antibacterial agent, in preparation for mechanical debridement, and would assist with the removal of superficial wound exudates. As the grafts age and stability improves, the duration and aeration may be increased.

TISSUE FLAPS

Whirlpool can also be used in the care of tissue flaps, whether they are cutaneous, muscular, or myocutaneous (free or pedicle type). Once again, consideration must be given to the viability and circulation of the flap. Is the flap free, where arteries have had to be anastomosed? Or is the flap a pedicle type, where the major circulatory supply to the flap has not been interfered with? If the whirlpool is too cold or if the patient should suffer a chill while in the whirlpool, this may cause vasoconstriction of the small infiltrating vessels, which could result in a portion or all the flap to undergo ischemia; leading to partial or full loss of the skin flap. Therefore, temperature of the whirlpool and of the hydrotherapy area, as well as agitation, are important considerations. In general, the younger the flap (in postoperative days), the less turbulence and shear force it will be able to tolerate.

PAINFUL OPEN LESIONS

When the open wound is painful, as in the case of an ischemic ulcer or burn, agitation should be gentle to avoid stimulating the neural tissue, thereby increasing pain. If used properly with the correct temperature and agitation, the whirlpool may actually help to relieve the discomfort created by the wound and provide a gentle method of debridement. Agitation should be kept at a minimal level and not directed at the wound. In the case of a pressure sore, stasis ulcer, or traumatic open wound, debridement may be the main objective and the maximal agitation level may be used.

SURROUNDING TISSUE CONDITION

A third and final consideration for the use of whirlpool to treat open wounds is the condition of the surrounding tissues or of the extremity being treated. The circulation, both arterial and venous, must be able to tolerate the increased temperature and turbulence created by the whirlpool. The surrounding soft tissue's neurologic status must also be considered. The sensation in the area must not be compromised to a level that would prevent the patient from being able to protect him- or herself from further injury (caused by the agitation or rise in tissue temperature). Traumatized tissues may not be able to tolerate whirlpool because of underlying fractures, joint injuries, or soft tissue damage.

In summary, the same indications and contraindications for superficial heating must be considered in addition to (1) the objectives of the whirlpool treatment; (2) the desired physiologic effect; (3) the condition and type of wound; and (4) the condition of the surrounding tissues or extremities.[1]

POOL THERAPY

Pool therapy combines the physical forces of water (buoyancy, pressure, and viscosity) with therapeutic exercise. Buoyancy can be used to assist with exercises, as a means of resistance to improve strength, or to reduce undue stress on joints providing support.[28] The general aims of pool therapy are to promote the patient's relaxation, improve circulation, restore mobility, strengthen muscles, provide gait training with less stress on the weight-bearing joints, and improve psychologic and emotional outlook (patients are often able to move or ambulate in water in ways they could not achieve without the aid of bouyancy).[29,30]

Buoyancy and Exercise

In order for buoyancy to assist with supporting the body part being moved, the body part must move in the same direction as the force of buoyancy. For example, in the sitting position abduction would be assisted by the water's buoyancy lifting (supporting) the arm. The limb is in essence moving through a gravity-eliminated range of motion. Resistance is achieved in this same manner, except the exercise is performed *against* the force of buoyancy (for example, hip flexion with the patient in the prone position).

Patient Selection

Proper patient selection for the use of pool therapy is very important. The patient should not be incontinent (feces or urine) unless catheterized. No patient for whom exposure to warm water or exercising is contraindicated (such as those with open or discharging wounds, upper respiratory infection or other febrile conditions, severe mental disorders, or cardiac or pulmonary conditions [especially with vital capacity below 1500 ml])[31] should be allowed to participate in pool therapy. Debilitated patients not usually suited to this treatment may be considered when the treatment for some reason is desirable and given for short periods of time. Pool therapy has been recommended for treatment of patients with rheumatoid arthritis,[29] orthopedic patients with joint injuries or replacements,[30] patients with neurologic disorders such as paraplegia, or those with poliomyelitis, polyneuritis, multiple sclerosis, and (in certain cases) cerebral palsy.[32]

Treatment Considerations and Equipment

Treatment should last from 15 to 45 minutes, while monitoring vital signs and not allowing either therapist or patients to remain in the pool for too long. High temperatures of 36°C to 37°C are most suitable for patients with arthritis. Lower temperatures of 30°C to 34.5°C are recommended for patients with spasticity and for any patient whose immersion may last for 20 to 45 minutes. The lower temperatures are chosen to reduce fatigue.[30]

The pool should be at least 12 feet by 16 feet in area, with a built-in filtration and chlorination system; and 3 to 4 feet in depth, with easy accessibility to either a ramp, ladder, or stairs and a mechanical overhead lift. Adequate room ventilation that does not allow condensation to accumulate on the walls or windows is important.[26] There should be a regular maintenance schedule for cleaning at least weekly and tests for water chlorine and pH levels should be performed twice a day.[30,33] Floats (such as rings for the trunk and extremities), paddle boards, slippers, parallel bars or hand rails, as well as weighted stools and chairs are necessary equipment. There must also be established safety rules and regulations, as well as established procedures for emergencies including at least one member of the staff present at all times being certified in cardiopulmonary resuscitation (CPR).

HOT TUBS AND JACUZZIS

With the increase in public awareness for physical fitness, health clubs have been increasing in number and have been including hot tubs or whirlpools as part of their facilities. In addition, Jacuzzis and hot tubs are becoming more popular in the home. One of the rising problems is infection with Pseudomonas aeruginosa causing folliculitis.[34] Organic contaminates reduce the effectiveness of the chlorine as a bactericidal agent. Heavy use of whirlpool increases the total organic carbon as well as ammonia and organic nitrogen. Since these events are accelerated by high temperatures and turbulence, there is an increased potential for pathogens to be present.

In order to prevent infection, the following steps should be taken. The pool should have a good filtration and chlorination system. Chlorine and pH levels should be monitored as often as hourly during periods of heavy use, and calcium hardness should be checked weekly. Superchlorination should be performed after each cleaning; and the water should be drained, cleaned, and refilled once every 3 months. Finally, the water temperature should not exceed 38.9°C to 40.5°C. Maintaining the appropriate temperature is also important because of the physiologic effects caused by total body heating and heat dissipation. High temperatures will put a greater demand on the cardiovascular and pulmonary systems. The same precautions and contraindications for any whirlpool should be observed.

SUMMARY

It is only with a thorough knowledge and understanding of (1) normal physiology and pathology; (2) the biophysical, thermal, and mechanical effects of whirlpool; and (3) the various physical properties of water and methods of heat transfer that the therapist can decide on the proper use of the whirlpool for treatment of the patient. This knowledge plays an important part in the decision-making process and assists with the recognition of the contraindications and precautions to be observed for the use of hydrotherapy. Knowledge of the contraindications and precautions (such as those to be considered with patients with medically compromising cardiovascular or pulmonary pathology, peripheral vascular disease including acute phlebitis, extremely debilitating or disorienting illness, severe infection or febrile process, renal failure, or gangrene), combined with general knowledge, will assist the therapist in problem solving in the borderline cases. Safe and effective operation of the whirlpool involves a combination of common-sense values and an understanding of the whirlpool's operation and components. Another aspect of this decision-making process requires recognition of the special consideration that must be observed when using whirlpool for various anatomic parts, such as upper and lower extremities, or full body immersion.

Wound management especially requires that we not only understand the aspects of hydrotherapy but also have a thorough knowledge of the nature of the wound, its physiology, and the condition of the surrounding tissues.

As we have seen in the example of pool therapy, hydrotherapy does not require agitation to be valuable. The inherent properties of water itself combine with therapeutic exercise effectively to treat a portion of the patient population. Finally, we have seen that the use of whirlpool outside the therapist's domain can create potential problems and dangerous situations. However, our knowledge can assist in properly educating those individuals

TABLE 6–3

Clinical decision making in hydrotherapy (clinical problems given with supporting rationale and treatment guidelines)*

Case	Rationale for Treatment with Hydrotherapy	Water Temperature and Tank Chosen	Additional Considerations
65-year-old diabetic female with draining ulcer on left heel.	Mechanical debridement of ulcer	At extremity skin temperature to avoid increase in metabolic needs of tissue; foot/ankle tank	Carefully dry and dress ulcer after treatment. Proper whirlpool sterilization, through evaluation of soft tissues, circulation, and neurologic status.
45-year-old male post–shotgun wound to dorsum of left wrist, with soft tissue loss; wound open, draining; motion of wrist, particularly in flexion, painful and limited	Mechanical debridement of wound Pain reduction to facilitate ease of exercise (buoyancy-assisted exercise)	34.4°C, neutral, comfortable; do not want to cause swelling; hand/arm tank	Carefully dry and dress wound after treatment; encourage patient to keep hand elevated and to do active exercise after whirlpool.
40-year-old female with flare-up of rheumatoid arthritis; ROM of all extremities limited, owing to pain; requires maximal assistance to transfer from supine to sit	Pain reduction; buoyancy-assisted exercise	37–38°C, Hubbard tank	Physical therapist present during session to supervise ROM exercises; overhead lift available; related medical problems of the pulmonary, cardiovascular, and peripheral vascular systems.

* The rationale should be covered over when the reader reviews problem, then uncovered to compare choices with those of the author.

no US
no heat
whirlpool

involved in preventing such situations from existing. The real challenge in hydrotherapy is not necessarily in its technical use but in the decision process that must occur before its use to achieve the end result of safe, effective treatment for the therapist's patient. Examples of clinical decision making in hydrotherapy are briefly outlined in Table 6–3.

REFERENCES

1. Holmes, G: *Hydrotherapy as a means of rehabilitation.* Br J Phys Med 5:93, 1942.
2. Zislis, J: *Hydrotherapy.* In Krusen, F (ed): *Handbook of Physical Medicine and Rehabilitation,* ed 2. WB Saunders, Philadelphia, 1971.
3. Beasley, R and Kester, N: *Principles of medical-surgical rehabilitation of the hand.* Med Clin North Am 53:645, 1969.
4. Abraham, E: *Whirlpool therapy for treatment of soft tissue wounds complicated by extremity fractures.* J Trauma 4:222, 1974.
5. Koepke, G: *The role of physical medicine in the treatment of burns.* Surg Clin North Am 50:1385, 1970.
6. Nave, CR and Nave, BC: *Physics For the Health Sciences,* ed 2. WB Saunders, Philadelphia, 1980.
7. Dawson, WJ, et al: *Evaluation of cardiac output, cardiac work, and metabolic rate during hydrotherapy exercise in normal subjects.* Arch Phys Med Rehabil 46:605, 1965.
8. Epstein, M: *Water immersion: Modern researchers discover the secrets of an old folk remedy.* The Sciences, November: 12, 1979.
9. Boyle, RW, Balisteri, F, and Osborne, F: *The value of the Hubbard tank as a diuretic agent.* Arch Phys Med Rehabil 45:505, 1964.
10. Abramson, D: *Physiologic basis for the use of physical agents in peripheral vascular disorders.* Arch Phys Med Rehabil 46:216, 1965.
11. Abramson, D, et al: *The effect of altering limb position on blood flow, O_2 uptake and skin temperature.* J Appl Physiol 17:191, 1962.
12. Abramson, D, et al: *Changes in blood flow, oxygen, uptake and tissue temperatures produced by a topical application of wet heat.* Arch Phys Med Rehabil 42:305, 1961.
13. Borrell, R, et al: *Comparison of in vivo temperatures produced by hydrotherapy, paraffin wax treatment, and Fluidotherapy.* Phys Ther 60:1273, 1980.
14. Nylin, J: *The use of water in therapeutics.* Arch Phys Med Rehabil 13:261, 1932.
15. Pope, C: *Physiologic action and therapeutic value of general and local whirlpool baths.* Arch Phys Med Rehabil 10:498, 1929.
16. Cohen, A, Martin, G, and Wakim, K: *The effect of whirlpool bath with and without agitation on the circulation in normal and diseased extremities.* Arch Phys Med Rehabil 30:212, 1949.
17. Hellerbrand, T, Holutz, S, and Eubank, I: *Measurement of whirlpool temperature, pressure and turbulence.* Arch Phys Med Rehabil 32:17, 1950.
18. Whitehall Hydrotherapy Equipment, Catalog No. 680, Hackensack, NJ.
19. Ascenzi, J: *The need for decontamination and disinfection of hydrotherapy equipment,* Vol 1. Asepsis Monograph, Surgikos, Inc, 1980.
20. Simonetti, A, Miller, R, and Gristina, J: *Efficacy of povidone-iodine in the disinfection of whirlpool baths and hubbard tanks.* Phys Ther 52:450, 1972.
21. Steve, L, Goodhart, P, and Alexander, J: *Hydrotherapy burn treatment: Use of chloramine-T against resistant microorganisms.* Arch Phys Med Rehabil 60:301, 1979.
22. Gieck, J: *Precautions for hydrotherapeutic devices.* Clinical Management 3:44, 1983.
23. Hunter, J and Mackin, E: *Edema and bandaging.* In Hunter, J, et al (eds): *Rehabilitation of the Hand,* ed 1, CV Mosby, St Louis, 1978.
24. Magness, J, Garrett, T, and Erickson, D: *Swelling of the upper extremity during whirlpool baths.* Arch Phys Med Rehabil 51:297, 1970.
25. Schultz, K: *The effect of active exercise during whirlpool on the hand.* Unpublished thesis. San Jose State University, San Jose, CA, 1982.

26. Walsh, M: *Relationship of hand edema to upper extremity position and water temperature during whirlpool treatments in normals.* Unpublished thesis. Temple University, Philadelphia, 1983.

27. Abston, S: *Burns in children.* Ciba Clinical Symposia 28:14, 1976.

28. Daggett, R and Gillespie, A: *Pool therapy in the treatment of rheumatoid arthritis.* In Lamont-Havers, RW and Hislop, HJ (eds): *Arthritis and Related Disorders.* American Physical Therapy Association, 1965.

29. Golland, A: *Basic hydrotherapy.* Physiotherapy 67:258, 1981.

30. Roberts, P: *Hydrotheraphy: Its history, theory and practice.* Occupational Health 235:5, 1981.

31. Harrison, RA: *Tolerance of pool therapy by ankylosing spondylitis patients with low vital capacity.* Physiotherapy 67:296, 1981.

32. Stewart, JB and Basmajian, JV: *Exercises in water.* In Basmajian, JV (ed): *Therapeutic Exercise,* ed 3. Williams & Wilkins, Baltimore, 1978.

33. Bickle, RJ: *Swimming pool management.* Physiotherapy 57:475, 1971.

34. Randt, GA: *Hot tub folliculitis.* Physician and Sports Medicine 11:75, 1983.

CHAPTER 7

THERAPEUTIC ULTRASOUND

MARVIN C. ZISKIN, M.D., M.S. Bm. E., AND
SUSAN L. MICHLOVITZ, M.S., P.T.

Heating agents are divided into two major types: superficial and deep. In Chapter 5, superficial heating agents were discussed. These agents produce temperature elevations in skin and underlying subcutaneous tissues to a depth of approximately 1 cm. In the next two chapters, deep heating agents are discussed. Deep heating agents are capable of causing temperature elevations in tissues to depths of 3 cm or more. Furthermore, these agents are capable of delivering the necessary energy to the deep structures without causing excessive heating of the overlying superficial tissues.

A deep heating agent is an appropriate adjunct to treatment of ailments such as those that (1) limit range of motion owing to a decrease in the extensibility of periarticular soft tissue; (2) cause skeletal muscle spasms that are not of an acute origin; or (3) produce pain secondary to chronic soft tissue dysfunction.

There are three different deep heating agents: ultrasound, shortwave diathermy, and microwave diathermy. Ultrasound is by far the most commonly used. Shortwave and microwave diathermy will be discussed in the next chapter.

Ultrasound has been employed in medicine for over 40 years. Biologic effects in tissues exposed to ultrasound (high-frequency sound waves) were first reported by Wood and Loomis in 1927.[1] They demonstrated lysis of red blood cells and decreased mobility in mice following exposure to high-frequency (300 kHz), high-intensity sound waves. The application of ultrasound for medical treatment was introduced in Germany in the late 1930s[2] and in the United States in the late 1940s.[3]

Ultrasound is used in medicine for diagnosis (imaging of internal structures), physical therapy (functional restoration and healing of soft tissue ailments), and tissue destruction (in surgery and hyperthermia for tumor irradiation). The intensity of ultrasound in each classification is different; the lowest intensity is used for diagnostic procedures and the highest for tissue destruction.

The objectives of this chapter are to (1) present the physical principles and biophysical effects of ultrasound; (2) discuss the clinical conditions for which ultrasound is effective; (3) discuss the clinical procedures for the application of ultrasound; and (4) present guidelines for the safe use of ultrasound, including a discussion of the contraindications and precautions for treatment with this agent.

PHYSICAL PRINCIPLES

The purpose of this section is to provide a basic foundation of the physics of ultrasound for the physical therapist. For a more complete and in-depth study, the excellent textbook by Wells[4] should be consulted.

Nature of Sound

Solids and liquids consist of molecules held together by elastic forces that behave like rubberbands connecting each molecule to each of its nearest neighbors. Thus, a molecule, if set into vibration, will cause its neighbors to vibrate, and in turn their neighbors, and so on until the vibration has propagated throughout the entire material. Each individual molecule vibrates back and forth a small distance about its initial position. However, the passage of vibrational energy travels over millions of molecules in propagating through tissue. The propagation of this vibratory motion is precisely what sound is.

Unlike electromagnetic waves such as light and x-rays, sound cannot travel in a vacuum. Very important for the patient is the fact that sound is non-ionizing and, therefore, its use does not impose the hazards attributed to ionizing radiation, such as cancer production and chromosome breakage.

FREQUENCY. The number of oscillations a molecule undergoes in 1 second defines the frequency of a sound wave and is expressed in units of hertz (Hz); that is, 1 Hz = 1 cycle/second, 1 kHz = 1000 cycles/second, and 1 MHz = 1 million cycles/second. Theoretically, frequency can vary from 0 Hz to infinity; however, the human ear is sensitive only to sound frequencies between 16 Hz and 20,000 Hz. Sound with a frequency greater than 20,000 Hz is called ultrasound.

For a given sound source, the higher the frequency, the less the emerging sound beam diverges. Sound at audible frequencies appears to spread out in all directions, whereas ultrasound beams are well collimated, similar to a light beam leaving a flashlight (Fig. 7–1). Ultrasound beams at frequencies greater than 800 kHz are sufficiently collimated to selectively expose a limited target area for physical therapy treatment.

Attenuation is the decrease in energy contained within a sound beam as it travels through tissue. It results from two processes: scattering and absorption. Scattering is the deflection of sound out of the beam that results

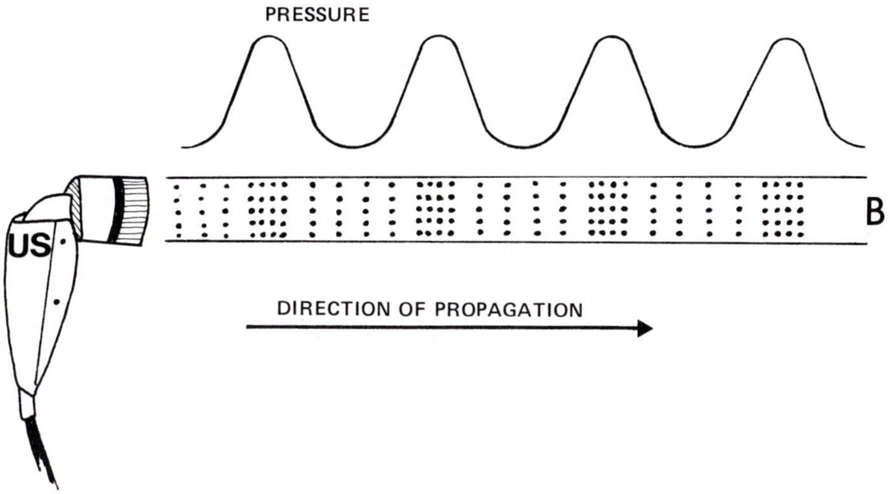

FIGURE 7–1

Diagram of a collimated ultrasound beam (B) coming from an ultrasound (US) applicator. The associated pressure wave is diagrammed above. Areas of increased molecular concentration (⁞⁞⁞⁞) are condensations. Areas of decreased molecular concentration are rarefactions (⁞ ⁞ ⁞ ⁞). (Adapted from Ziskin, MC: *Basic principles.* In Goldberg, BB, Kotler, MN, Ziskin, MC, and Waxham, RD (eds): *Diagnostic Uses of Ultrasound.* Grune & Stratton, New York, 1975.)

when it strikes a reflecting surface. Absorption is the transfer of energy from the sound beam to the surrounding tissues.

Absorption of sound, and therefore attenuation, increases as the frequency increases. Absorption occurs in part because of the internal friction in tissue that needs to be overcome in the passage of sound. The higher the frequency, the more rapidly the molecules are forced to move against this friction. As the absorption increases, there is less sound energy available to propagate further through the tissue (Fig. 7–2). At frequencies greater than 20 MHz, superficial absorption becomes so great that less than 1 percent of the sound penetrates beyond the first centimeter.

For physical therapy applications, 1.0 MHz is the frequency most often used, because it offers a good compromise between sufficiently deep penetration and adequate heating under customary exposure levels.

SOUND VELOCITY. This velocity is the speed at which the vibratory motion is propagated through a material. The more rigid the material, the greater the velocity of sound passing through it. Sound travels through average soft tissue at 1540 m/sec and through compact bones at 4000 m/sec. The depth of a structure beneath the skin can be determined by measuring the time required for sound to travel to the structure and return. This ability to chart the position of reflecting surfaces forms the basis of the extensive use of ultrasound in medical diagnosis.

WAVELENGTH. A finite period of time elapses before the vibration of a molecule causes its neighbor to vibrate. Because of this delay, the first

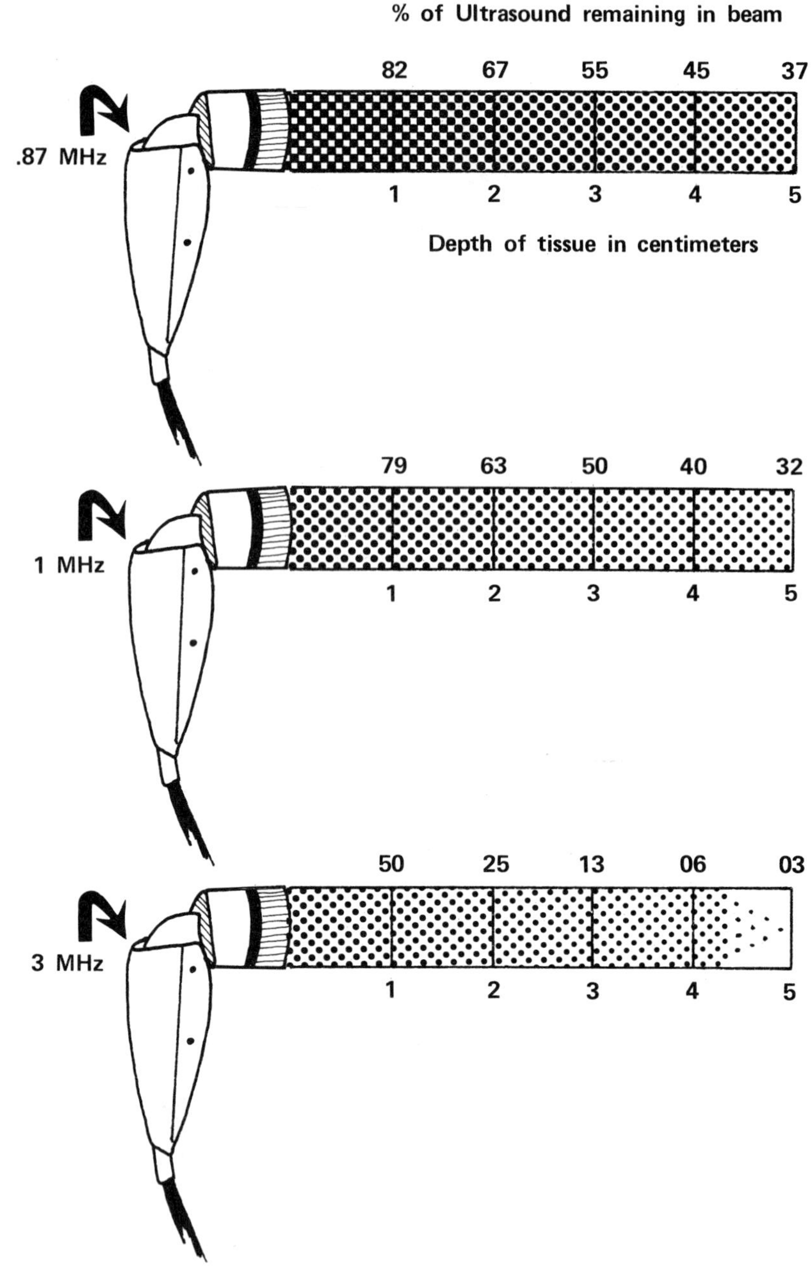

FIGURE 7–2

Attenuation of the sound beam in soft tissue at various frequencies, assuming that uniform attenuation approximately 1 dB/cm/MHz.

molecule will reach its point of maximal excursion before its neighbor does, and as long as they continue to vibrate the second molecule will lag behind the first. These molecules are said to oscillate asynchronously, or be out of phase, and the time delay is called the *phase shift*. There is an equal phase shift between each of the successive molecules in the path of sound propagation. Because of this overall asynchrony, the concentration of molecules increases in regions called *condensations* and decreases in alternating regions called *rarefactions* (Fig. 7–1). The local pressure is proportional to the molecular concentration and, as shown in Figure 7–1, varies sinusoidally along the direction of propagation with its peak values occurring at regions of condensations. Wavelength is defined as the distance between two successive peaks in the pressure wave.

Wavelength is inversely related to frequency, as indicated in the fundamental equation, Velocity = Frequency × Wavelength. Using the value of 1540 m/sec for velocity and 1 MHz for frequency, which are typical values applicable in therapeutic situations, this equation enables one to show that the corresponding wavelength of ultrasound is 1.5 mm.

Types of Waves

Sound waves are classified as longitudinal or transverse, according to the direction of motion of the molecules of the medium through which they travel. A *longitudinal wave* is one in which the direction of motion of the molecules is parallel to the direction of wave propagation (Fig. 7–3). In a *transverse wave,* the direction of molecular motion is perpendicular to the direction of wave propagation.

Since gases and liquids are not able to sustain transverse vibrations, transverse sound waves do not occur in these substances. In solids, both longitudinal and transverse waves occur. With the exception of compact

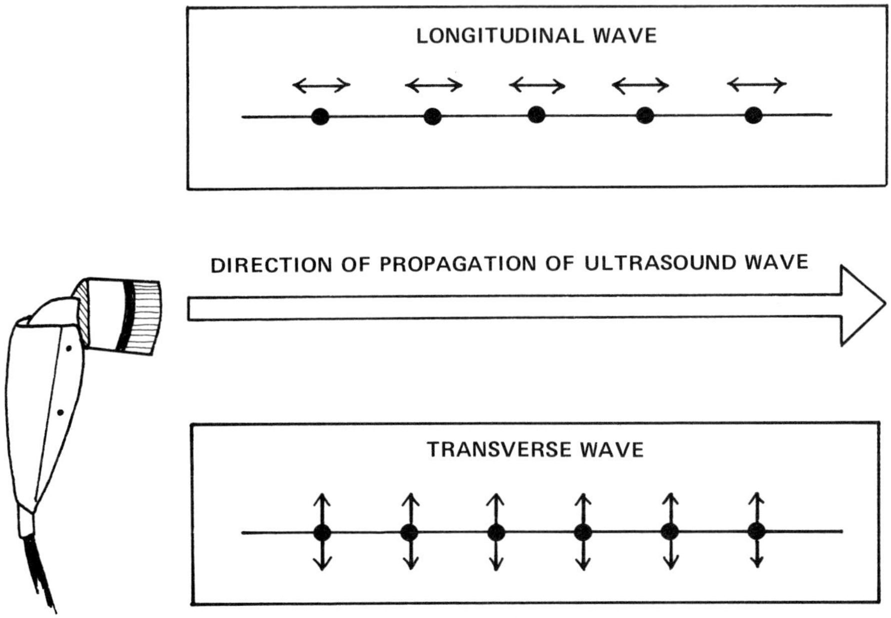

FIGURE 7–3
Types of ultrasound waves are schematically depicted.

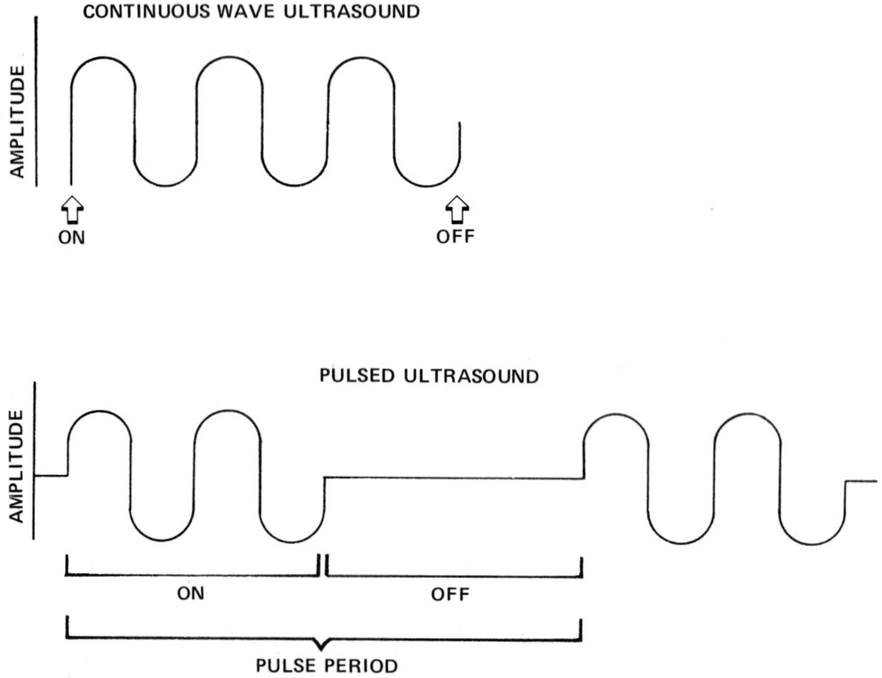

FIGURE 7–4

Continuous wave and pulsed wave ultrasound. The duty cycle of the pulsed wave mode illustrated is $\frac{2\ \text{msec}}{4\ \text{msec}} = 0.5 = 50\%$.

bone, the tissues of the body behave acoustically as though they were liquids and support only longitudinal waves. Within the body, therefore, transverse waves are found only in bone.

Sound waves can be produced as *continuous wave* (CW) or *pulsed wave*. A continuous wave is one in which the sound intensity remains constant (Fig. 7–4), whereas a pulsed wave is intermittently interrupted. Pulsed waves are further characterized by specifying what fraction of the time the sound is present over one pulse period. This fraction is called the *duty cycle* and is calculated using the following equation:

$$\text{Duty cycle} = \frac{\text{Duration of pulse (time-on)}}{\text{Pulse period (time-on + time-off)}}$$

Typical duty cycles for therapy machines when in the pulsed mode range from 0.2 (20 percent) to 0.5 (50 percent).

Intensity

The strength of an ultrasound beam is determined by its intensity. Intensity is the rate at which energy is delivered per unit area and is expressed in units of watts per square centimeter (W/cm^2). Intensities employed in physical therapy range from about 0.5 to 3.0 W/cm^2. With all other factors held

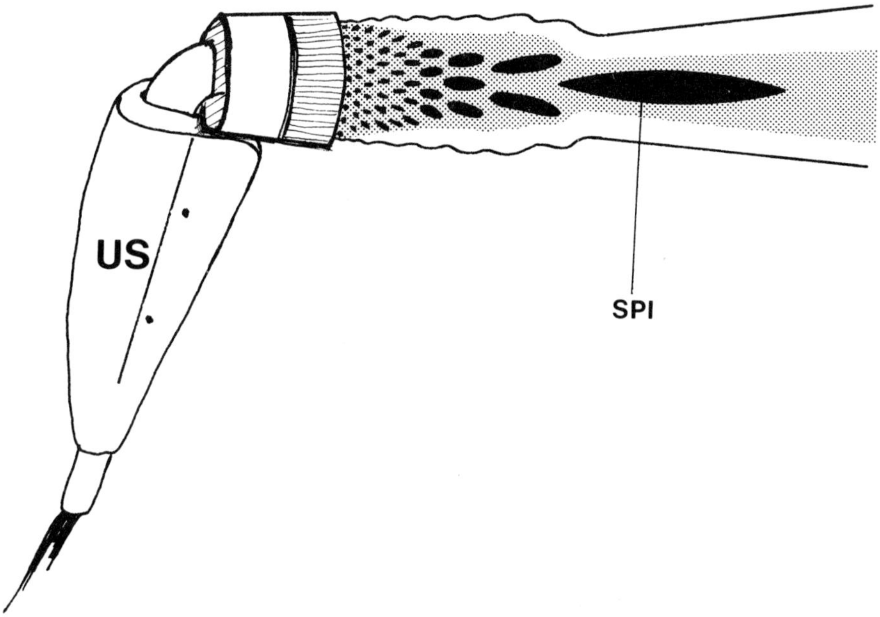

FIGURE 7–5
Schematic diagram of ultrasound beam. The darkest areas indicate more intense regions. The greatest intensity within the beam is the spatial peak intensity (SPI). (Adapted from Stewart, HF and Stratmeyer, ME (eds): *An Overview of Ultrasound: Theory, Measurement, Medical Applications, and Biological Effects.* HHS Publication FDA 82-8-90, 1982.)

constant, the greater the intensity, the greater the resulting temperature elevation.

The measurement of intensity is performed by measuring the total power output (in watts) of the ultrasound applicator and dividing by the area* (in cm^2) of the applicator face. Because the ultrasound beam is not uniform, some regions of the beam will be more intense than other regions. The above measurement of intensity gives an average intensity and is referred to as the *spatial average* intensity. Occasionally, it is desirable to know the greatest intensity anywhere within the beam. This is called the *spatial peak* intensity (Fig. 7–5).

In the case when the sound beam is pulsed, the intensity will be zero when the sound is off and at its maximum during the pulse (Fig. 7–6). This maximum intensity is called the *temporal peak* intensity or the *pulse average* intensity. The *temporal average* intensity is obtained by averaging the intensity over both the on and off periods. For example, a pulsed sound beam with a duty cycle of 0.5 (50 percent) and a temporal peak intensity of 2.0

---

* Since not all of the applicator face is actually emitting sound, the value to be used in this computation is reduced to that corresponding to just the effective radiating area (ERA) of the crystal. The ERA of a typical therapeutic applicator is approximately 80 percent of the total area of the transducer face.

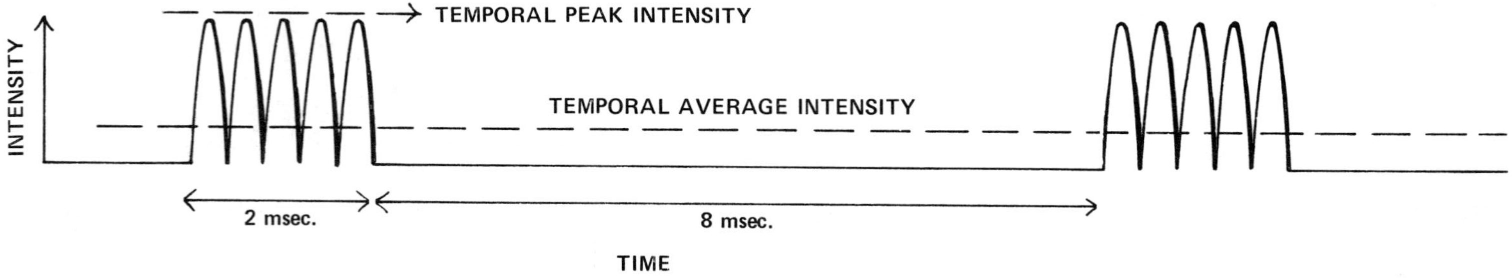

FIGURE 7–6

A typical pulsing pattern. The total pulse period is 10 msec. The pulse duration is 2 msec. The duty cycle is 0.20 (20 percent).

W/cm^2 would have a temporal average intensity of 1.0 W/cm^2 (2.0 W/cm^2 $\times$ 0.5 = 1.0 W/cm^2); if the duty cycle had been 0.25 (25 percent), the temporal average intensity would be 0.5 W/cm^2. In this chapter, unless stated otherwise, all pulsed intensities quoted will be spatial average, temporal peak values along with the duty cycle.

The amount of heating depends on the temporal average intensity rather than the temporal peak. By interrupting (pulsing) a continuous wave sound beam, the temporal average intensity is decreased proportionately to the amount of time the sound is off. Thus, less heating will occur even though the temporal peak intensity is unchanged. Pulsing would be of benefit when the desired effect is due to a nonthermal mechanism and when heating is to be minimized, such as in the treatment of stasis ulcers.

When recording the ultrasound exposure administered to a patient, it is important to specify clearly the intensity, the duty cycle and the total duration. For continuous wave exposures, the spatial average intensity and the duration are reported.

Spatial average intensities ranging from 0.5 to 3.0 W/cm^2 are used in therapeutic applications. Intensities above 10.0 W/cm^2 are used to destroy tissue surgically, and intensities (temporal average) below 0.1 W/cm^2 are used for diagnostic purposes.

Generation of Ultrasound

Sound within the audible frequency range is normally produced by vibrating membranes, such as the vocal cords or the diaphragm of a loudspeaker. Movement of these membranes sets up corresponding vibrations in the surrounding air molecules, and when this vibration pattern reaches our ears we perceive it as sound. The frequency of the sound is precisely the frequency of the membrane vibration. Because of their inertia, these membranes cannot vibrate rapidly enough to generate ultrasonic frequencies. However, ultrasound can be generated by replacing these membranes with special crystals that are able to vibrate very rapidly and possess the property of piezoelectricity.

THE PIEZOELECTRIC EFFECT. There are two forms of the piezoelectric effect—direct and reverse (indirect) (Fig. 7–7). The *direct piezoelectric effect* is the generation of an electric voltage across a crystal when the crystal is compressed. If the crystal is expanded instead of compressed, a voltage of opposite polarity is induced. A sound wave impinging on a piezoelectric crystal will cause the crystal to expand and contract at the same frequency as the sound wave and in turn induce an oscillating voltage across the crystal face. The direct piezoelectric effect is utilized for converting ultrasound into an electrical signal that replicates the sound pattern and can be conveniently and accurately processed and analyzed.

The *reverse piezoelectric effect* is the contraction or expansion of a crystal in response to a voltage applied across its face. A change in the polarity of the applied voltage causes a contracted crystal to expand, and vice versa.

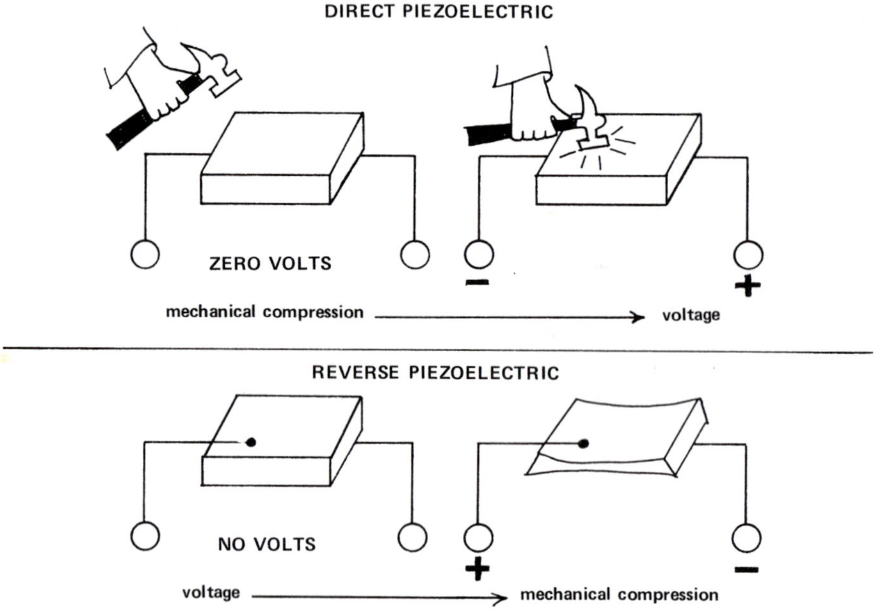

FIGURE 7–7

The direct and indirect (reverse) piezoelectric effects are shown. (Adapted from Ziskin, MC: *Basic principles*. In Goldberg, BB, Kotler, MN, Ziskin, MC, and Waxham, RD (eds): *Diagnostic Uses of Ultrasound*. Grune & Stratton, New York, 1975.)

An alternating voltage makes the crystal vibrate at the frequency of the electrical oscillation. In this manner, a piezoelectric crystal can be used to generate ultrasound at any desired frequency.

THE TRANSDUCER. A transducer is any device that converts one form of energy into another. The piezoelectric crystal is a transducer that converts electrical energy into sound energy, and vice versa.

Many naturally occurring crystals, such as quartz, possess the property of piezoelectricity, but synthetic ceramic crystals, such as barium titanate or lead zirconate titanate (PZT), are almost always used because of their superior mechanical and electrical properties. These crystals are sliced into wafers approximately 2 to 3 mm thick. The diameter may vary from 1 to 3 cm depending on the intended use. Because of their small size and mechanical fragility, these crystals must be mounted in an applicator to be clinically useful and durable and to facilitate electrical connections. The entire applicator is commonly referred to as the transducer.

Therapeutic Ultrasound Units

The basic components of therapeutic ultrasound units include a power supply, oscillator circuit, transformer, coaxial cable, and ultrasound applicator. The purpose of the therapeutic ultrasound unit is to produce a sound beam at a specific frequency. The frequency is generated by an oscillator circuit carefully tuned by the manufacturer to the preferred frequency for the transducer. Occasional tuning adjustments may be necessary, particularly when a transducer is replaced. These adjustments are best left to the biomedical technician. The intensity is determined by the electrical voltage applied to the transducer. The voltage is controlled by the setting of the intensity control which adjusts a variable gain transformer.

A circuit can be added that interrupts the oscillator to produce a pulsed mode. The duty cycle control selector on the face of the machine can change the on/off times by controlling a pulse timing circuit. The treatment timer limits how long the instrument is energized. In many units, the timer also serves as the on-off switch.

To work properly, the unit is supplied with appropriate voltages obtained through a transformer to which electrical power from the wall receptacle is applied. Appropriate power can also be supplied through a battery.

A coaxial cable connects the ultrasound applicator to the generator (console). The purpose of the coaxial cable is to maximize transmission of the electrical energy and to minimize frequency distortion and interference with the external environment.

All units have a power meter calibrated to read in both watts (acoustic power) and W/cm^2 (acoustic intensity). For any given applicator, the ratio of the acoustic power to the intensity is a constant, the effective radiating area (ERA). A typical ultrasound unit is pictured in Figure 7–8.

BIOPHYSICAL EFFECTS

The biophysical effects resulting from the interaction of ultrasound with tissue can be grouped into two classifications: (1) thermal—those effects produced by the ability of ultrasound to elevate tissue temperature; and (2) nonthermal—those effects that must be attributed to mechanisms other than an increase in tissue temperature. The mechanism of some of the biologic changes produced by ultrasound may be thermal or nonthermal, or a combination of both. For many responses, such as the pain reduction reported following sonation, the underlying physiologic or physical mechanism has not been thoroughly identified and is only speculative at this time.

Thermal Effects

The major reason for the use of ultrasound as a therapeutic agent is based on the knowledge that ultrasound can elevate tissue temperature to depths of 5 cm or more. The physiologic responses attributed to a thermal mechanism include increase in collagen tissue extensibility, alterations in blood flow, changes in nerve conduction velocity, increase in pain threshold, increased enzymatic activity, and changes in contractile activity of skeletal

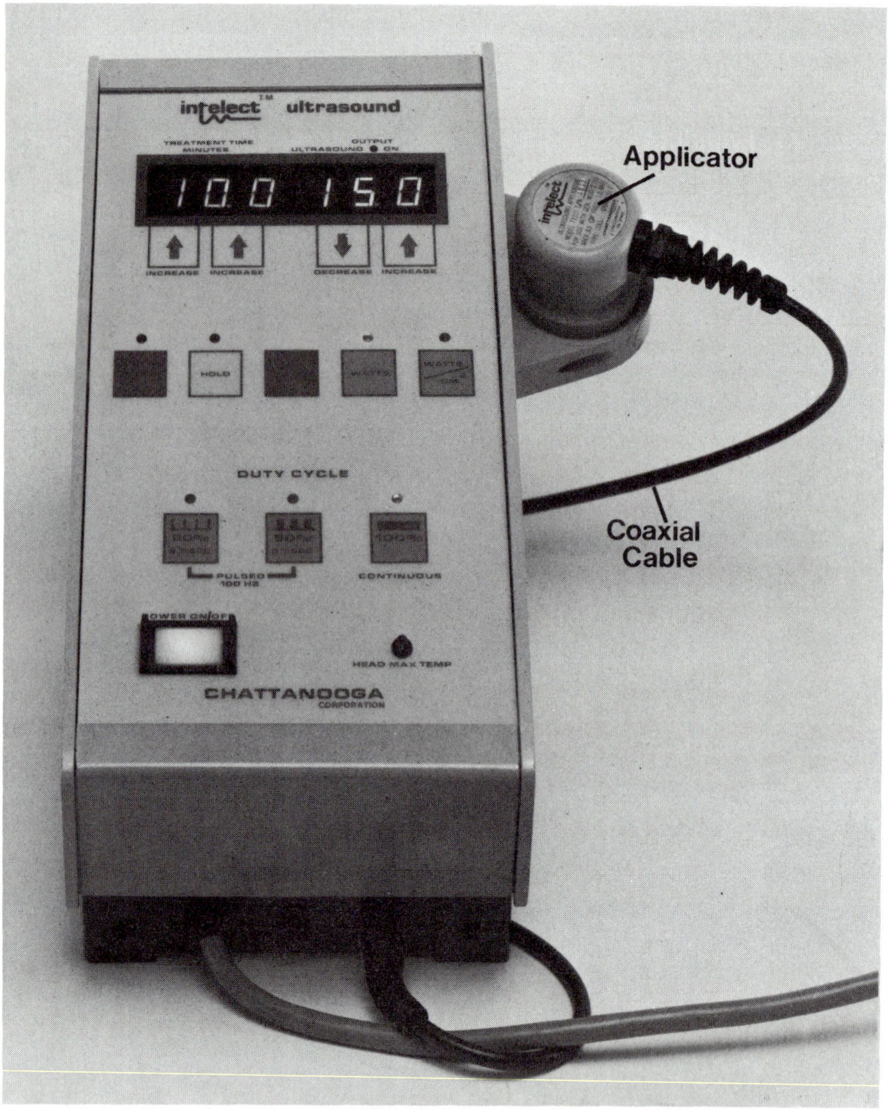

FIGURE 7–8

A therapeutic ultrasound generator is pictured. (Photo courtesy of Chattanooga Corp., Chattanooga, TN.)

muscle. Physiologic changes such as these are reviewed in Chapter 5. Ultrasound intensities at ranges higher than those used for therapeutic application have been demonstrated to retard growth of long bones, damage spinal cord tissue, and destroy various other tissues.

Tissues of high collagen content absorb a large amount of the ultrasound beam and thus are affected to a greater extent by ultrasound energy. The amount of heat produced will depend on the intensity of ultrasound, the duration of exposure, and the size of the area sonated. Bone and joint capsular structures have a very high collagen content and are thus the structures that absorb the most ultrasound energy. Ultrasound penetrates

TABLE 7–1
Attenuation of a 1 MHz ultrasound beam

Tissue	Attenuation (%/cm)
Blood	3
Fat	13
Muscle	24
Blood vessel	32
Skin	39
Tendon	59
Cartilage	68
Bone	96

through skin and subcutaneous fat with small to moderate attenuation (Table 7–1).

Ultrasound energy absorption and the subsequent tissue temperature elevation are frequency dependent. The higher the frequency, the greater the attenuation of energy in superficial structures. At 3.0 MHz, most of the energy is absorbed within a depth of 1 to 2 cm. At lower frequencies, ranging from 800 kHz to 1.0 MHz, there is less attenuation in the superficial tissues, allowing more energy to be available for absorption in deeper tissues. These latter frequencies are commonly used in the United States in the treatment of musculoskeletal dysfunctions, when an increased depth of penetration and subsequent absorption are desired.

Ultrasound can be used as a deep heating agent to increase selectively the temperature of periarticular structures[5] and muscle at the bone-muscle interface.[6,7] Intensities required to elevate tissue temperature to a range of 40°C to 45°C vary from 1.0 to 2.0 W/cm^2 for a duration of 5 to 10 minutes. A residual increase in length of tendons in amphibians has been demonstrated by elevating tissue temperature with ultrasound and then applying a stretch during the time the temperature remains elevated.[8] In mammalian preparations, similar increases were reported when tissue temperature was elevated by a water bath and a stretch was applied.[9,10] This effect has been attributed to the change in viscous properties of the tissues irradiated, producing a change in the plastic deformation of collagen tissues. This information has been applied clinically to increase range of motion of contracted joints (see section on clinical application).

With an increase of tissue temperature, a mild inflammatory response and an increase in blood flow would be expected. Numerous investigators have measured blood flow in limbs following ultrasound irradiation, some reporting an increase, some a decrease, and some no changes. Intensities, frequencies, and exposure durations of ultrasound application and the methods of measuring changes in blood flow were not consistent among the experimenters. Therefore, drawing clinically useful conclusions is difficult. However, the following statements appear to summarize this information accurately. Following 10 to 20 minutes of ultrasound at intensities greater than 2.0 W/cm^2, skeletal muscle temperature and blood flow increases have been found.[11–13] At lower intensities and for shorter durations, either no change or inconsistent changes in blood flow were noted.[13–15]

Changes in motor and sensory nerve conduction velocity after ultrasound exposure have been reported. Five minutes of ultrasound at 1.5 W/cm^2 over the lateral cutaneous branch of the femoral[16] and superficial cutaneous branch of radial nerves[17] decreased latency. No changes were found in the amplitude or duration of the nerve action potential. When sensory nerve latency is decreased, an increase in conduction velocity is implicit. In a similar experimental set-up, latency was decreased in the superficial radial nerve following 1.0 W/cm^2 varying from 5 to 20 minutes.[18] Two groups of investigators compared ultrasound with infrared heating.[17,18] Because latencies were reduced with both agents and temperature increases were similar, the investigators attributed their findings to thermal mechanisms.

Ulnar motor nerve conduction velocity (NCV) increased 3.0 m/sec with continuous wave ultrasound at 1.5 W/cm^2 for 5 minutes and infrared radiation.[19] Placebo ultrasound and pulsed ultrasound at 1.5 W/cm^2 (1:5 pulse ratio) for 25 minutes caused a decrease in NCV. The decrease was proposed to be correlated with the reduction of temperature caused by a cool coupling medium. The thermal effects rather than the nonthermal effects were thought to produce the increased NCV.

Pain threshold was elevated following increases in tissue temperature with continuous wave ultrasound at 1.5 W/cm^2.[20] These findings are consistent with what would be expected when tissue temperature is elevated by a thermal agent.

Nonthermal Effects

Some effects of ultrasound cannot be explained by a thermal mechanism. These nonthermal effects include cavitation and mechanical and chemical alterations. *Cavitation* is the vibrational effect on gas bubbles by an ultrasound beam. Changes in local pressure produced by ultrasound can cause the expansion and compression of small gas bubbles that may be present in the blood or tissue fluids. During the period of rarefaction, the small bubbles will expand; during condensations, these bubbles will be compressed. The pulsation of the bubbles in the ultrasound field, if sufficiently intense, can cause changes in cellular activity and tissue damage. If the bubbles in the field pulse but do not increase much in overall amplitude, stable cavities result. These stable cavities can result in diffusional changes along cell membranes and thus alter cell function.[21] *Unstable* or *transient cavitation* refers to the violent collapse of bubbles within the sound field, resulting in tissue destruction. Transient cavitation may be responsible for blood vessel damage.[22] The threshold intensity for unstable cavitation is higher than for stable cavitation. The intensity threshold for cavitation may be within the intensity range used in therapy, and although many questions remain, there is some evidence to suggest that cavitation may occur in therapeutic applications. We do not know which, if any, of the beneficial nonthermal effects are due to cavitation.

Acoustical streaming refers to the movement of fluids along the boundaries of cell membranes as a result of the mechanical pressure wave. This streaming has been implicated in the changes in ion fluxes and subsequent changes in cellular activity found with ultrasound application. Increases in cell membrane and vascular wall permeability have been found within the range of therapeutic intensities. Potassium leakage from red blood cells in vitro resulted following sonation at ranges from 0.5 to 3.0 W/cm^2.[23] Increases in fibroblastic activity (for example, protein synthesis)[24] and increases in calcium fluxes across smooth muscle membranes of the mouse uterus were found using pulsed ultrasound.[25] These changes may be a result of the mechanical action of ultrasound on cell membranes, rather than by a thermal mechanism.

On the other hand, changes in the diffusion of ions across epithelial cells in isolated frog skin have been attributed to both thermal and mechanical components.[26] Using a stationary applicator, ultrasound at 1.5 W/cm^2 applied to the small blood vessels in the hamster cheek pouch resulted in areas of petechiae and demonstrable increases in vascular permeability at the level of the postcapillary venules.[27] The results could have been due to thermally induced changes in permeability or to cavitation resulting in damage to vessel endothelial cells. Petechiae in mice were also found after abdominal exposure to ultrasound.[22] Cavitation was implicated as the mechanism producing the observed results.

Other adverse reactions, including stasis of blood flow and endothelial damage, have been demonstrated in chick embryos.[28] Platelet aggregation in blood vessels was shown to occur in guinea pig ears.[29] These responses were attributed to nonthermal mechanisms, because either pulsed ultrasound or very low intensity continuous wave ultrasound was administered. A stationary transducer was used for all applications. The investigators speculated that such results would not be produced with a moving sound head.

To further elucidate the effects of ultrasound on the microcirculation, Hogan and associates[30,31] have recently studied the effects of ultrasound on circulation in the rat in an ischemic muscle preparation. When pulsed ultrasound was applied at 2.5 W/cm^2 for 5 minutes on alternating days, an increase in capillary density and improved blood flow to medium-sized arterioles was found. At higher intensities of pulsed ultrasound, increased vasomotion of small arterioles and decreased flow was found. Although the underlying mechanisms for all the changes seen were not known, they probably were not thermal in origin, because similar findings were not observed when the skeletal muscle was heated in the absence of ultrasound.

In summary, a review of the literature shows that ultrasound can cause many effects. Most of these effects are intensity dependent. With appropriate care to control intensities ultrasound can be applied to patients in a safe and effective manner.

CLINICAL APPLICATIONS OF ULTRASOUND AT THERAPEUTIC INTENSITIES

Ultrasound is commonly used in rehabilitation as an adjunct in the management of various soft tissue dysfunctions including joint contracture, scar tissue, tendonitis, bursitis, skeletal muscle spasm, and pain. In addition, ultrasound at therapeutic intensities has been included in treatment regimens for the management of stasis ulcers, pressure sores, and plantar warts and as a noninvasive technique to drive medication through the skin (phonophoresis). The basis for the clinical application of ultrasound as a therapeutic agent was developed in the previous section. In this section, the procedures and rationale for the clinical utilization of ultrasound will be discussed.

Joint Contracture and Scar Tissue

Joint contracture is a debilitating consequence of immobilization or trauma. If range of motion is limited owing to periarticular connective tissue changes, stretching exercises are usually employed to increase motion. Elevation of tissue temperature up to 45°C preceding or during a gentle passive or active stretch will be more effective in gaining motion than when either is done in isolation. This concept of "heat and stretch" has been demonstrated in well-designed in vitro laboratory studies.[9,10,32] A greater residual increase in tissue length with less potential damage is produced when preheating or simultaneous heating is employed. Length-tension analyses revealed that tissue extensibility was increased when Gersten[8] applied ultrasound at intensities of 1.0 to 3.0 W/cm^2 resulting in tissue temperatures ranging from 39°C to 47°C.

Heating has been postulated to alter the viscoelastic (plastic) properties of collagen tissue and collagen molecular bonding, thus facilitating ease of stretch. Deep tissues responsible for decreasing the range of motion at a joint are rich in collagen. Therefore, ultrasound is a logically chosen thermal agent to selectively heat these deep structures.

Lehmann and associates[33] demonstrated that ultrasound was effective in increasing the temperature of the hip joint when applied within therapeutic intensities for at least 5 minutes. A combination of ultrasound and exercise was compared with infrared and exercise for increasing range of motion of the hips of elderly patients following internal fixation of fractures.[34] Ultrasound was applied to the anterior, lateral, and posterior hip joint at intensities of 1.0 to 2.5 W/cm^2 for 5 minutes per field. The other group received infrared heating for 30 minutes. Results of treatment were evaluated by range-of-motion measurements. Individuals receiving ultrasound improved in range of motion. Those receiving infrared showed less or no gain when compared with those receiving ultrasound. Information obtained from these studies can certainly be applied to the treatment of joint contracture in other areas of the body. Joints with a smaller amount of soft tissue coverage such as the elbow, wrist, or ankle are usually treated at intensities averaging 1.0 W/cm^2 or less.

Ice and ultrasound applications were compared for the treatment of painful "frozen shoulder."[35] Ultrasound therapy was administered to one group at an intensity of 0.5 W/cm^2 for 5 to 8 minutes, three times a week for a total of 15 treatments. Iced towels were applied to the other group for 15 minutes three times a week for a total of 12 treatments. Both groups were placed on a program of passive and active range-of-motion exercises following thermal agent application. All patients reported a decrease in pain and had an increased range of motion that was attributed to their treatment with no apparent differences between the groups. The intensity of ultrasound used for treatment, though, was less than that which has been demonstrated to elevate joint structure temperature at the knee,[5] a joint with approximately as much soft tissue coverage as the shoulder. This observation points out that unless a sufficient intensity is used, one should not expect any greater benefit from the use of ultrasound than with superficial heating or cooling.

Scar tissue is more dense than surrounding tissue and can be selectively heated by ultrasound energy prior to friction massage and range-of-motion exercises. Bierman[36] reported successfully increasing the range of motion in a small series of patients who had scar tissue secondary to lacerations, x-ray burns, and Dupuytren's contracture. Ultrasound was administered at intensities of 1.0 to 2.0 W/cm^2 for 6 to 8 minutes every other day. On the other hand, Wright and Haase[37] found that ultrasound at a lower intensity than used by Bierman was not effective in reducing the size of keloids. The low intensity used may have accounted for the unsuccessful treatment they reported.

Ultrasound has a definite role in the treatment of joint contractures and scar tissue. However, in order to be effective, exposures must be sufficient in intensity and duration.

Reduction of Pain and Muscle Spasm

Following ultrasound application, pain threshold is usually increased. Although the mechanism of pain reduction is not clear, the heat produced by ultrasound could result in counterirritation, heat activation of large-diameter fibers, or an altering of the response to stimulation of the pain receptors (free nerve endings). Pain threshold was elevated following ultrasound application to the arm at 1.5 W/cm^2 for 2 minutes.[20] Because similar changes were found with infrared and microwave diathermy applications (both surface and deep heating agents), the implicated mechanism of action is through the ability of all three agents to elevate the threshold for activation of the free nerve endings.

Ultrasound combined with exercise was compared with exercise alone by Munting[38] for patients with shoulder pain. The patients included in the study had no evidence of tendinitis, fracture, or degenerative joint changes. Over a 3-week period, ultrasound was applied for a total of 10 treatments each, at an intensity of 1.5 W/cm^2 for 3 to 5 minutes, to the anterior, inferior, and posterior aspects of the shoulder. The patients who received ultrasound reported a higher percentage of pain relief (81 percent) than those who received only exercise (44 percent). In addition, the gains in active and passive range of motion were greater in the ultrasound-treated groups. At 3-month followup, 73 percent of the patients who had received ultrasound reported no pain, compared with 55 percent of the "exercise-only" group.

Patients with hemiplegia who had painful shoulders were treated using three different regimens: (1) range-of-motion exercises, positioning, and ultrasound at 0.5 to 2.0 W/cm^2; (2) range-of-motion exercises, positioning, and sham ultrasound; or (3) range-of-motion exercises and positioning.[39] No statistically significant difference in range of motion was reported among the groups. The authors concluded that in this patient sample, ultrasound was probably not a useful adjunct to treatment with the dosages they administered.

Neuromas in amputation stumps can be sources of pain and can delay the rehabilitation process. Ultrasound has been used in the conservative management of neuromas. When Soren[40] applied ultrasound to patients' painful neuromas, at intensities averaging 1.5 W/cm^2, five of the six patients studied had decreased pain and improved function.

Ultrasound therapy is often included in the care of patients with low back dysfunction of various etiologies. Considering the extent of use, little had appeared in the literature to support or refute its efficacy in the management of this clinical condition. The technique that is generally employed is paravertebral application with or without sonation along the involved nerve trunk(s). There appears to be only three reports on such application, two from the 1950s and one from the 1980s. Kuiwert[41] described six patients with referred pain secondary to osteoarthritis of the spine, damage to vertebral bodies, and/or herniated intervertebral discs. Doses of 0.5 to 1.5 W/cm^2 were applied paravertebrally on a daily basis for 6 to 12 sessions, averaging 10 minutes per session. Five patients reported decreased pain and muscle spasm, and improved motion. One patient had no change. No other treatments were compared with ultrasound.

Two hundred and nine cases of low back pain secondary to herniated intervertebral disc syndrome were reported by Aldes and Grabin.[42] Symptoms were relieved in 86 percent of the patients when treated with a 12-session course of ultrasound at intensities ranging from 0.3 to 0.8 W/cm^2. Sonation was administered paravertebrally and along the gluteus maximus, hamstring, and gastrocnemius muscles in patients with radiculitis. Since hot packs and massage were also included in treatment regimens, the relief experienced by the patients may have been produced by these superficial heating agents rather than by the ultrasound. The ultrasound intensities used by the investigators were lower than those customarily used for an area with such a large amount of soft tissue.

Low back pain resulting from herniated intervertebral discs from L4 to S2 were treated by Nwuga[43] using three different protocols. All patients were seen within 2 weeks after onset of pain. The three groups designated received (1) analgesics and bed rest, (2) sham ultrasound and bed rest, and (3) ultrasound at 1.0 to 2.0 W/cm^2 for 10 minutes and bed rest. Ultrasound and sham ultrasound were given three times a week over a 4-week period. Straight leg raising (Lasèque test) and lumbar spinal flexion, extension, side-flexion, and rotation were measured. Subjective assessments of pain were made. The group treated with ultrasound obtained the best results, with the greatest improvement in flexion, extension, and straight leg raising and a reduction in pain.

Skeletal muscle temperature can be elevated by ultrasound. Temperature measurements of thighs were made, using implanted thermistors.[7] Ultrasound produced temperature elevations at the bone/muscle interface. The ability of ultrasound to elevate tissue temperature may partially explain the basis for the use of this agent in treating skeletal muscle spasm. Ultrasound did seem to reduce muscle spasms in patients with neck dysfunction and with muscle spasms of the lower extremity secondary to poliomyelitis.[44]

The mechanism of action for reduction of skeletal muscle spasm with ultrasound is not clear but may be due to thermal effects that alter the skeletal muscle contractile process directly, reduce muscle spindle activity, or reduce pain resulting in a break in the pain-spasm-pain cycle.

Ultrasound used alone was not as effective as ultrasound used in conjunction with occlusive splint therapy, acupuncture, and muscle-conditioning exercises in patients with temporomandibular joint (TMJ) dysfunction and associated muscle spasms. When administered for TMJ dysfunction, coupling was achieved through a small water-filled plastic bag. Intensities were kept below 0.6 W/cm^2.[45] Of interest is the suggestion that a higher intensity of ultrasound may have produced even more beneficial results.

Bursitis and Tendinitis

Another common use of ultrasound is with patients having bursitis and tendinitis. There is little statistically significant supportive documentation that demonstrates the efficacy of this modality for patients with these problems. Decreased pain, increased range of motion and decreased tenderness have been reported in patients receiving ultrasound therapy for subacromial bursitis.[46–48] Similar success was found in patients with bicipital tendinitis.[48] None of these reports, though, compared ultrasound with other forms of therapy.

In a recent study,[49] the combination of sham ultrasound and exercise was compared with real ultrasound and exercise in patients with subacromial bursitis of greater than 1 month's duration. Ultrasound was administered at an intensity averaging 1.0 to 2.0 W/cm^2 for 6 minutes, three times a week for 4 weeks. Intensity levels were determined by increasing power until the patient reported a dull aching or pricking sensation, then reducing the ultrasonic intensity by 10 percent. Therefore, intensity was determined individually for each case.[49a] All medications were held constant during the time of the study. No differences between the groups could be found in pain relief, range of motion of the shoulder, or overall condition. The authors concluded that ultrasound was probably not a useful adjunct in the conservative management of subacromial bursitis.

Although there is little scientific evidence to support the application of ultrasound for tendinitis and bursitis, its use is widespread. Perhaps the subjectively determined good effects that have been reported could be due to the temporary symptomatic relief of pain.

Calcium Deposits

Some clinicians have stated that ultrasound can be a valuable agent in assisting in the reabsorption of calcium deposits in soft tissue. Although case reports[50] have concluded that ultrasound facilitates calcium reabsorption, no controlled studies or follow-up studies using radiographic analysis have appeared in the literature. Therefore, statements that ultrasound exposure results in calcium reabsorption may be incorrect. Nevertheless, ultrasound may help relieve the inflammation around a calcium deposit, thus relieving a patient's pain and improving function.

Phonophoresis

Ultrasound energy has been used to drive anti-inflammatory drugs (cortisol, dexamethasone, salicylates) and local analgesics (lidocaine) through the skin to underlying tissue. The technique of delivering medication by ultrasound has been termed *phonophoresis*. The rationale for this technique is that it delivers the drug directly to the site where the effect is sought. Cortisol has been driven to depths of 5 to 6 cm subcutaneously into skeletal muscle and peripheral nerve following phonophoresis.[51] More lidocaine was extracted from rabbit tissue following ultrasound than when the lidocaine was applied topically and not followed by ultrasound.[52]

The implicated mechanism that allows the medication to be driven across the skin to underlying tissues could be due to the changes in tissue permeability following heating with ultrasound. Furthermore, the radiation pressure of the ultrasound beam could force the medication away from the transducer into the body. Diffusion rates could possibly be enhanced by acoustic streaming. Thus, the medication can follow the well-focused pattern of the ultrasound beam.

Ultrasound has also been used to enhance the effects of hydrocortisone injection.[53] Griffin and associates[54] studied the effects of ultrasound and a placebo cream versus those of ultrasound and hydrocortisone ointment on patients with osteoarthritis, periarticular arthritis, and rheumatoid arthritis. Sixty-eight percent of the group treated with hydrocortisone and ultrasound (at less than 1.5 W/cm^2 for 5 minutes, once a week) had improved range of motion and decreased pain. Of those treated with placebo cream and ultrasound at the same dosage, only 25 percent had marked improvement in the measured characteristics. All patients received other forms of therapy during the experimental period.

Moll[55] treated a series of trigger points comparing three groups treated with (1) a placebo solution and sham ultrasound, (2) a water-based solution and ultrasound, or (3) a decadron-lidocaine solution and ultrasound. The ultrasound dosage was less than 1.5 W/cm^2 for 5 minutes, twice a week for 3 weeks. While greatest improvement was found in those patients receiving the phonophoresis with decadron-lidocaine solution, the number of subjects in the study was too small to show a statistically significant difference.

More well-controlled studies on the efficacy of phonophoresis are warranted. This technique may provide the clinician with a means of administering medication locally in a relatively easy and painless fashion. Phonophoresis may be the method of choice in patients who are apprehensive about receiving injections with hypodermic needles.

Wound Healing

Low-intensity continuous wave or pulsed wave modes have been used in the treatment of acute and chronic wounds to enhance the reparative process.

During the first 24 to 48 hours following trauma, edema prevention or reduction is an important goal. Persistent edema can prolong the inflammatory process and increase pain, thereby reducing function. Using an animal model, Fyfe and Chahl[56] induced edema in abdominal tissue with an intracutaneous injection of silver nitrate. (The release of histamine and prostaglandins, and other chemical mediators of inflammation, can be induced by silver nitrate.) The animals treated for 2 to 4 minutes with pulsed ultrasound, 0.5 W/cm^2, at a 20 percent or 50 percent duty cycle at 0.79 MHz had less leakage from the capillaries into the interstitial space than did untreated animals. Determining the clinical effectiveness of this technique in humans during the acute phase following trauma would be beneficial.

Dyson and associates[57] reported that ultrasound facilitated a greater increase in growth of tissue in rabbit ears, compared with that in untreated control subjects following excision of a small amount of tissue. Ultrasound was initiated 2 weeks after the wound occurred and continued three times a week. The dosages found to be most effective were 0.25 and 0.5 W/cm^2 pulsed (20 percent duty cycle) and 0.1 W/cm^2 continuous wave at 3.5 MHz for 5 minutes. With higher intensities—4.0 to 8.0 W/cm^2 pulsed (25 percent duty cycle)—swelling resulted. Because tissue temperature increases were only 0.53°C to 1.35°C in the successfully treated wounds, the investigators suggested that acoustical streaming may have been part of the mechanism with facilitated repair. Streaming may in fact alter ion fluxes across membranes.

This work of Dyson and associates on tissue regeneration has served as an impetus for further studies on the use of ultrasound for fresh-wound healing. Roberts[58] applied ultrasound through a "window" in the casts of animals with surgically repaired tendons. The dosage given was 0.8 W/cm^2 pulsed for 5 minutes, 5 days a week for 6 weeks. The control animals with tendon repairs were treated only by cast immobilization for 6 weeks. In the casted-only group, tensile strength of the tendons (as measured by breaking strength) at 6 weeks was within the range of values reported by Lundborg and Rank[59] following tendon repair. In the ultrasound group, none of the tendons showed evidence of healing; the breaking strength was less than that of the casted-only group. Therefore, the use of ultrasound in the early period after tendon repair was considered to be detrimental to healing. The investigators stated that the intensity of ultrasound chosen for the experiment was similar to that which would be administered to the human hand.

These preliminary studies on wound healing suggest that the time in the course of healing at which ultrasound therapy is administered is important. When therapy is initiated during the early stages of wound healing, within the first week, repair may be hindered. On the other hand, if therapy at low intensities is initiated after 2 weeks, during the proliferative phase (fibroblastic infiltration and collagen formation) and early into the remodeling phase, ultrasound at low intensities may be beneficial. Further well-designed and well-controlled investigations are needed to determine the efficacy of ultrasound in facilitating wound repair.

Ultrasound has been employed in the treatment of chronic skin ulcers, especially when other methods of therapy have failed. Paul and associates[60] used dosages of 0.5 to 1.0 W/cm^2 three times a week in managing pressure sores in patients with spinal cord injuries. Thirteen of the 23 ulcers treated with ultrasound healed, five improved, and the remainder did not benefit from the treatment. Previous methods of treatment had failed.

In a later paper, Dyson and Suckling[61] reported on a series of patients with chronic varicose ulcerations. Sham ultrasound was compared with ultrasound at 1.0 W/cm^2, pulsed at a 20 percent duty cycle, for 5 to 10 minutes three times a week. The frequency of the ultrasound generator used was 3.0 MHz. At 28 days after the initiation of treatment, the average size of the ultrasound-treated ulcers was 66 percent smaller compared with a 10 percent reduction of size in the sham ultrasound group.

If ultrasound is chosen as an adjunct treatment in ulcer care, coupling can be direct or indirect in water, depending on the location of the ulcer. The ultrasound energy can be applied around the periphery of the ulcer for 5 minutes, or increased to 10 minutes in ulcers greater than 2.5 cm^2 in size. It is important to emphasize that other aspects of ulcer care should not be ignored. Prior to ultrasound application, the wound should be cleansed and debrided if necessary. Between ultrasound treatments, the wound should be kept as free of moisture as possible, and pressure should be kept off the area. All of these measures should aid in preventing further skin breakdown and facilitate healing.

Plantar Warts

Plantar warts (verruca plantaris) are skin lesions containing thrombosed capillaries in a soft whitish core covered by hyperkeratotic epithelial tissue.[62] They occur most often in children and young adults and are usually found on the weight-bearing areas of the feet. These often painful lesions are probably of viral origin, but traumatic and psychogenic etiologies have also been proposed. A multitude of treatments, including electrodesiccation and curettage, surgical excision, x-ray, and cryosurgery with liquid nitrogen or dry ice, have been performed to eradicate plantar warts. Ultrasound has also been employed in the management of these lesions by some clinicians during the past 25 years. The proponents of such treatment feel that ultrasound causes no discomfort during application, leaves the patient more comfortable between treatment sessions than other forms of treatment, and is less likely to result in scar formation.

Ultrasound at intensities averaging 0.6 W/cm^2, for 7 to 15 minutes, has most commonly been recommended for wart removal.[63] The suggested number of treatment sessions has ranged from 2 to 15. Both direct and indirect contact methods have been suggested.

The reported efficacy of treatment has varied. In a preliminary report, Kent[64] found 90 percent success as measured by pain relief and necrosis of the warts using ultrasound at 0.6 W/cm^2 for 15 minutes, for 1 to 11 treatment sessions. Similar results have been cited by Rowe[65] and Cherup and their associates.[66] In a series of 15 patients using ultrasound at 1.0 W/cm^2 for 15 minutes two times a week. Quade and Radzyminski[67] found complete remission of the plantar warts in three patients, almost complete remission in two patients, some remission in eight patients, and no improvement in two patients. This investigator felt the best results were in patients who had no previous treatment and had lesions of the shortest duration.

The direct versus indirect methods of coupling were compared by Vaughn.[68] With the direct technique at 0.69 W/cm^2 for 15 minutes, 83 percent success was found with an average of 7.8 treatment sessions. A lower percentage of success, 51 percent, was reported with the underwater coupling method at an intensity of 0.75 W/cm^2.

Only one double-blind study using ultrasound to treat plantar warts has been reported. Braatz and co-workers[69] compared sham ultrasound with actual ultrasound, at an intensity of 0.8 W/cm^2 for 12 minutes, with underwater coupling. No previous treatment had been given, and all patients had lesions of less than 6 months' duration. All lesions were soaked in tepid water and swabbed with hydrogen peroxide, and the calluses were shaved prior to actual or sham ultrasound treatments. Both groups demonstrated disappearance of the plantar warts, after an average of 9.7 weeks (85 percent of the patients) for the sham ultrasound–treated group and after 7.6 weeks (82 percent of the patients) for the ultrasound-treated group. Braatz concluded that ultrasound was probably of little benefit in the care of plantar warts.

None of the investigators reported an exacerbation of pain, an increase in size of the lesion or any other adverse reactions when ultrasound was given for the conservative management of plantar warts. Additional studies (for instance, those that use control subjects and those that compare ultrasound with other methods of care) are warranted, to demonstrate the role of ultrasound in the treatment of plantar warts.

GUIDELINES FOR CLINICAL ADMINISTRATION

The therapeutic aim with continuous wave ultrasound is to elevate the tissue temperature for a given duration at a specific anatomic location. The pulsed wave mode, or a continuous wave mode of very low intensity, can be chosen if the goal of treatment is to facilitate soft tissue healing and when a significant increase in tissue temperature is not desired (for example, in the case of stasis ulcers). The average intensity for a given power output machine-setting is less with the pulsed wave mode than with the continuous wave mode.

To achieve the therapeutic goal that has been delineated, certain protocols should be followed when applying ultrasound. The ultrasound generators for patient care should be properly calibrated and electrically safe (see Chapter 3). Even though the operation of all units is similar, the instructions provided by the manufacturer should be carefully reviewed prior to the use of a machine. The therapist should be present during treatment. Having patients administer their own ultrasound should be discouraged.

Coupling Techniques

Unlike electromagnetic energy, which can travel well through air, ultrasound energy is markedly attenuated in air and is totally reflected at air/tissue interfaces. Therefore, a coupling medium must be used to transmit ultrasound energy from the transducer to the irradiated surface. When the surface area being treated is larger than the applicator surface and is relatively regular or flat in contour, a direct method of coupling can be employed. With this technique, a thin layer of water-soluble gel or mineral oil is spread over the area to be treated, and the sound head is placed in contact with the gel. The objective of the coupling is to eliminate as much air as possible between the transducer and the skin and thereby to maximize the amount of sound entering the body.

The choice of a coupling agent for the direct contact technique is based on viscosity, ease of application, cost, and therapist preference. Substances that may irritate or be driven through the skin should be avoided. The viscosity of the gel should be high enough to prevent any "run-off" during treatment and low enough to permit ease of movement of the transducer across the skin surface. The gel or oil can feel very cold to the patient as it comes directly out of its storage container and, therefore, some therapists preheat the gel purely for patient comfort. However, over-zealous heating of the gel will decrease viscosity and often make the gel "runny." Lehmann and co-workers[70] have suggested that coupling agents such as mineral oil, when applied at a lower temperature (18°C to 20°C), will be more effective in transmitting ultrasound energy to deeper tissues without heating superficial tissues than they will be at a temperature of 24°C. However, the differences produced in deep tissue temperature elevation were found to be minimal. Therefore, in the interest of patient comfort, it may be best to preheat the gel.

Although a number of agents have been suggested in the past, commercially available gels for ultrasound therapy are usually more practical to use in a busy clinic. The salt found in gels used for electrocardiogram (ECG) or surface electromyogram (EMG) may damage the transducer face, so if these gels are used, they should be wiped from the transducer face very carefully using tap water, after the treatment is complete.

If there are bony prominences in the area (for example, over the lateral epicondyle of the humerus in a small-framed person) or if the surface is small and irregular in contour (for example, a distal extremity), other methods of coupling may be selected.

For treatment of the hand and wrist or foot and ankle areas, a basin can be filled with room-temperature water and the part can be immersed in the bath. Ideally, degassed water is the medium of choice, but its preparation and maintenance render it impractical for clinical use. Tap water is a reasonable alternative. If treatment is given in a metal basin or whirlpool, some of the ultrasound energy will be reflected off the metal, thus increasing intensity in certain areas near the metal. A plastic or rubber basin will not cause as much reflection. In addition, water in a whirlpool often has a large number of air bubbles, which tend to reduce the transmission of ultrasound. This situation can be particularly troublesome if the turbine has been used before the ultrasound is to be given.

Both mineral oil and glycerin have been tested as couplants for the immersion technique. The use of either can result in greater surface heating and an increase in couplant temperature, compared with a water medium.[71] When coupling is done with the immersion technique, the recommended medium for the bath is water.

When the immersion technique is employed, the transducer should be held 0.5 to 3.0 cm from the body surface area to be treated. Small air bubbles tend to accumulate on the face of the applicator and the skin surface when this method is utilized. However, the operator can wipe off the accumulated bubbles during exposure, as long as this is done quickly to prevent the therapist's being unduly exposed to the ultrasound energy.

Another alternative for the irradiation of an irregular surface has been suggested.[72] A rubber balloon or condom is filled with water and the entry closed. The sac is then placed between the skin surface and the transducer, with layers of coupling gel between the transducer and the balloon and the balloon and the skin surface. Another choice is to secure the open end of the water-filled balloon to the transducer and put a layer of coupling gel between the balloon and the skin surface.

Moving Versus Stationary Applicator

Two treatment methods have been used to deliver ultrasound energy to the tissue to be irradiated: (1) stationary applicator and (2) moving applicator.

Some clinicians have preferred to hold the transducer stationary over the area to be irradiated. This technique has usually been done when the treated area was very small (e.g., over a plantar wart) or when the intensity delivered was very low (less than 0.5 W/cm^2). Because of the nonuniformity of the sound beam, the distribution of energy to the tissue is uneven; therefore, some areas within the beam may receive a large amount of energy and other areas effectively none. This situation predisposes the patient to "hot spots" and potential tissue damage. Various effects due to a stationary sound beam have been noted in laboratory studies using animal models. In particular, stasis of blood flow,[28] venular endothelial damage, and platelet aggregation[29] have occurred at therapeutic intensities.

With the moving technique, the transducer is slowly moved over the underlying tissue approximately 4 cm/sec.[19] The purpose of the motion is to distribute the energy as evenly as possible throughout the tissue. Longitudinal stroking or overlapping circular movements can be used. The total area covered is usually two to three times the size of the irradiating crystal for every 5 minutes of exposure.[73] If a larger area is covered, the effective dosage delivered to any one region is decreased and the tissue temperature rise will be less. With the moving technique, the energy delivered to the target tissue should be evenly distributed, causing no hot spots within the sound field. For this reason, the moving technique is preferred over the stationary technique.

Exposure Factors

Although the dosage delivered to the patient cannot be precisely controlled or calculated, an estimate can be made and duplicated for subsequent treatments if the exposure factors are recorded. These factors include the power output of the ultrasound beam, the effective radiating area (ERA) of the crystal, the ultrasound frequency, and the duration of exposure. The surface area of the body that is irradiated should also be reported.

As mentioned earlier in this chapter, the intensity is recorded in watts per square centimeter, or W/cm^2 (power/effective radiating area of the crystal). With the continuous wave mode, the usual method of recording intensity is by the spatial average (the average power across the beam/ERA). With pulsed wave ultrasound, the duty cycle should also be included.

The intensity selected for ultrasound therapy is based upon the objective of the treatment and the amount of soft tissue being treated. When vigorous heating is desired, Lehmann and de Lateur recommend increasing the ultrasound power until the patient reports a dull, deep ache (indicating elevation of tissue temperature at the periosteum) and then reducing the power by 10 percent.[74] A mild sensation of warmth should be felt by the patient during the treatment. When using the continuous wave mode to elevate tissue temperature over an area such as the hip or low back (where there is a large quantity of soft tissue), intensities as high as 1.5 to 2.0 W/cm^2 are typically used. This intensity should be effective in increasing tissue temperature and should result in the desired physiologic response. For vigorous heating of the same areas, intensities as high as 3.0 to 4.0 W/cm^2 have been recommended;[74] however, many of the available generators are capable of a maximum acoustical output of only 2.5 to 3.0 W/cm^2, and many patients will find intensities as high as 3.0 to 4.0 W/cm^2 uncomfortable.

A lower intensity on the order of 0.5 to 1.0 W/cm^2 is employed over areas where there is less soft tissue coverage and where bone is closer to the skin surface (for example, over the wrist).

The higher intensities are usually chosen when the purpose of treatment is to elevate tissue temperature of periarticular structures during or preceding a slow, sustained stretch with limited range of motion. A lower intensity can be employed when the desired temperature rise is not as high, for pain reduction and relief of muscle-guarding spasms. The best guideline, though, for determining a maximal, tolerated intensity that will not produce a burn or other tissue damage is patient tolerance, or the patient's report of a feeling of deep warmth underlying the transducer. For that reason, when ultrasound is used for heating, it is important that the patient's pain and temperature sensations are intact. Furthermore, patients should be instructed not to "rough it." Should the patient report deep aching (periosteal pain), either the power can be reduced or a larger area can be covered.

Occasionally, a patient will report an increase in temperature of the transducer—a feeling of surface heating. This sensation can be indicative of inadequate coupling or of loosening of the crystal in its mounting. If coupling appears to be adequate, then the transducer should be tested by a qualified service technician.

The aforementioned intensities are appropriate for typical-sized transducers and would need to be modified if transducers with smaller or larger effective radiating areas were used. For example, suppose we wish to heat a 10 cm^2 tissue area using a transducer with an effective radiating area of 10 cm^2, and emitting ultrasound at an intensity of 1 W/cm^2. If the transducer is held stationary, the 10 cm^2 area of skin immediately beneath the transducer crystal would receive a total exposure of 10 W (1 W/cm^2 $\times$ 10 cm^2). In contrast, a transducer with a smaller effective radiating area—say 5 cm^2—emitting the same ultrasonic intensity would have to be applied with a moving technique in order to cover the 10 cm^2 area of skin. In this latter case, the total exposure would be 5 W (1 W/cm^2 $\times$ 5 cm^2). Consequently, heating of this area of skin would be reduced by a factor of two. Thus, in order to produce the same therapeutic effect, the intensity of the smaller transducer would have to be raised to 2 W/cm^2.

When pulsed wave ultrasound is applied, the spatial average intensity read from the meter will appear to be the same as in the continuous wave mode. But the time-averaged intensity will be less, because the energy is delivered in periodic bursts, with the power on for a fixed duration and then off for a fixed duration. The time the power is on is sometimes referred to as the "mark" and the time off as the "space." Thus a mark:space ratio can be reported. Both time on and time off are measured in milliseconds.

A more common way of providing the same information is by reporting the duty cycle. As defined previously, the duty cycle is the percentage of the time the power is on during one pulse period (time on + time off). Some generators are equipped with variable duty cycles. As duty cycle increases (for example, from 20 percent to 50 percent), the time-averaged intensity will increase. With a low duty cycle, there will be minimal if any detectable rise in tissue temperature. As duty cycle increases, a rise in tissue temperature can be expected.

If the desired response from the treatment is nonthermal, then a small duty cycle should be chosen. At present, not enough data have been provided by well-designed clinical studies to suggest a given duty cycle for a particular pathology. There is a need for more studies establishing the clinical indications and the efficacy of pulsed wave ultrasound.

Technique of Phonophoresis

When performing phonophoresis, coupling can be direct or indirect using water. The medication (such as hydrocortisone ointment) is rubbed directly onto the surface of the skin. Coupling gel is then spread over the medication, and sonation is initiated. With the indirect technique, the ointment is spread over the area to be sonated, then the part is placed in a water bath.

A 10 percent hydrocortisone ointment is preferred by some clinicians,[75] rather than a 1 percent ointment. Results obtained in treating humeral epicondylitis and subdeltoid bursitis were better with the 10 percent ointment than with the 1 percent ointment. The 10 percent hydrocortisone ointment should be prepared by a pharmacist.

When hydrocortisone is prepared pharmaceutically it may have air trapped in it; therefore, massaging the ointment into the skin may reduce air bubbles and improve transmissivity. In fact, it has been demonstrated in laboratory studies that the transmission of ultrasound energy through hydrocortisone ointments is less than through other coupling media.[76]

Patient Positioning and Field Selection

Because ultrasound energy can be well focused at a delineated target, careful patient positioning and determination of areas to be treated is often critically important in producing an effective treatment. The anatomic structures to be treated and the treatment goal should be well delineated by careful evaluation. The site of soft tissue involvement, whether muscle, joint capsule, tendon, or bursa, should be determined. Depending on the particular pathology, the position of the patient can vary for each joint or body surface area affected.

As a representative example, dysfunction about the shoulder will be discussed. Three different examples of shoulder dysfunctions include (1) capsular shortening/contracture, (2) supraspinatus tendinitis, and (3) muscle-guarding spasm and pain secondary to degenerative joint disease. In the

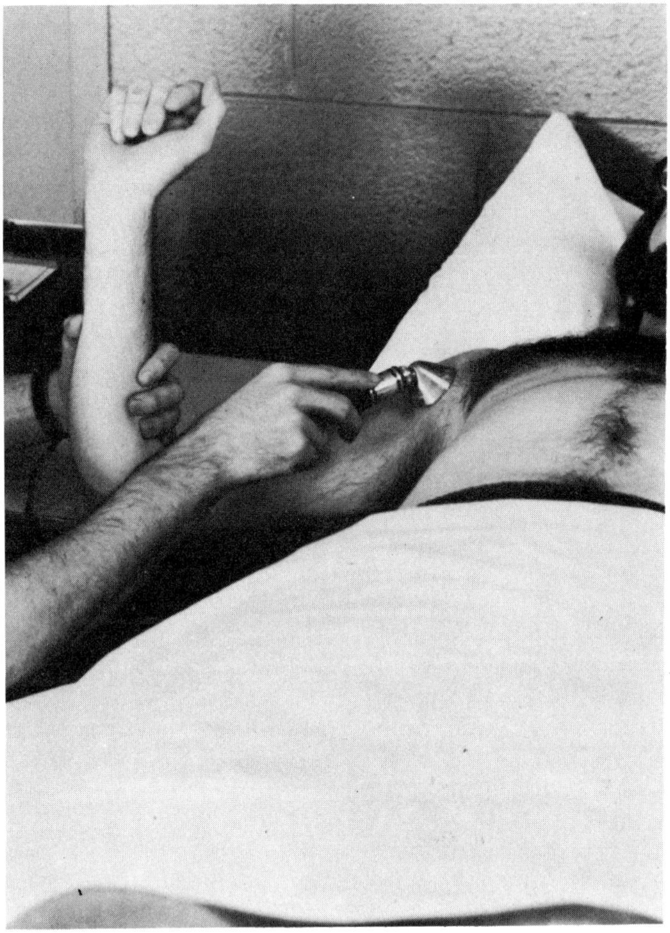

FIGURE 7–9
Ultrasound being applied to a patient with adhesive capsulitis of the shoulder. Note the position of the arm in abduction.

first case, the area of the joint capsule around the glenohumeral joint, which is not likely to shorten or develop tightness, is the anterior-inferior aspect. The resulting limitations in motion affect predominantly abduction and external rotation. To facilitate an increase in range of motion, while elevating joint capsular temperature with ultrasound, the therapist can externally rotate and abduct the patient's shoulder and simultaneously apply ultrasound over the anterior and inferior axillary areas (Fig. 7–9).

If the intention is to elevate temperature at the site of the insertion of the supraspinatus, as in the second example, the position of choice for ultrasound application would be with the arm adducted and internally rotated. This position is chosen in order to expose the supraspinatus tendon from under the acromion process (Fig. 7–10).

In the third case, the patient with muscle spasm is in pain and is therefore guarding motion. The position of choice would be that in which the patient is comfortable and as relaxed as possible.

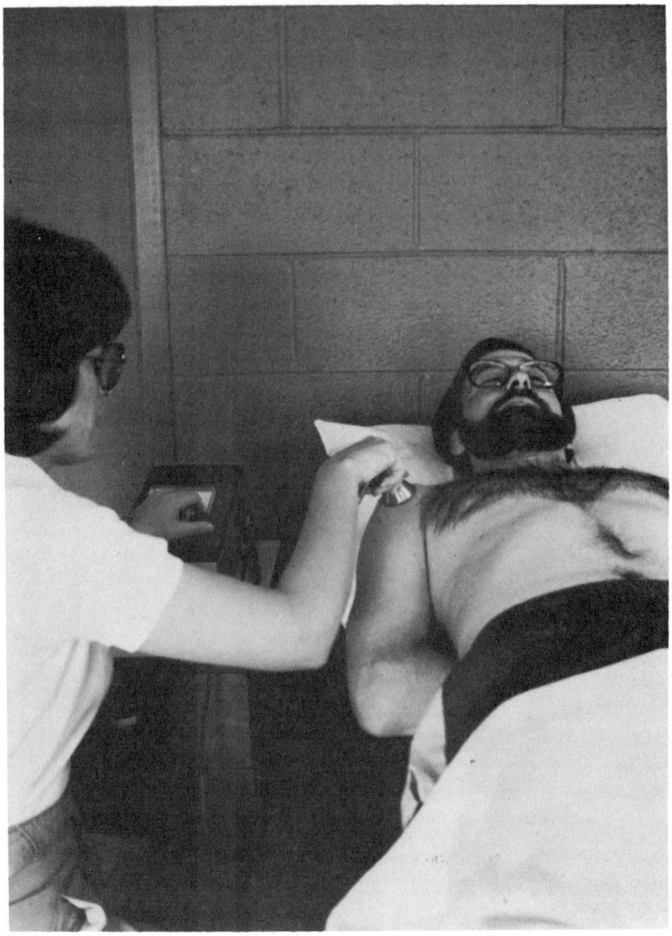

FIGURE 7–10
Ultrasound being applied to a patient with supraspinatus tendinitis. Note the position of the arm in adduction and internal rotation.

In all of these examples, the patients have shoulder dysfunction, but in each case a different anatomic site has been delineated as being problematic. Therefore, ultrasound can be well focused over an area to achieve a particular therapeutic goal if anatomic relationships are appreciated.

TREATMENT PRECAUTIONS

Therapeutic ultrasound should not be applied over the eye. The blood supply to the lens is poor, so that heat applied to that area is not dissipated adequately. Temperature elevations can result in cataract production.[77] Most of the sound entering the eye will reach the retina, because the aqueous humor and the vitreous humor minimally attenuate the ultrasound energy. Local destruction of areas of the retina can result.

Irradiation over the heart should be avoided. In preliminary laboratory experimentation, one of this chapter's authors (MZ) found ECG changes (S-T segment elevation) in dogs following direct exposure at 2.5 W/cm^2 to the heart. At all costs, cardiac pacemakers should be protected from direct ultrasound exposure because of the possibility of the sound's interference with the electrical circuitry of the pacemaker.

One should not apply therapeutic ultrasound over the pregnant uterus. The fetus should not be exposed to the therapeutic ultrasound beam, because temperature elevation of the fetus has been shown to cause abnormalities such as low birth weight, brain size reduction, and various orthopedic deformities in experimental animals.[78] Unless reassured by the patient that she is not pregnant, it is probably prudent to avoid exposing a woman over the abdominal region or low back during the reproductive years except during the first 10 days following onset of menses.[79]

Ultrasound should not be applied over the testes. Prolonged temperature elevation in this area can produce temporary sterility.

Except in the special case of treatment for cancer (hyperthermia), ultrasonic irradiation to malignant tissue should be avoided. Research done under in vitro conditions has suggested that this may increase cellular detachment and the possibility of metastasis.[80,81]

A major safeguard for patients undergoing therapeutic ultrasound is their ability to perceive accurately any changes in pain and temperature. For this reason, the therapist must be very cautious when applying ultrasound over areas of impaired pain and/or temperature sensation. This concern is particularly pertinent in areas where sensory nerves may have been severed immediately following surgery (for instance, on the extremities or spine).

Caution should be used in applying ultrasound over areas with reduced circulation, because of possible excessive temperature elevation. Owing to the reduced circulation, the heat generated cannot be adequately dissipated. Ultrasound should not be administered over areas of thrombophlebitis, because the possibility of clotting or of dislodging a thrombus could be increased.

Epiphyseal areas (growth areas of bone) in children should be exposed to ultrasound only minimally. Literature in the field suggests that intensities used therapeutically would be safe.[82] But at intensities above 3.0 W/cm^2 there is some evidence of demineralization of bone, damage to epiphyseal plates, and retardation of bone growth when using a stationary transducer for periods of 3 minutes or greater.[83–85]

There are no reasons to avoid ultrasound application over fracture sites. In fact, recent animal studies by Dyson and Brookes[86] have demonstrated that pulsed ultrasound may accelerate fracture healing. Certainly, this subject warrants further investigation.

CLINICAL DECISION MAKING

After treatment goals and plans have been established, if a heating agent is desired, the choice of which one to use can depend on a number of factors.

These factors include (1) stage of inflammation and repair, (2) site of pathology (including depth and anatomic location), (3) total amount of tissue to be heated, and (4) presence or absence of orthopedic metal implants.

During the subacute stages of healing, a mild heat would be the logical choice. Surface heating agents, such as hot packs or infrared, may provide the desired response. If the site of pathology is in deep-seated structures, such as the hip joint, then low-intensity ultrasound at less than 1.0 W/cm^2 may be best. With a chronic condition in which pain and limited range of motion are the key problems, a deep heat–like ultrasound treatment at a higher intensity may be used.

The site of pathology is also important. If the goal of application is to deliver a deep heat to a well-defined area, then ultrasound should be the therapeutic agent of choice. For example, a knee flexion contracture secondary to capsular tightness may respond best to ultrasound followed by a slow, gentle stretch. If a larger area with a large muscle mass is to be heated, then the agent chosen should be shortwave diathermy. For example, limited motion and pain secondary to chronic hamstring strain may be best heat-treated by an agent that can apply heat to the entire muscle belly in the most efficient manner. Of course, ultrasound is capable of elevating hamstring temperature, but only a small area at a time can be heated using ultrasound.

Many patients seen for rehabilitation have surgical metal implants either for stabilization of fractures or replacement of damaged joint surfaces. In these cases, ultrasound can be safely employed over the area of the metal implant using the moving technique.[87,88] Shortwave and microwave diathermy, however, may not be given over areas of metal implants. Many of

TABLE 7–2
Clinical decision making: Ultrasound vs diathermy for deep heating

Case Problem	Decision	Rationale
70-year-old female, 2 months post–open reduction and internal fixation of intertrochanteric hip fracture with a nail and plate; now has pain on hip flexion and abduction; muscle-guarding spasms contribute to decreased ROM	Continuous ultrasound	Pain reduction; able to increase temperature of joint structures and overlying muscle; can focus energy to target areas; can apply over metal implant
45-year-old bricklayer 1 month post–lumbar injury; L5–S1 herniated intervertebral disk with paravertebral muscle-guarding spasms	Shortwave diathermy with induction drum	Capable of increasing temperature of paravertebral musculature; can cover a relatively large area

Case examples are provided with supporting rationale for treatment with the chosen deep heat agent. (Readers should cover the authors' decision and rationale while formulating their own, then uncover and compare with their own decision.)

the implants used for prosthetic joint replacements have high-density polyethylene components and are fixed in place by methylmethacrolate cement. If the moving technique is employed, ultrasound can be applied over these joints.[89]

Often ultrasound is used in conjunction with other physical agents, such as hot packs, cold packs, and electrical stimulation. Hot packs may provide additional pain relief and encourage relaxation of the patient. Cold packs should not be given prior to ultrasound, because cold alters the patients' perception of pain and temperature, which thereby limits their ability to tell the therapist if the ultrasound intensity is too high.

Ultrasound and electrical stimulation have been used in combination, to treat trigger points and muscle spasm. The authors are not aware of any physiologic rationale for using the two in combination or of any controlled clinical studies that have addressed this issue.

Clinical decision-making examples are provided in Table 7–2.

SUMMARY

Ultrasound, high-frequency acoustical energy, can be employed in a physical rehabilitation program to increase tissue temperature to depths of up to 5 cm. The physiologic effects of ultrasound, including increasing collagen tissue extensibility, decreasing pain and muscle spasm, and facilitating tissue healing, serve as the rationale for its use as a therapeutic agent. In order to maximize effectiveness and appropriateness of treatment with ultrasound, the therapist should be knowledgeable about the physics, biophysical effects, and possibly adverse consequences of ultrasonic energy at therapeutic intensities.

REFERENCES

1. Wood, RW and Loomis, AL: *The physical and biological effects of high frequency waves of great intensity.* Philosoph Mag 4:417, 1927.
2. Buchtala, V: *The present state of ultrasonic therapy.* Br J Phys Med 15:3, 1952.
3. Kuitert, JH and Harr, ET: *Introduction to clinical application of ultrasound.* Phys Ther Rev 35:19, 1955.
4. Wells, PNT: *Biomedical Ultrasonics.* Academic Press, London, 1977.
5. Lehmann, JF, et al: *Heating of joint structures by ultrasound.* Arch Phys Med Rehabil 49:28, 1968.
6. Lehmann, JF, et al: *Heating produced by ultrasound in bone and soft tissue.* Arch Phys Med Rehabil 48:397, 1967.
7. Lehmann, JF, et al: *Therapeutic temperature distribution produced by ultrasound as modified by dosage and volume of tissue exposed.* Arch Phys Med Rehabil 48:662, 1967.
8. Gersten, JW: *Effect of ultrasound on tendon extensibility.* Am J Phys Med 34:662, 1955.
9. Lehmann, JF, et al: *Effect of therapeutic temperatures on tendon extensibility.* Arch Phys Med Rehabil 51:481, 1970.
10. Warren, CG, Lehmann, JF, and Koblanski, JN: *Heat and stretch procedures: An evaluation using rat tail tendon.* Arch Phys Med Rehabil 57:122, 1976.
11. Paul, ED and Imig, CJ: *Temperature and blood flow studies after ultrasonic irradiation.* Am J Phys Med 34:370, 1955.

12. Abramson, DI, et al: *Changes in blood flow, oxygen uptake and tissue temperatures produced by therapeutic physical agents. I. Effect of ultrasound.* Am J Phys Med 39:51, 1960.
13. Bickford, RH and Duff, RS: *Influence of ultrasonic irradiation on temperature and blood flow in human skeletal muscle.* Circ Res 1:534, 1953.
14. Wyper, DJ, McNiven, DR, and Donnelly, TJ: *Therapeutic ultrasound and muscle blood flow.* Physiotherapy 64:321, 1978.
15. Paaske, WP, Hovind, H, and Seyerson, P: *Influence of therapeutic ultrasonic irradiation on blood flow in human cutaneous, subcutaneous and muscular tissues.* Scand J Clin Lab Invest 31:389, 1973.
16. Currier, DP, Greathouse, D, and Swift, T: *Sensory nerve conduction: effect of ultrasound.* Arch Phys Med Rehabil 59:181, 1978.
17. Currier, DP and Kramer, JF: *Sensory nerve conduction: heating effects of ultrasound and infrared.* Physiotherapy Canada 34:241, 1982.
18. Halle, JS, Scoville, CR, Greathouse, DG: *Ultrasound's effect on the conduction latency of superficial radial nerve in man.* Phys Ther 61:345, 1981.
19. Kramer, JF: *Ultrasound: Evaluation of its mechanical and thermal effects.* Arch Phys Med Rehabil 65:223, 1984.
20. Lehmann, JF, Brunner, GD, and Stow, RW: *Pain threshold measurements after therapeutic application of ultrasound, microwaves and infrared.* Arch Phys Med Rehabil 39:560, 1958.
21. Lehmann, JF and Guy, AW: *Ultrasound therapy.* In Reid, J and Sikov, MR (eds): *Interaction of Ultrasound and Biological Tissues.* DHEW Pub (FDA) 73-8008, Session 3:8, 141–152, 1971.
22. Lehmann, JF and Herrick, JF: *Biologic reactions to cavitation, a consideration for ultrasonic therapy.* Arch Phys Med Rehabil 34:86, 1953.
23. Lota, MJ and Darling, RC: *Change in permeability of the red blood cell membrane in a homogeneous ultrasonic field.* Arch Phys Med Rehabil 36:282, 1955.
24. Harvey, W, et al: *The stimulation of protein synthesis in human fibroblasts by therapeutic ultrasound.* Rheumatol Rehabil 14:237, 1975.
25. Dyson, M and ter Haar, GR: *The response of smooth muscle to ultrasound* (abstr). In Proceedings from an International Symposium on Therapeutic Ultrasound, Winnipeg, Manitoba (Canada), September 10–12, 1981.
26. Lehmann, JF and Biegler, R: *Changes of potentials and temperature gradients in membranes caused by ultrasound.* Arch Phys Med Rehabil 35:287, 1954.
27. Michlovitz, SL, Lynch, PR, and Tuma, RF: *Therapeutic ultrasound: Its effects on vascular permeability* (abstr). Fed Proc 41:1761, 1982.
28. Dyson, M, et al: *The production of blood cell stasis and endothelial damage in the blood vessels of chick embryos treated with ultrasound in a stationary wave field.* Ultrasound Med Biol 11:133, 1974.
29. Zarod, AP and Williams, AR: *Platelet aggregation in vivo by therapeutic ultrasound.* Lancet 1:1266, 1977.
30. Hogan, RD, Burke, KM, and Franklin, TD: *The effect of ultrasound on microvascular hemodynamics in skeletal muscle: Effects during ischemic.* Microvasc Res 23:370, 1982.
31. Hogan, RD, et al: *The effect of ultrasound on microvascular hemodynamics in skeletal muscle: Effect on arterioles.* Ultrasound Med Biol 8:45, 1982.
32. LaBan, MM: *Collagen tissue: Implications of its response to stress in vitro.* Arch Phys Med Rehabil 43:461, 1962.
33. Lehmann, JF, et al: *Comparative study of the efficiency of shortwave, microwave and ultrasonic diathermy in heating the hip joint.* Arch Phys Med Rehabil 40:510, 1959.
34. Lehmann, JF, et al: *Clinical evaluation of a new approach in the treatment of contracture associated with hip fracture after internal fixation.* Arch Phys Med Rehabil 42:95, 1961.
35. Hamer, J and Kirk, JA: *Physiotherapy and the frozen shoulder: A comparative trial of ice and ultrasonic therapy.* NZ Med J 83:191, 1972.
36. Bierman, W: *Ultrasound in the treatment of scars.* Arch Phys Med Rehabil 35:209, 1954.
37. Wright, ET and Haase, KH: *Keloids and ultrasound.* Arch Phys Med Rehabil 52:280, 1971.
38. Munting, E: *Ultrasonic therapy for painful shoulders.* Physiotherapy 64:180, 1978.
39. Inaba, MK and Piorkowski, M: *Ultrasound in treatment of painful shoulders in patients with hemiplegia.* Phys Ther 52:737, 1972.

40. Soren, A: *Nature and biophysical effects of ultrasound.* Journal of Occupational Medicine 7:375, 1965.
41. Kuiwert, JH: *Ultrasonic energy as an adjunct in the management of radiculitis and similar referred pain.* Am J Phys Med 33:61, 1954.
42. Aldes, JH and Grabin, S: *Ultrasound in the treatment of intervertebral disc syndrome.* Am J Phys Med 37:199, 1958.
43. Nwuga, VCB: *Ultrasound in treatment of back pain resulting from prolapsed intervertebral disc.* Arch Phys Med Rehabil 64:88, 1983.
44. Fountain, FP, Gersten, JW, and Sengu, O: *Decrease in muscle spasm produced by ultrasound, hot packs and IR.* Arch Phys Med Rehabil 41:293, 1960.
45. Grieder, A, et al: *An evaluation of ultrasonic therapy for temperomandibular joint dysfunction.* Oral Surg 31:25, 1971.
46. Bearzy, HJ: *Clinical applications of ultrasonic energy in the treatment of acute and chronic subacromial bursitis.* Arch Phys Med Rehabil 34;228, 1953.
47. Bundt, FB: *Ultrasound therapy in supraspinatus bursitis.* Phys Ther Rev 38:826, 1958.
48. Echternach, JL: *Ultrasound: An adjunct treatment for shoulder disability.* Phys Ther 45:865, 1965.
49. Downing, D and Weinstein, A: *Ultrasound therapy of subacromial bursitis* (abstr). Arthritis Rheum 26 (Suppl):587, 1983.
49a. Downing, D: Personal communication, 1983.
50. Cline, PD: *Radiographic follow-up of ultrasound therapy in calcific bursitis.* Phys Ther 43:16, 1963.
51. Griffin, JE, Touchstone, JC, and Liu, A: *Ultrasonic movement of cortisol into pig tissue. II. Peripheral nerve.* Am J Phys Med 44:20, 1965.
52. Novak, EJ: *Experimental transmission of lidocaine through intact skin by ultrasound.* Arch Phys Med Rehabil 45:231, 1964.
53. Newman, MK, Kill, M, and Frampton, G: *Effects of ultrasound alone and combined with hydrocortisone injections by needle or hydrospray.* Am J Phys Med 37:206, 1958.
54. Griffin, JE, et al: *Patients treated with ultrasonic driven cortisone and with ultrasound alone.* Phys Ther 47:594, 1967.
55. Moll, MJ: *A new approach to pain: Lidocaine and decadron with ultrasound.* USAF Medical Service Digest, May-June, 8, 1977.
56. Fyfe, MC and Chahl, LA: *The effect of ultrasound on experimental oedema in rats.* Ultrasound Med Biol 6:107, 1980.
57. Dyson, M, et al: *The stimulation of tissue regeneration by means of ultrasound.* Clin Sci 35:273, 1968.
58. Roberts, M, Rutherford, JH, and Harris, D: *The effect of ultrasound on flexor tendon repairs in the rabbit.* Hand 14:17, 1982.
59. Lundborg, G and Rank, F: *Experimental intrinsic healing of flexor tendons based upon synovial fluid nutrition.* J Hand Surg 3:21, 1978.
60. Paul, BJ, et al: *Use of ultrasound in the treatment of pressure sores in patients with spinal cord injury.* Arch Phys Med Rehabil 41:438, 1960
61. Dyson, M and Suckling, J: *Stimulation of tissue repair by ultrasound: A survey of mechanisms involved.* Physiotherapy 64:105, 1978.
62. Isselbacher, KJ: *Harrison's Principles of Internal Medicine,* ed 9. McGraw-Hill, New York, 1980.
63. Delacerda, FG: *Ultrasonic techniques for treatment of plantar warts in athletes.* Journal of Orthopedics and Sports Physical Therapy 1:100, 1979.
64. Kent, H: *Plantar wart treatment with ultrasound.* Arch Phys Med Rehabil 40:15, 1959.
65. Rowe, RJ and Gray, JM: *Ultrasound treatment of plantar warts.* Arch Phys Med Rehabil 46:273, 1965.
66. Cherup, N, Urben, J, and Bender, LF: *The treatment of plantar warts with ultrasound.* Arch Phys Med Rehabil 44:602, 1963.
67. Quade, AG and Radzyminski, SF: *Ultrasound in verruca plantaris.* J Am Podiatry Assoc 56:503, 1966.
68. Vaughn, DT: *Direct method versus underwater method in treatment of plantar warts with ultrasound.* Phys Ther 53:396, 1973.

69. Braatz, JH, McAlistar, BF, and Broaddus, MD: *Ultrasound and plantar warts: A double blind study.* Milit Med 139:199, 1974.

70. Lehmann, JF, de Lateur, BJ, and Silverman, DR: *Selective heating effects of ultrasound in human beings.* Arch Phys Med Rehabil 46:331, 1966.

71. Griffin, JE: *Transmissiveness of ultrasound through tap water, glycerin, and mineral oil.* Phys Ther 60:1010, 1980.

72. Summer, W and Patrick, MK: *Ultrasonic Therapy.* American Elsevier, New York, 1964.

73. Reid, DC and Cummings, GE: *Factors in selecting the dosage of ultrasound with particular reference to the use of various coupling agents.* Physiotherapy Canada 63:255, 1973.

74. Lehmann, JF and de Lateur, BJ: *Therapeutic heat.* In Lehmann, JF (ed): *Therapeutic Heat and Cold,* ed 3. Williams & Wilkins, Baltimore, 1982.

75. Kleinkort, JA and Wood, F: *Phonophoresis with 1 percent versus 10 percent hydrocortisone.* Phys Ther 55:1320, 1975.

76. Warren, CG, Koblanski, JN, and Sigelmann, RA: *Ultrasound coupling media: Their relative transmissivity.* Arch Phys Med Rehabil 57:218, 1976.

77. Sokoliu, A: *Destructive effect of ultrasound on ocular tissues.* In Reid, JM and Sikov, MR: *Interaction of Ultrasound and Biological Tissues.* DHEW Pub (FDA) 73-8008, 1972.

78. Edwards, MJ: *Congenital defects in guinea pigs: Prenatal retardation of brain growth of guinea pigs following hyperthermia during gestation.* Teratology 2:329, 1969.

79. NCRP Report No 74: *Effects of Ultrasound: Mechanisms and Clinical Implications.* National Council on Radiation Protection and Measurements, Bethesda, MD, 1983, p 197.

80. Conger, AD, Ziskin, MC, and Wittels, H: *Ultrasonic effects on mammalian multicellular tumor spheroids.* J Clin Ultrasound 9:167, 1981.

81. Siegel, E, et al: *Cellular attachment as a sensitive indicator of the effects of diagnostic ultrasound exposure on cultured human cells.* Radiology 133:175, 1979.

82. Vaughen, JL and Bender, LF: *Effects of ultrasound on growing bone.* Arch Phys Med Rehabil 40:158, 1959.

83. Bender, LF, Janes, JM, and Herrick, JF: *Histologic studies following exposure of bone to ultrasound.* Arch Phys Med Rehabil 35:555, 1954.

84. Cerino, LE, Ackerman, E, and Janes, JM: *Effects of ultrasound on experimental bone tumor.* Surg Forum 16:466, 1965.

85. DeForest, RE, Herrick, JF, and Janes, JM: *Effects of ultrasound on growing bone: An experimental study.* Arch Phys Med Rehabil 34:21, 1953.

86. Dyson, M and Brookes, M: *Stimulation of bone repair by ultrasound* (abstr). Ultrasound Med Biol 8 (Suppl 50):50, 1982.

87. Gersten, JW: *Effect of metallic objects on temperature rises produced in tissues by ultrasound.* Am J Phys Med 37:75, 1958.

88. Lehmann, JF, et al: *Ultrasonic effects as demonstrated in live pigs with surgical metallic implants.* Arch Phys Med Rehabil 40:483, 1959.

89. Lehmann, JF, et al: *Ultrasound: Considerations for use in the presence of prosthetic joints.* Arch Phys Med Rehabil 61:502, 1980.

CHAPTER 8

SHORTWAVE AND MICROWAVE DIATHERMY

LUTHER KLOTH, P.T., M.S.

In contrast to ultrasound, which introduces mechanical energy into the tissues, the application of diathermy involves transmission and absorption of electromagnetic (EM) energy by the body, with subsequent conversion of the non-ionizing radiation into therapeutic heat by the resisting tissues.

In the late 1800s, d'Arsonval[1,2] reported that alternating current (AC) at a frequency greater than 10 kHz produced perceptible warming of the skin without evoking the muscular contractions that occurred when lower frequencies were used. Since the early 1900s, methods of generating higher-frequency, shorter-wavelength currents have been developed with sufficient power to enable the energy to be absorbed by subcutaneous and deep tissues.

Shortwave diathermy (SWD) uses high-frequency alternating currents that oscillate at specified frequencies between 10 and 50 MHz. SWD is most commonly used for thermotherapy at a frequency of 27.12 MHz. Microwave diathermy (MWD), another form of EM radiation, has qualities that allow it to be beamed or directed toward the body and reflected from the skin, owing to its ultra-high frequency (UHF) and spectral proximity to radiant energy. The frequency most commonly used with therapeutic microwave is 2450 MHz.

Clinical application of diathermy was introduced in Germany in the late 1920s. Therapeutic applications of microwave heating began in the United States in the late 1940s. The utilization of diathermy in medicine can be categorized into three groups: (1) functional restoration and analgesia, (2) facilitation of healing of recently injured soft tissue, and (3) hyperthermia for tumor eradication. Clinical effectiveness in therapeutic applications of diathermy is dependent upon the intensity and time of exposure and ultimately on the extent of tissue temperature elevation.

The objectives of this chapter are to (1) provide a basic understanding of the physical principles and effects of diathermy, (2) discuss the clinical methods for applying diathermy, (3) discuss the clinical conditions for which diathermy is effective, and (4) discuss potential hazards related to the use of diathermy.

PHYSICAL PRINCIPLES

Electromagnetic (EM) Radiation

As discussed in Chapter 3, EM radiation is emitted in wave form from the natural source of the sun and from artificial sources, such as heated objects and electronic oscillators that generate high-frequency alternating currents. The energy available from EM waves exists in separate packets called photons. The quantum energy from the diathermies is not great enough to break chemical bonds by knocking electrons off atoms or molecules when absorbed. The diathermies are forms of non-ionizing EM radiation. Thus, quanta of EM radiation from shortwave and microwave diathermy are restricted to thermal and nonthermal effects on tissues causing atoms and dipole molecules (especially water) to vibrate and rotate, rather than directly breaking chemical bonds. When heat gain produced by shortwave or microwave diathermy is greater than heat loss and the tissue temperature rise is greater than the therapeutically desirable range of 40°C to 45°C, deleterious changes in tissue may occur from a thermal overload.

The frequencies used for shortwave and microwave diathermy are not capable of depolarizing motor nerves or eliciting a contractile response from innervated or denervated skeletal muscle. Excitation of these tissues resulting in depolarization does not occur with diathermy because the wavelength (duration) of the high-frequency alternating current is not sufficiently long to cause mobilization or migration of ions through cellular membranes of nerve or muscle.

It is evident that shortwave and microwave diathermy are forms of EM radiation that are physically distinguishable from other types of EM radiation only by the fact that their frequencies are different. However, only when the radio frequency portion of the total spectrum of EM waves is considered can the terms "shortwave" and "microwave" be placed into perspective (see Fig. 3–2). Then it becomes obvious that the wavelengths of frequencies used for shortwave diathermy are indeed shorter than those used in standard (AM) radio broadcasting and that microwaves are even shorter than the wavelengths employed in FM radio, television, and shortwave diathermy. Therefore, the terms "shortwave" and "microwave" only correctly denote the relative shortness of these waves when compared with the lengths of other waves of lower frequency in the radio frequency portion of the EM spectrum.

FEDERAL COMMUNICATIONS COMMISSION (FCC) REGULATIONS FOR CLINICAL DIATHERMY. Therapeutic diathermy generators are essentially weak radio transmitters with a patient applicator/electrode that functions as a broadcast antenna. The EM energy delivered to the patient from diathermy equipment is within the wavelength and frequency ranges spec-

TABLE 8–1
Shortwave and Microwave Diathermy Frequencies (FCC approved)

Frequency	Wavelength	Type of Diathermy
13.56	22 m	SWD
27.12*	11 m	SWD
40.68	7.5 m	SWD
915.00	33 cm	MWD
2450.00*	12 cm	MWD

* Most widely used frequency.

ified by the FCC for commercial and military radio and television broadcasts. Frequencies must be closely controlled to prevent the transmitted energy from interfering with the reception and operation of nearby electrically powered nonmedical devices, such as AM/FM radios, television, and police and military radio communications. The FCC is responsible for assigning industrial, scientific, and medical frequencies and for monitoring the air space to ensure that stray energy does not interfere with communications.

In the late 1940s, the FCC designated specific operating frequencies for short- and microwave diathermy (Table 8–1). At present, an additional microwave frequency of 915 MHz (wavelength 33 cm) is permitted, because studies[3–5] have shown that greater depth of penetration and absorption as well as increased blood flow occur with the lower frequency. The microwave frequency of 433.9 MHz (wavelength 69 cm) is currently under investigation for application in oncology using hyperthermia.

TYPE OF WAVES. All EM waves are classified as transverse waves because the wave displacement is perpendicular or transverse to the direction of propagation. These waves consist of two components—a transverse sinusoidal electric (E) field and a transverse magnetic (B) field. The first step in generating these two fields in a shortwave diathermy device is the application of an alternating voltage to the primary windings of a power transformer.

The voltage induced across the secondary coil of the transformer is used to place an electric charge on the transmitting antenna (diathermy applicator/electrode). Since the charging potential applied to the transformer of the shortwave generator alternates at a high frequency (for example, 27.12 million times per second), the charge on the applicator constantly reverses polarity at that frequency. Clearly, if the polarity of the applicator constantly reverses, then charge must flow up and down the applicator wire. This oscillating flow of charge constitutes a current, which creates an electric field that constantly reverses direction in the air space surrounding the applicator. Simultaneously, the changing electric field creates a changing magnetic field about the applicator. The magnetic field is propagated through air space in phase with the electric field but is perpendicular to it (Fig. 8–1). This combined electric and magnetic field is a wireless, electromagnetic radio frequency wave that originates in the accelerated motion of

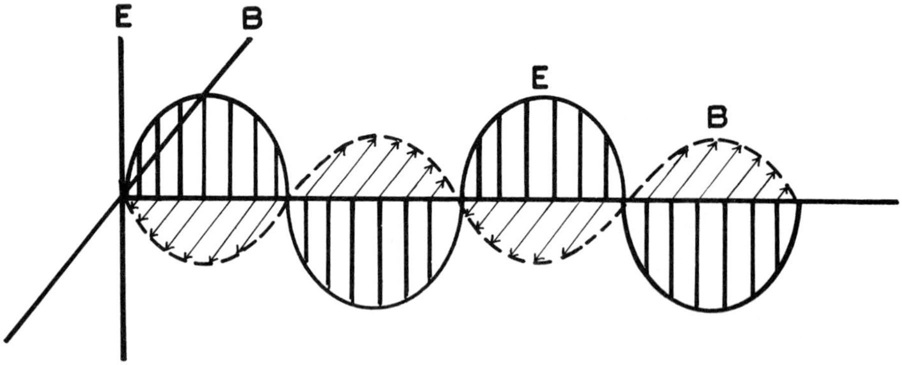

FIGURE 8–1

The changing electric field (E) creates a changing magnetic field (B) that is propagated through space in phase but perpendicular to it. (Adapted from Bueche,[6] p 446.)

charges and travels away from the source through space at 3 x 10^8 m/sec (the speed of light in a vacuum).

Most shortwave diathermy devices deliver their high-frequency EM energy as a continuous wave in which the amplitude and frequency remain constant. Pulsed shortwave is produced by some devices that deliver interrupted trains of high-frequency, constant-amplitude waves.

Microwaves are transmitted at much higher frequencies than shortwaves, and, because they occupy the region of the EM spectrum between radio waves and infrared, they possess optical qualities resembling radiant energy. This means that they are more easily reflected and refracted than shortwaves. In contrast to shortwave diathermy, the frequencies and wavelengths of microwave diathermy are such that the electric field predominates and not much magnetic field is generated or transmitted. The high-frequency microwaves are emitted from special applicators that emit a collimated (well-focused) beam.

ELECTRIC AND MAGNETIC FIELDS

ELECTRIC FIELD. Electric charges having similar polarity repel each other, while charges of opposite polarity attract. The electric force of attraction or repulsion is given by Coulomb's law, which states that the force (F) between two charges (q and q′) is proportional to the magnitude of each charge and varies inversely with the square of the distance (r) between them:

$$F \propto q \cdot q'/r^2$$

Thus, all charged bodies are surrounded by an electric (electrostatic) field of force that is represented by imaginary lines of force. The intensity at any point in the electric field (E) is equal to the force per unit positive charge at that point. The number of lines of force surrounding a charged

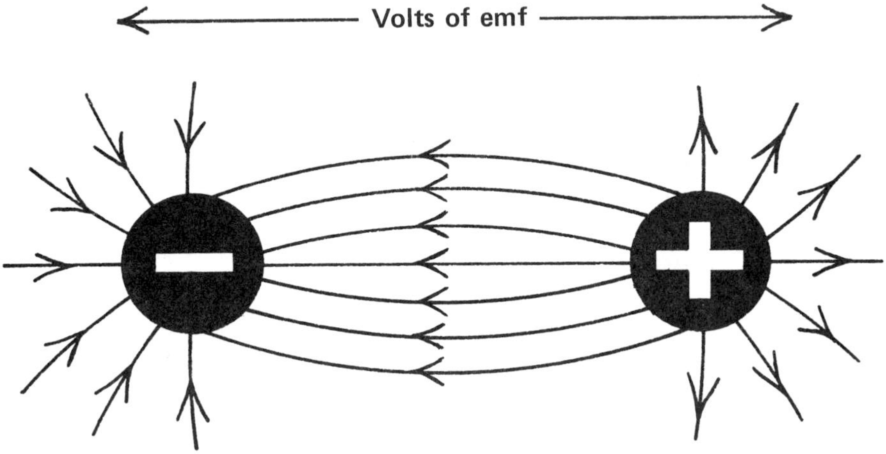

FIGURE 8–2
The electrical field pattern around charged bodies. (Adapted from Grob, B: *Basic Electronics,* ed 4. McGraw-Hill, New York, 1977, p 289.)

body represent the field intensity and vectors indicate the direction along which the electric force acts at any point.[6] Figure 8–2 shows vector patterns of electric force fields around paired charged bodies. Positive charges move along the lines of force away from the isolated positively charged body, while negative charges move in the opposite direction. Electric fields are always generated by separation of charges, and field lines that originate on charges can only terminate on charges having opposite polarity. In the paired charges shown in Figure 8–2, the field intensity is greatest near the point charges as indicated by the proximity of the field lines to each other. The spacing between field lines increases as the distance from the point charges increases, which indicates that the field density and therefore the intensity decreases.[7]

The principle that electric fields are generated by separation of charges should help to conceptualize how electric field line patterns are arranged when air-spaced plate (electrostatic/capacitive) applicators are used to apply shortwave diathermy. Air-spaced plate applicators are shown in Figure 8–3 as two flat metal surfaces of opposite charge. The arrangement shown in Figure 8–3 constitutes a capacitor; and the electric field lines originate and terminate perpendicular to the positive and negative capacitor plates, respectively. The uniformity of spacing between the field lines and their perpendicular orientation are influenced by the size of the capacitor plates and the distance between them. Only if the plates had infinitely large surface dimensions would all field lines be evenly spaced and straight. However, toward the edges of the plates in Figures 8–3*A* and *B* there is a loss of space uniformity between field lines and a loss of their right-angle orientation. This indicates a weakening of the field intensity at the periphery of the plates, especially when the distance between them is increased, as seen in Figure 8–3*B*. The field intensity also changes when capacitive (air-spaced)

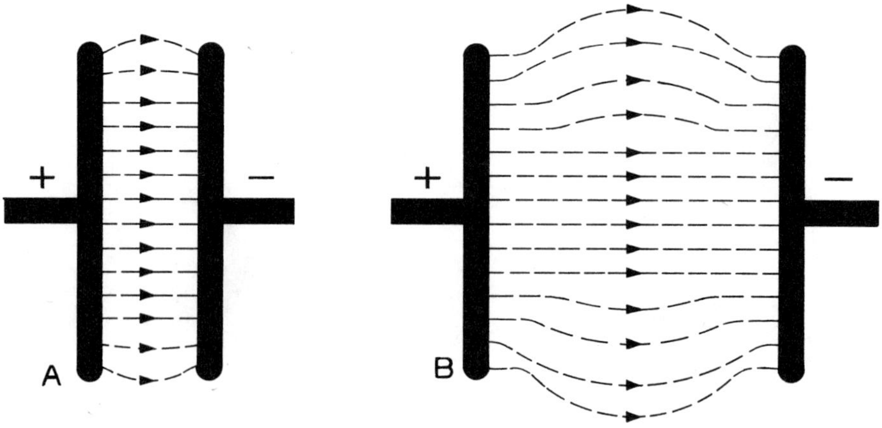

FIGURE 8–3
The electric field created between parallel, equal-sized capacitor plates with narrow spacing (A) and wide spacing (B). (Adapted from Ward,[7] p 115.)

plate applicators are no longer parallel or when the plates are of different sizes. Greater field intensity occurs when plate edges are closer together. If two plates are different sizes, the field intensity will be greater under the smaller plate. More will be said about the relationship of these concepts to electrode application in a later section of this chapter (see Fig. 8–11).

MAGNETIC FIELD. When current is passed through two isolated strands of wire arranged so that each strand has one side lying close to the other, the wires are attracted if the current passing through them is in the same direction. When the current travels through the wires in opposite directions the wires are repelled (Fig. 8–4). Ampère's law ($F \propto I_1, I_2/r$) states that this magnetic force (F) of attraction or repulsion is proportional to the current (I_1, I_2) and length of each wire and inversely proportional to the distance (r) between them. A more intense magnetic field may be produced by passing current through a conducting wire or cable that is formed into a loop or spiral (solenoid) turns, as shown in Figure 8–5. This coil configuration resembles a type of shortwave diathermy applicator that provides magnetic field heating in clinical practice.

The main differences between electric forces and magnetic forces are that magnetic forces are attracted by similar currents, that is, currents that flow in the same direction while the electric forces are repelled by similar charges. In addition, the force lines of the magnetic field are oriented perpendicular to the direction of current flow, while forces between electrostatically charged bodies are parallel to the lines of force. Table 8–2 summarizes the features of electric and magnetic forces.

Effects of Materials in Electric and Magnetic Fields

DIELECTRIC MATERIALS IN THE ELECTRIC FIELD. As a basis for understanding how EM energy from diathermy interacts with various tissues

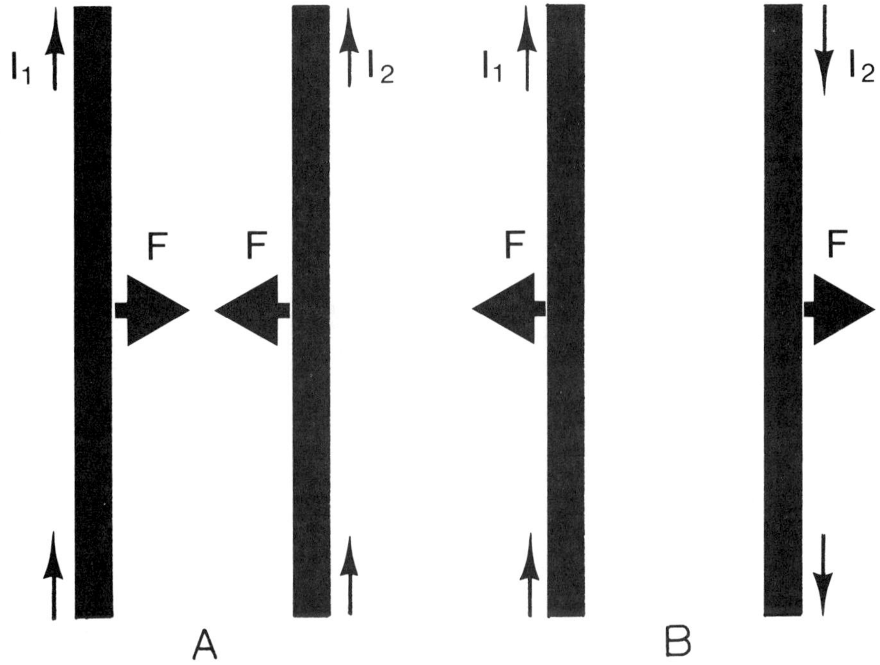

FIGURE 8–4

Current (I_1, I_2) traveling through two wires in the same direction causes the wires to be attracted (A). Repulsion of the wires occurs when current in them travels in opposite directions (B). (Adapted from Ward,[7] p 119.)

of the body a discussion of the electric and magnetic properties of different materials of biologic and nonbiologic origin is necessary.

Electron movement of different substances varies greatly. When *conductors* such as metals (aluminum and copper) are electrically charged, their free electrons move readily. However, materials that are poor conductors do not allow free movement of electrons. These latter materials are known as *insulators* or *dielectrics*. Examples of ideal dielectrics that retain a charge indefinitely are glass and plastics. In comparison, biologic substances are neither good insulators nor good conductors. While the terms "insulator" and "dielectric" may be used to describe materials having poor conduction properties, the terms "good insulator" and "good dielectric" have different meanings. A good insulator provides a very high resistance to current flow. Such a flow of current relates to the ease of movement of charges through a material but says nothing about dielectric constant. A good dielectric material contains very polar molecules and has a high dielectric constant. A good conductor has a very low resistance to current flow.

Figure 8–3 showed the orientation of electric field lines between the plates of a capacitor. Certain clinical methods of applying diathermy use air-spaced applicators that form a capacitor system with the patient's tissues placed in the electric field between the capacitor plates.

A capacitor is a device designed to store and release large amounts of charge and consists of two conductive plates separated by some material

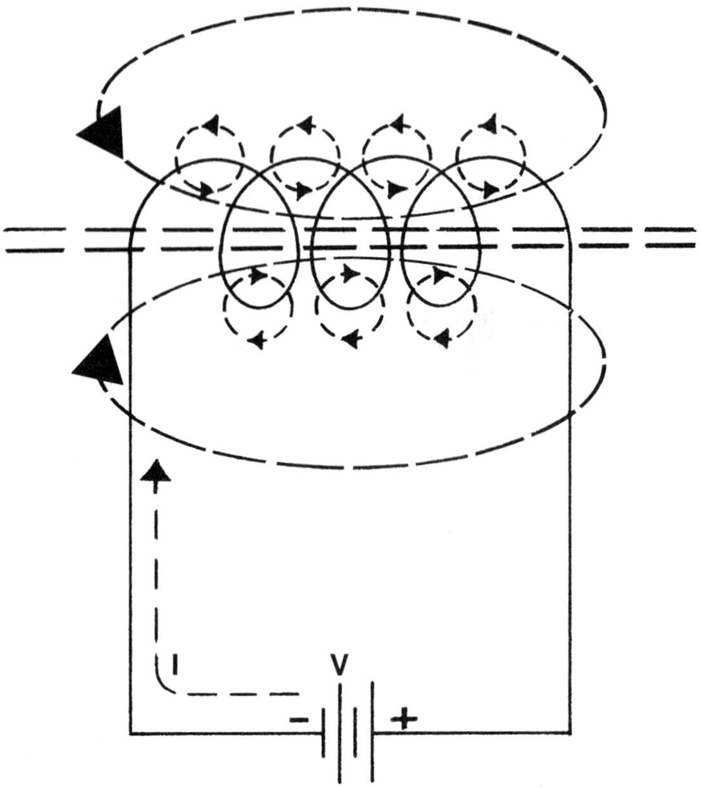

FIGURE 8–5

Current passed through a coiled cable produces a total field pattern consisting of an electrostatic field (large dashed lines and circles) and an electromagnetic field (small circles). (Adapted from Grob, B: *Basic Electronics,* ed 4. McGraw-Hill, New York, 1977, p 297.)

known as a *dielectric.* The relative ease with which a capacitor acquires and stores charge for each volt of applied potential difference is called its *capacitance.* Capacitance depends on the area of the plates and the distance between them. Larger plates and plates with narrow distances between them hold more charge than do smaller plates or plates with greater distances between them. In clinical SWD units, the diameters of air-spaced

TABLE 8–2

Summary of Features for Electric and Magnetic Field Forces

Electric Force	Magnetic Force
Force parallel between charges	Force perpendicular to current direction
Repulsion of similar charges	Attraction by currents flowing in same direction
Between two charges	Between two currents
Dependent on charge size	Dependent on current size
Proportional to $1/r^2$	Proportional to $1/r$

r = distance between two wires.

plate applicators are fixed during a treatment procedure. The distance between the plates and the patient's skin may vary between 0.5 and 3.0 cm.

Capacitance also depends on the type of dielectric material placed between the plates. Nonconductive or dielectric materials such as oil, glass, or water placed between the plates will increase the capacitance and the strength of the electric field between them. The increased capacitance depends on a property called the *dielectric constant* of the material. Dielectric constant is the ratio of a capacitor's ability to store charge in a vacuum to its ability for charge storage when the space between the plates is occupied by a dielectric material. Thus, the ratio only depends on the kind of dielectric material between the capacitor plates. A substance with a low dielectric constant (for instance, air) produces a very small increase in capacitance, whereas water, with a high dielectric constant produces a large increase in capacitance.

The polarity of molecules that make up a substance also plays an important role in determining the magnitude of its dielectric constant. A polar substance like water has a high dielectric constant and can be classified as being a good dielectric. Polar tissues of the body containing high water content will, therefore, respond differently when exposed to EM waves from diathermy than will tissues that are either weakly polarized or nonpolarized. For example, when a material consisting of polar molecules is placed in the electric field between two charged capacitor (air-spaced) plates, the dipoles consisting of positive and negative regions will be oriented by attraction of unlike charges in the direction of the field lines (Fig. 8–6). This polarization of the material affects the magnitude of the externally applied electric field, because each dipole has its own weak electric

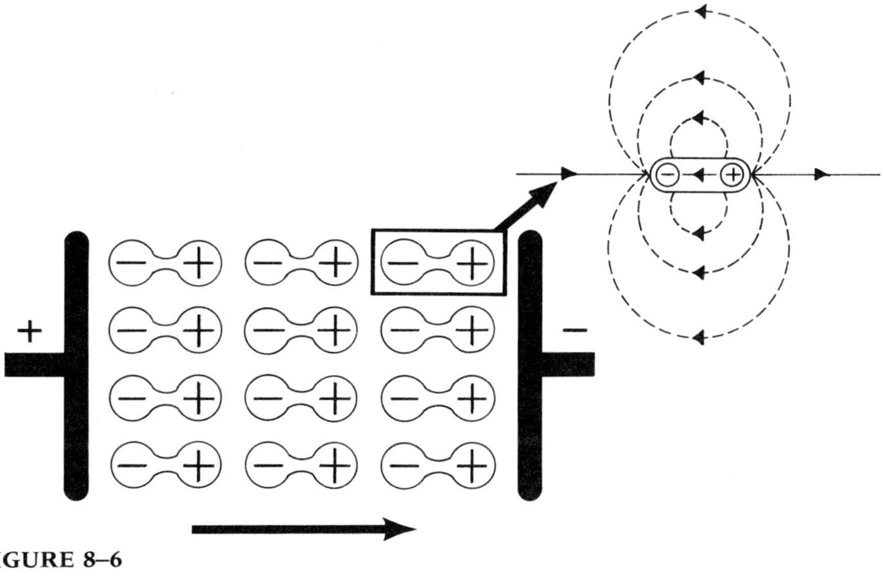

FIGURE 8–6

In the polarized dielectric, the dipoles orient themselves in the direction of the field lines. (Adapted from Thom,[38] p 42.)

field with field lines directed from the positive to the negative end of the molecule.[7] The cumulative effect of many polarized dipoles with their field lines oriented opposite to the direction of the externally applied electric field is to cancel part of the applied field, thereby weakening it. As a result, the field within the dielectric material will be less than the field being applied externally.

Individual nonpolar molecules contained in dielectrics like oil or fat have a symmetrical electron cloud around them instead of the electric field of the polar molecule. When an external electric field is applied to a dielectric substance containing nonpolar molecules, the electron cloud of the individual molecules can undergo distortion, creating induced dipoles and thus becoming polarized.

However, nonpolar molecules do not weaken the externally applied electric field to the extent that polar molecules do, because induced dipoles from nonpolar substances are weaker than dipoles from polar substances. *The clinical significance of this fact is that an electric field applied to nonpolar tissues (fat) may be more intense, resulting in a tendency toward undesirable heating, especially in subcutaneous fat.*

When an electric field from diathermy is applied to water that may be present on the skin or in a wound or wound dressing, a strong surface charge of polarization may occur as a result of many field lines terminating on the surface of the dielectric (water). When Figure 8–6 is studied again, we observe that the polarized dipoles within the dielectric water molecule are oriented so that for any positive charge in a given dipole, there is a negative charge on an adjacent dipole, which cancels it. The only place cancellation of charges does not occur is on the surfaces of the molecule that are perpendicular to the external field. Thus, one surface has a positive charge imbalance and the opposite surface a negative charge imbalance. The imbalance of charges creates a surface charge of polarization on which many field lines converge and terminate (Fig. 8–7). *Because of this occurrence, applications of diathermy in the presence of localized surface moisture may result*

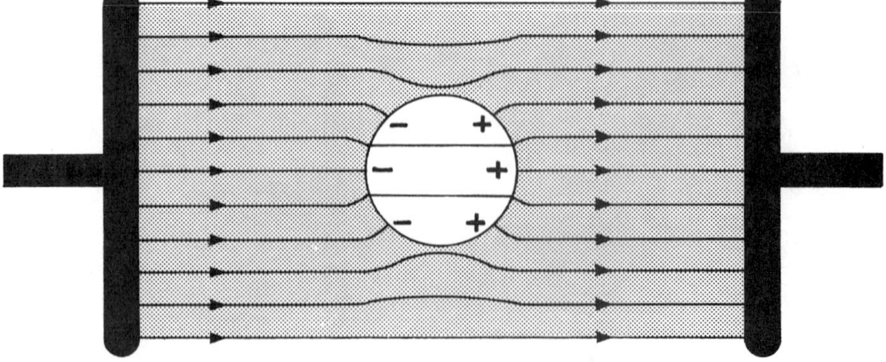

FIGURE 8–7

A more intense electric field occurs on the surfaces of objects that are perpendicular to the field lines due to the surface charge of polarization. (Adapted from Ward,[7] p 129.)

in undesirable heating of the moisture, with subsequent burning of adjacent tissues.

MATERIALS IN THE MAGNETIC FIELD. A more intense magnetic field is produced when a current is passed through a wire coiled into either a single loop or a succession of loops called a solenoid (see Figs. 8–5, 8–8). In addition, when certain materials such as iron are placed within the confines of a solenoid, an increase in inductance results in a considerable increase in strength of the magnetic field around the coiled inductor. The ability of a conductive material to change the inductance of a solenoid is determined by the property known as *permeability.* The effect of permeability on a magnetic field is analogous to the effect on an electric field created by placing a dielectric material between the plates of a capacitor. Permeability is the ratio of the inductance produced by a material to the inductance produced without the material. Unlike the dielectric constant, which is always greater than one, permeability of most materials is very close to one.[6]

Of practical significance is the fact that the permeability of tissues is so close to one that an insignificant distortion of field lines occurs when magnetic field energy is transmitted through them. Therefore, tissues can be considered to be "transparent" to the magnetic field. However, when a high-frequency alternating current from shortwave diathermy is induced from a solenoid coil applicator into a large-volume conductor such as a human extremity, the current in the extremity forms circular paths perpendicular to the magnetic field. *These "eddy currents" shown in Figure 8–8 are responsible for heating tissues when any of the magnetic (inductive) field coil applicators are used with shortwave diathermy.* More will be said about magnetic field methods of applying shortwave diathermy later in the chapter.

REFRACTION OF FIELD LINES AT INTERFACES. Closer inspection of Figure 8–7 reveals that some electric field lines end at the dielectric surface,

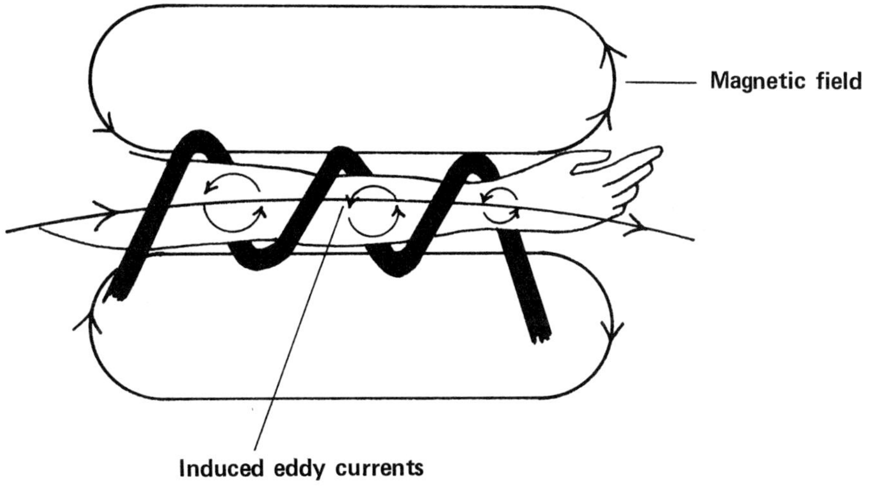

FIGURE 8–8
Eddy currents are induced in the tissues by magnetic field shortwave applicators.

TABLE 8–3*

Dielectric Constants and Conductivities of Select Tissues and Materials

Tissues/Materials	Conductivity (σ)	Dielectric Constant (ϵ)
0.9% saline	11.7	80
Muscle	0.7–0.9	85–100
Kidney	0.7–1.1	120–130
Bone marrow	0.02–0.04	7–8
Fat tissue	0.04–0.06	11–13
Distilled water	2×10^{-4}	80
Oil	10^{-11}	2
Metals	10^{6}–10^{7}	—

* Values are given for tissues and materials at 37°C and 50 MHz. The values are temperature and frequency dependent.

whereas others arrive at the surface at an angle, pass through the dielectric, and emerge at an angle. This change in direction of field lines at an interface is called *refraction.* Refraction occurs at interfaces of different dielectrics and materials having different conductivities (Table 8–3). When a dielectric material is placed in an electric field, the capacitance increases, resulting in greater accumulation of charge on the capacitor plates and an increase in field intensity between each plate and the dielectric surface. The intensity of the field within the dielectric decreases, owing to surface charge of polarization and to refraction, which angulates and disperses the remaining field lines.

The presence of an ideal conductor such as metal in an electric field also causes refraction and surface charge accumulation of field lines. *Therefore, diathermy exposure of implanted or surface metal lying adjacent to tissues of the body will produce selective over-heating of the metal, which in turn will cause thermal necrosis of the tissues in contact with it.*

Thus, we can conclude that electric field lines undergo significant refraction when they pass the boundary from a poor conductor to a better conductor or from a medium with a low dielectric constant to one with a high dielectric constant.

Conduction and dielectric properties of saline, muscle, and kidney are similar, since these tissues contain approximately 80 percent water by weight. The lower conductivity and dielectric constant values of fat and bone marrow relates to their lower water content. Metals are very good conductors, while oil and distilled water are good insulators.

REFLECTION OF FIELD LINES AT INTERFACES. EM wave energy depends on the amplitude and frequency of oscillations as well as on the impedance of the medium the wave passes through. Generally, when waves cross a boundary into a new medium, they maintain a constant frequency; however, complete transfer of energy occurs only when the electrical impedance of each medium is the same.

When EM waves cross a boundary or interface between tissues with different impedances, not all of the incident radiation arriving at the boundary will be transmitted—some will be reflected. As the incident transverse

EM wave hits the boundary between tissues with different impedances, a reflected wave traveling in the opposite direction is produced. The reflected wave may add to the incident wave to form a standing wave (for example, a separate stationary wave pattern).

Standing waves may occur at either a fat-muscle or tissue-metal interface. They are more likely to occur with microwave than with shortwave diathermy because of the greater tendency of microwaves to be reflected. The result of standing wave formation will be an increase of field intensity in that area.

Therapeutic microwaves undergo greater reflection than do shortwaves. This is true because reflection is due to differences in electrical impedance at tissue boundaries. Electrical impedance (determined by dielectric constant and conductivity of tissue) depends on the frequency of the applied alternating field. At higher frequencies dielectric constant is lower, but conductivity is higher and reflection is greater. Dielectric constants and conductivities at different frequencies are shown in Table 8–4 for tissues with high and low water content. Notice that these values differ significantly at microwave frequencies compared with shortwave frequencies.

Since fat and bone are tissues with low water content and muscle and skin contain a high water content, considerable reflection of microwave will occur at the skin-fat, fat-muscle, and muscle-bone interfaces.

According to Schwan and co-workers,[8–10] the percentage of total energy reflected ranges between 60 and 70 percent at frequencies below 1000 MHz. Above 3000 MHz, nearly 60 percent is reflected. In the frequency range between 1000 and 3000 MHz, reflection is dependent on skin and fat thickness and may vary between 0 and 80 percent. An important implication is that at the 2450 MHz frequency customarily used for therapeutic microwave a strong tendency for development of standing waves occurs, which may create intense heating in subcutaneous fat tissue because of reflection at the fat-muscle interface. Moreover, the difference in electrical properties of air and skin augments the unwanted heating of fat owing to reflection of the incident microwave energy that strikes the skin from spaced applicators. The use of direct-contact microwave applicators at the 915 MHz frequency significantly reduces reflection at the air-skin interface, allowing a greater percentage of microwave energy to be absorbed in deeper tissues.

TABLE 8–4

Dielectric Constant and Conductivity of Tissues with High and Low Water Content at Shortwave and Microwave Frequencies

	Dielectric Constant (ϵ)		Conductivity (σ)		
	Water Content		Water Content		
Frequency (MHz)	High	Low	High	Low	SWD/MWD
27.12	113	20	0.602	27.1	SWD
40.68	97.3	14.6	0.680	32.7	SWD
433	53	5.6	1.18	77.9	MWD
915	51	5.6	1.28	101.3	MWD
2450	47	5.5	2.17	154.7	MWD

BIOPHYSICAL EFFECTS

The primary use of diathermy is to raise the temperature of exposed tissues to a therapeutically effective level. This section provides a more thorough coverage of how diathermy induces endogenous tissue heating. When high-frequency AC electrical signals are applied to the patient, corresponding high-frequency oscillating electric and magnetic fields are produced in the tissues.

MOLECULAR ACTIVITY. Three types of tissue molecules (ions, water, and fat), each with its own electrical properties, are influenced in different ways when they encounter therapeutic EM fields. The charged ionic particles (such as potassium), oscillate back and forth along field lines colliding with other molecules. In doing so, kinetic energy is lost, resulting in heat production. Polar molecules (such as water) rotate in an alternating manner and create some heat by frictional drag between themselves and adjacent molecules. The nonpolar molecules (such as fat) become polarized in alternate directions, and some heating is produced from the back-and-forth shifting of the electron clouds to opposite ends of the molecule. The back-and-forth movement of each type of molecule constitutes an alternating flow of current in the tissues. The amount of thermal energy that results from conversion of this alternating tissue current is different for the three molecular types. Ionic oscillations are the most efficient for producing heat. Less heat is generated by the rotational activity of polar molecules and the least efficient means of heat production is from nonpolar molecules.

REAL VERSUS DISPLACEMENT CURRENT. The electrical impedance of different materials and tissues varies with resistance (reciprocal of conductance) and capacitance (dependent on dielectric constant). It is important to distinguish between real current in tissues, which is related to heat production, and displacement current, which is current flow that does not produce tissue heating.

When real current flows through tissue resistances the rate of conversion of electrical energy to heat energy is expressed by Joule's law:

$$P = VI$$

where P is the power dissipated in watts or electrical energy dissipated per second (1 watt [w] = 1 joule/sec), V is voltage, and I is the real current flowing through the tissues. Displacement current is associated with current that flows through tissue capacitance.

For a capacitor to be ideal, the material between its plates must be an ideal dielectric. An ideal dielectric is a material that is capable of polarizing and repolarizing in an electric field without loss of energy due to dielectric absorption. Most gases and some oils are close to being ideal dielectrics. Therefore, any heat produced in them by displacement current would be zero. Water is not an ideal dielectric, so dielectric absorption and heating caused by displacement currents in tissues of high water and ion content occurs with contributions from both real and displacement currents. Tissues with high ionic content receive considerable heating, primarily by real current. Nonpolar tissue such as fat, which comes close to being an ideal dielectric, receives displacement current flow and therefore heats the actual fat tissue somewhat because of its high resistance. Thus, current flow in tissues with high water content (muscle) is primarily real, while current flow in tissues of low water content (fat and bone) is predominantly displacement.[7]

Based on these facts we might expect that the potential for heat production in fat would be less than for muscle, but this is not true. Adipose tissue consists not only of homogeneous nonpolar molecules but also of pervasive lymphatic and blood vessels. Both blood and lymph have higher values of conductivity and dielectric constant (owing to electrolyte and fluid content) which causes field lines to focus on them, resulting in high local field intensities with high rates of heating of the vessels permeating through fat. This fact, together with the knowledge that muscle has a higher dielectric constant than fat, helps to explain why burning of subcutaneous tissues at the fat-muscle boundary as well as within the fat layer may occur with diathermy if adequate precautions are not taken.

Figure 8–9 illustrates field line directions and relative proportions of real and displacement current in capacitive and inductive electrode applications to a limb model. Notice that in both diagrams there is an air space between the applicator and the outer (skin) surface of the model. This space must be maintained to avoid the risk of burning the superficial tissues. Recall that the field intensity increases as the distance between the diathermy applicators decreases. The field intensity is higher in the fatty tissue than in muscle (Fig. 8–9*A*). This is due to the high resistance of fat, selective heating of vessels owing to focusing, refraction of field lines at the fat-muscle boundary, and termination of some field lines at the fat-muscle boundary.

TRANSMISSION, ABSORPTION, AND PENETRATION OF EM WAVES. In Chapter 7, it was emphasized that a material medium is required for transmission of ultrasonic waves. EM waves that travel through a vacuum or through space at the velocity of light do not require a material medium for transmission. However, when EM waves do travel through a medium, their velocity is slowed; their transmission into the medium and their ultimate depth of penetration depend on how much wave energy is absorbed. Absorption depends on the amount, density, and electric and magnetic properties of the absorbing material, as well as on the wave frequency. EM wave energy from diathermy is absorbed by tissue molecules. Energy is given up by the molecules and converted to heat during their high-frequency oscillations and collisions with each other. Muscle and other tissues with high dielectric constant and conductivity will absorb EM energy to a greater extent than will fatty tissue, which has low dielectric and conductivity values. *Therefore, clinically diathermy can be used to increase the temperature of skeletal muscle.*

Penetration depth of EM energy also depends on wave frequency and the properties of the medium the wave travels through. As waves of any

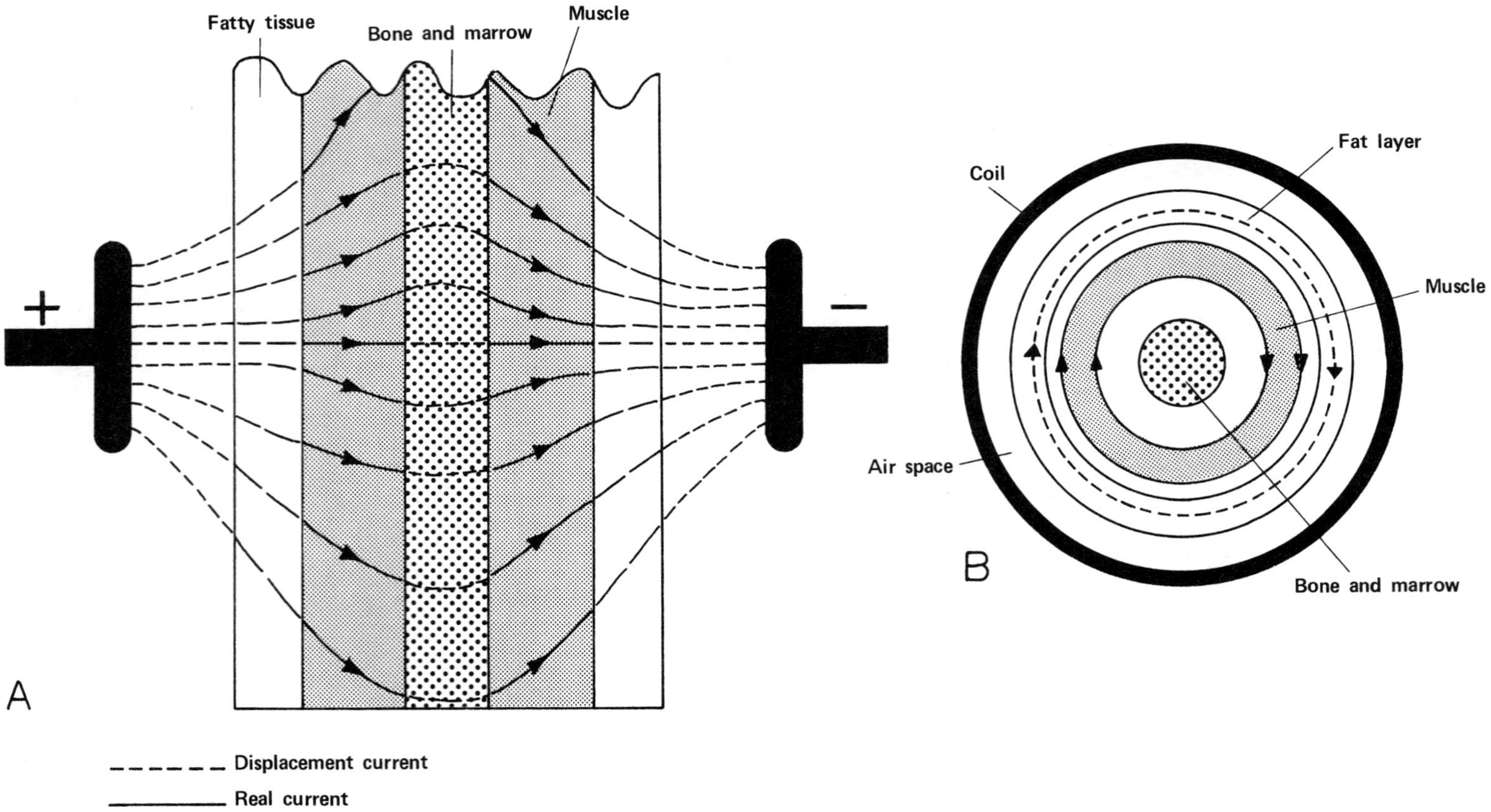

FIGURE 8–9

Relative distributions of real and displacement currents in a limb model for capacitive field (A) and magnetic (coil) field (B) applicators. (Adapted from Ward,[7] pp 158–159.)

frequency travel through an absorbing medium, their energy decreases exponentially with distance. As a wave travels through a medium, it progressively releases energy. Penetration depth is the depth required to absorb 63 percent of the original wave energy. Penetration depth of therapeutically desirable temperatures (between 40°C and 45°C) for inductively applied shortwave diathermy at 27.12 MHz usually does not exceed 3 cm.[11,12]

When the subcutaneous fat layer is 1 cm thick, the effect of frequency and applicator-skin distance on penetration depth is particularly influential in the therapeutic microwave range. At microwave frequencies, dielectric and conductivity values, especially for muscle, are considerably higher than they are at shortwave frequencies. With spaced MW applicators this results in a greater rate of microwave absorption in superficial muscle (and fat), with less penetration in muscle than can be obtained with shortwave diathermy. To substantiate this, Lehmann and associates[12] applied microwave diathermy at 2450 MHz with a C applicator spaced 2 cm from the skin of a human thigh in which the fat-muscle interface was 0.8 cm below the skin surface. In this case, therapeutically desirable temperatures were recorded at a depth of only 1.85 cm with the power output adjusted to the point at which discomfort or mild pain was felt temporarily on the skin surface. In contrast, DeLateur and colleagues[5] used a direct skin contact aperture MW applicator at 915 MHz with surface cooling to the skin of a human thigh. Applied to an area having a subcutaneous fat thickness of 2.1 cm, therapeutically desirable temperatures were recorded at a tissue depth of 4.5 cm with skin heating elevated to only 37°C during the last 2 minutes of a 20-minute treatment.

The effect of mismatches in impedance at tissue boundaries also influences the total percentage of diathermy energy that is absorbed. Since microwave is easily reflected at tissue interfaces, the reflected waves will result in a tendency toward excessive heating in subcutaneous fat and superficial bone.

When microwave diathermy is used, frequencies below 1000 MHz are required to effectively heat tissues located beneath a few centimeters of subcutaneous fat. For microwave heating of structures close to the skin surface that are not covered by a thick layer of soft tissue a frequency of 2450 MHz is adequate. Very deep structures like the hip joint cannot be heated with either shortwave or microwave diathermy at therapeutic frequencies.

PHYSIOLOGIC EFFECTS

Specific Absorption Rate (SAR)

In 1981, the National Council on Radiation Protection and Measurements (NCRP Report No. 67, March 1, 1981) recommended the use of the quantity SAR, expressed in units of watts per kilogram (W/kg), to quantify the rate of energy absorbed per unit tissue mass exposed to EM fields. SAR is proportional to the electrical conductivity of the tissue being exposed. Since it is necessary to elevate tissue temperature to between 40°C and 45°C for therapeutic effectiveness,[13] the therapist should be assured that the diathermy equipment is sufficiently powerful to do this. The SAR required to reach the upper end of this range is approximately 170 W/kg.[14–16] At this SAR, there is an increase in blood flow up to nearly 30 ml/100 g tissue/min, which results in a vigorous physiologic response. The response is comparable to blood flow increases obtained in response to maximal exercise, which may produce a flow of 30 to 35 ml/100 g tissue/min.

Vasculated and contracted tissue may be safely treated with SWD or MWD that produces initial time-rates of temperature change of 0.8°C to 2.7°C per minute corresponding to a SAR of 50 to 170 W/kg. Less vasculated tissues or tissues that are in a resolving (subacute) inflammatory stage would tolerate a SAR and time-rate of temperature increase that is toward the lower end of this range to avoid undesirable rapid temperature increases.[17]

Therefore, the rate of heating is related to the rate at which power is applied. If necrosis of well-vasculated tissue occurs when a temperature of 45°C is maintained for a brief time period, then for vigorous heating the critical temperature of 44°C should be reached within 10 minutes to maintain the temperature for achieving maximum therapeutic benefits.[11]

Thermal Effects

The effects of shortwave heating on skin blood flow in humans was studied by Millard,[18] who showed that clearance of radioactive sodium increased nearly 150 percent after exposure, resulting in an average temperature rise of 5.3°C. In the same study, muscle clearance rates increased by 36 percent with a muscle temperature rise of 5.2°C. Using 2450 MHz microwave diathermy, McNiven and Wyper[19] produced a 400 percent increase in vastus lateralis muscle blood flow in five subjects. This occurred after an 8-minute exposure at a power output adjusted to a comfortable level.

The effect of SWD application on the circulation of knees resulted in a 100 percent increase according to Harris[20] in a study of radio-sodium clearance from the knee joint. Similar SWD treatment of chronic (quiescent) rheumatoid knees showed a circulation increase of 60 percent, whereas with most acute rheumatoid knees treated there was a resultant decrease in circulation. This decrease was comparable to decreases found with intra-articular hydrocortisone. Harris suggests that this provides some rationale for using local heat therapy in rheumatoid arthritis (see Hazards of Shortwave and Microwave Diathermy, on use of diathermy with acutely inflamed joints).

The physiologic effects obtained with other forms of therapeutic heat are also produced with shortwave and microwave diathermy. Generally, the power of EM fields from diathermy modalities allows greater depth of heating than occurs with superficial heating agents. Logically then, the selection of shortwave or microwave diathermy is correct when the desired treatment outcome is to increase extensibility of deep collagen tissue, decrease joint stiffness, relieve deep pain and muscle spasm, increase blood flow, and assist in resolution of inflammatory infiltrates and exudates.

Nonthermal Effects

Only one, poorly understood nonthermal effect can be attributed to diathermy. The effect, referred to as pearl-chain formation, is produced when micro-organisms, unicellular organisms, fat globules in milk, or red blood cells in serum become oriented in chain formation parallel to the lines of force in the EM field. The effect is produced by either continuous or pulsed shortwave of the same average output[21,22] and by microwave diathermy.[23]

Pulsed shortwave diathermy was originally developed to produce nonthermal effects in contrast to the thermal effects of continuous diathermy. The equipment operates at a frequency of 27.12 MHz. The individual pulse duration is 65 microseconds, and the pulse rate varies from 100 to 5200 pulses per second. The peak power is 1000 watts, and the average power is 40 watts. Despite many scientific attempts to demonstrate the efficacy of pulsed diathermy for therapeutic purposes, there is not sufficient evidence to support its use clinically. No clearly identified therapeutic responses can be attributed to the nonthermal effects of diathermy.[13] Therefore, pulsed diathermy devices are clinically useful only if they have sufficient power to produce a measurable temperature rise in exposed tissues.

INSTRUMENTATION AND METHODS OF APPLICATION

Shortwave Diathermy

Figure 8–10 illustrates the basic components of a shortwave diathermy device, which include (1) power supply that converts AC wall current to DC for the power amplifier and frequency generator circuits, (2) oscillator that produces the high-frequency (27.12 MHz) sine wave AC, (3) power amplifier that amplifies AC produced by the generator to give a sufficiently strong signal for therapeutic applications, and (4) patient tuning circuit with applicators that allow transfer of energy from the device to the patient. The patient circuit will either require manual tuning or will automatically tune the resonant frequency of the device to equal the resonant frequency of the patient circuit.

The patient circuit of SWD emits either a stronger electric field or a stronger magnetic field, or both fields may be nearly equal depending on the type of applicator (electrode) used. Absorption of electric and/or magnetic field energy leads to increased tissue temperature when a patient is exposed to SWD.

TYPES OF APPLICATORS/ELECTRODES. The treatment applicators used in SWD are classified as either capacitive or inductive. For the most effective

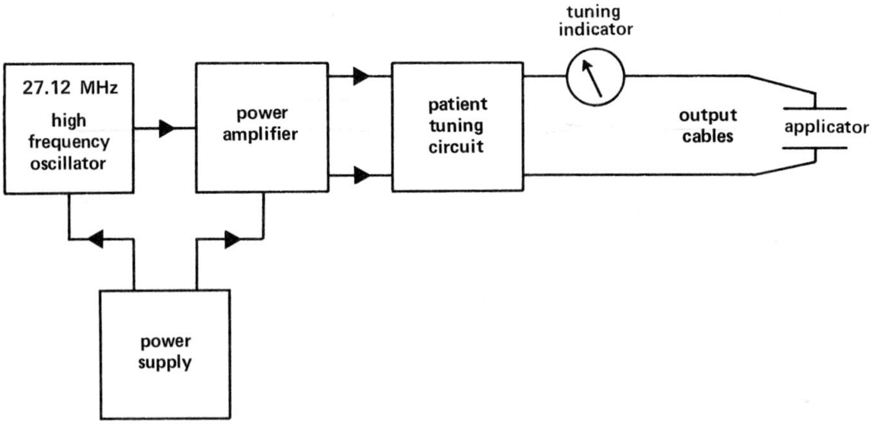

FIGURE 8–10

A schematic diagram of shortwave diathermy components showing the patient circuit. In this case, the high-frequency current is capacitively coupled to the patient.

treatment in a given patient situation, it is the therapist's responsibility to know whether the applicator to be used provides predominantly electric or magnetic field or an equal proportion of the two different types of energy. Capacitive applicators deliver mostly electric field energy to the tissues,[7,9] whereas inductive applicators deliver primarily magnetic field energy, plus any residual electric field energy. Electric field energy is readily absorbed by the skin and subcutaneous fat while magnetic field energy is absorbed by tissues with a high electrolyte content, such as blood and muscle.

The capacitive applicator system employs two air-spaced metal plates that range from 7.5 to 17.5 cm in diameter. The high-frequency alternating current allows the energy to oscillate from one plate to the other. The intervening air and the patient's tissues placed between the plates constitute the dielectric. Since the electrodes are physically connected to the oscillating circuit this means that the patient is an integral part of the circuit in the capacitive electrode system.

A glass or plastic plate guard surrounds each plate to prevent contact between the plate and the patient's skin. A severe electrical burn may occur if either the therapist's or patient's skin contacts the bare metal plate with the diathermy device in operation. To prevent focusing of the electric field on moisture that may accumulate on the skin from perspiration, a single layer of terrycloth toweling is placed between the plate applicators and the skin to absorb the moisture. Most plates are manually movable through a distance of about 3 cm within the guard. In some older models, the plate is not movable but the plate guard can be manually adjusted so the plate to skin distance is 2 to 3 cm. For optimum heating, the guard should be as close to the skin as possible and the plate as far away from the skin as the plate guard allows. This positioning of the plate and guard with reference to the skin provides for increased relative depth and heating depth of the tissues absorbing the energy.[24] In fact, when applied correctly and to patients whose subcutaneous fat layer is less than 1 cm thick the capacitive field

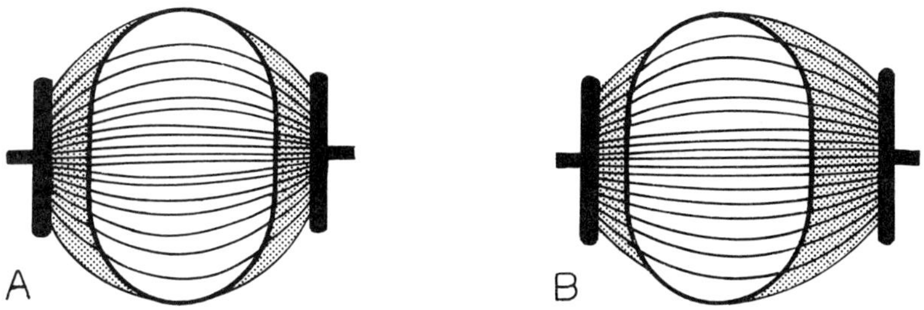

A. Even distribution of the lines of force in electrodes of equal size and equal electrode-skin distance.

B. Stronger heating with an electrode located closer to the body.

C. If the edge of an electrode is positioned close to the skin, undesirable strong field and heat concentration are created under the edge of the electrode closest to the body surface.

D. Relatively uniform heating of a total body section with the application of large electrodes, at a large distance. Heating achieved at a depth is greater with this arrangement.

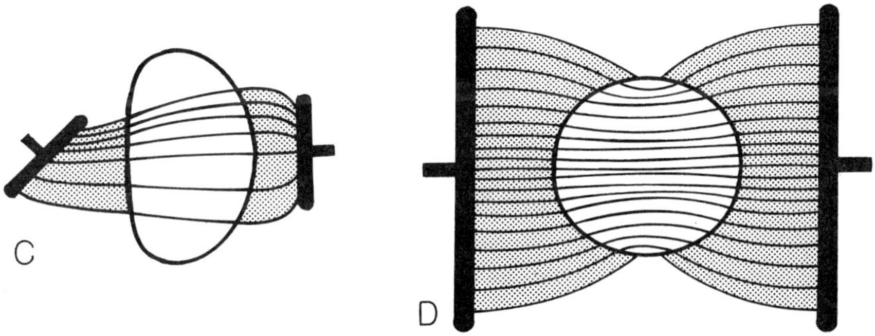

FIGURE 8–11

Air-spaced applicator positions. (Adapted from Thom,[35] pp 46, 48.)

technique may be capable of delivering energy into tissue depths that correspond to the depths heated with inductive applicators.[25] This is achieved with shortwave devices that are engineered with deep field efficient circuitry that automatically increases wattage (power) output as the plate-skin distance increases, and decreases output as plate-skin distance decreases. In reality, most SWD devices maintain constant power output with changes in plate-skin distance. Thus, power will be high when the plate-skin distance is small, which may lead to selective and even deleterious heating of skin and subcutaneous fat.

Air-spaced plates should always be positioned so that the distance between any part of the two plates is at least as great as the diameter of the plate. Figure 8–11 shows some placements of capacitive applicators, with the resulting heating patterns.

Magnetic field or inductive short-wave applicators are available in two forms—the more widely and frequently used drum, and the cable (Fig. 8–12). The drum may be a single or multiple unit. The single-drum unit is intended to treat only one surface. A smaller version of the single-drum unit called the "minode" and a larger version called the "monode" consist primarily of an induction coil arranged in either a monoplanar or multiplanar configuration and contained within a rigid insulator housing. The housing allows propagation of electric and magnetic field energy only from the applicator treatment surface which is placed in contact with a single layer of terrycloth toweling on the patient's skin. Therefore, the treatment surface of the applicator housing serves the same function as the plate guard in the air-spaced applicator: to space the inductive coil away from the skin.

The multiple-unit drum called a "diplode" is hinged so that one or more body part surfaces can be treated simultaneously. The diplode consists of a rectangularly arranged induction coil contained within an insulator housing that also serves to space the coil away from the patient's skin. Because of the coil's proximity to the treatment surface within the diplode, approximately 1 cm of terrycloth toweling must be used to separate the applicator from the patient's skin to prevent excessive surface heating.

The cable electrode (Fig. 8–12) may vary in length from 2 to 5 meters and may be wound in a monoplanar or helical fashion around the patient part. Hence, the cable electrode can be used to treat one or more surfaces simultaneously. However, its greater flexibility compared with that of the drum requires more time to position the cable properly for each treatment. Because there is no rigid housing as with the drum or a capacitive electrode, the user must always add a dielectric material such as terrycloth between the cable insulation and the patient's skin. This dielectric is needed to absorb perspiration, which could cause a superficial skin burn. For ideal energy transfer to the patient, the intervening dielectric material should be 1 to 2 cm thick, except when the body weight is resting on the cable and then a dielectric 2 to 3 cm thick is required. The radiated energy can travel from coil to coil along the surface of the skin. Therefore, when the cable turns are less than 3 cm apart, there is increased energy exchange between adjacent coil turns. This causes inefficiency in bringing about an increase in deep tissue temperature because of the undesired loss of energy between cable turns.

All diathermy units have external cables that conduct the EM energy from the high-frequency oscillating circuit to the patient applicator. Most SWD devices do not use a coaxial (shielded) cable, which prevents stray radiation emission because of power loss owing to earth-referenced grounding back into the chassis of the device. Therefore, because these cables are usually rubber-insulated and do emit radiation in all directions when the applicators are energized, care must be taken to prevent them from directly contacting the patient or any metal or synthetic materials.

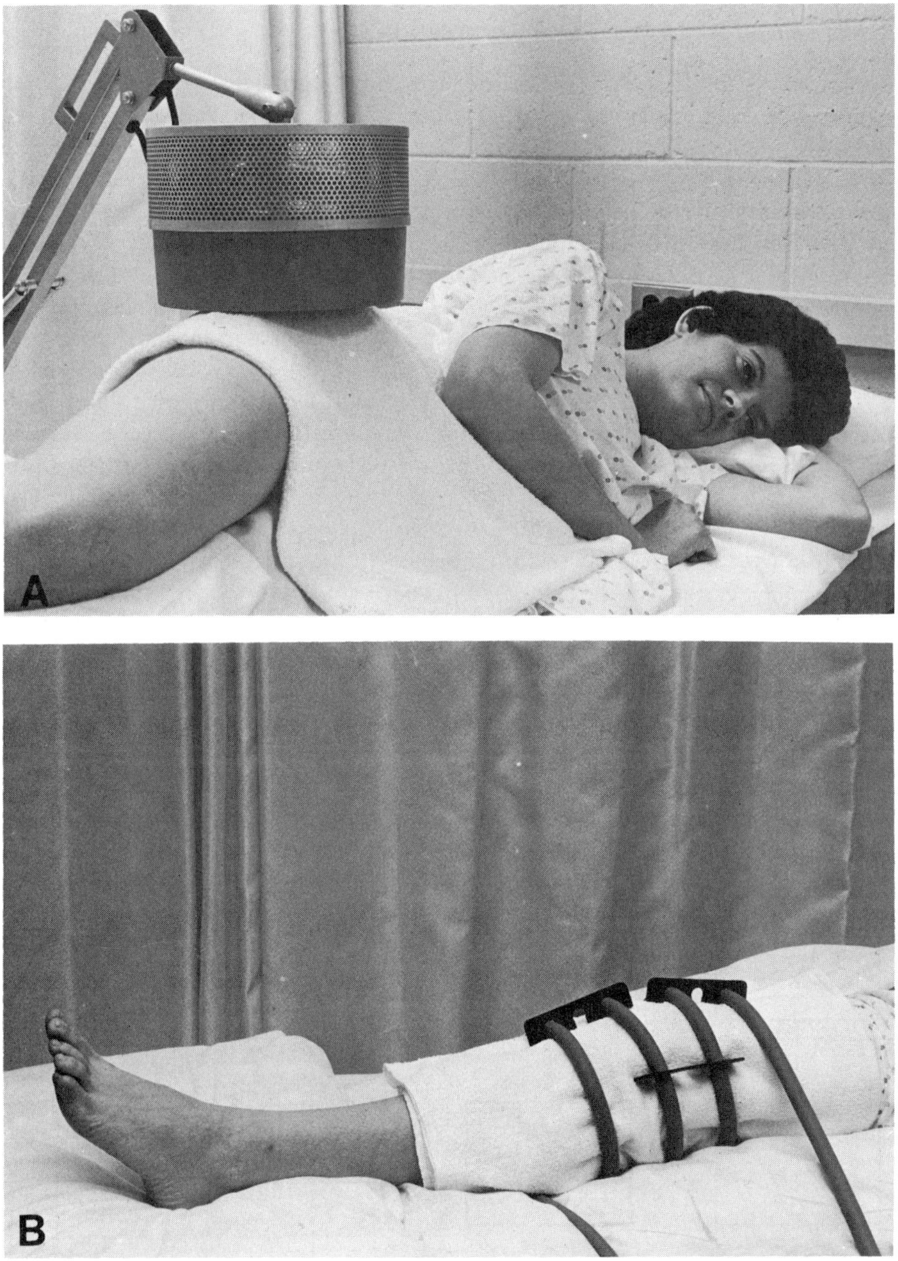

FIGURE 8–12

Magnetic field (inductive) shortwave diathermy. *A,* Single-drum unit applied to lateral hip. Note layer of toweling for spacing. *B,* Induction coil applicator around a knee joint. Induction coils are separated by spacers. Spacing between coil and skin is maintained by toweling.

Microwave Diathermy

The basic components of microwave diathermy are (1) power supply, (2) magnetron oscillator, and (3) various treatment applicators (Fig. 8–13). The standard frequency in clinical microwave diathermy use is 2450 MHz. This high frequency allows microwave energy to be directed or beamed from the applicator toward the patient. This is in contrast to any shortwave frequency, with which focusing or beaming is not possible at practical cost. A therapeutic MWD device consists of a power supply, magnetron tube to generate the UHF energy, and a variable power control. The E field of MWD is oriented parallel to the body surface, which reduces fat heating while providing deep heating. Several types of applicators can be used with this generator.

Microwave diathermy is absorbed by high–water content tissues such as muscle and blood in a greater quantity than SWD is absorbed. Since microwave energy may be reflected from high dielectric tissues (at boundaries between dissimilar tissues), increased thermal concentration may occur at interfaces between fat and muscle and between bone and adjacent soft tissues. Reflection from bone surfaces may cause concentration from standing waves. In studies on the effects of microwaves on bone, muscle, and nearby tissue,[26] temperature increases of 4.3°C in subcutaneous fat, 4.6°C in muscle overlying bone, 3.8°C in bone itself, and 3.6°C in bone marrow were recorded.

Temperature differences in muscle and fat have been reported for various frequencies.[3] Studies by Schwan and associates led other researchers to compare heating patterns of various microwave frequencies.[13,27–29] These studies clearly indicate the superiority of frequencies lower than 2450 MHz for deep heating (>1 cm). Comparison of the 915 and 2450 MHz

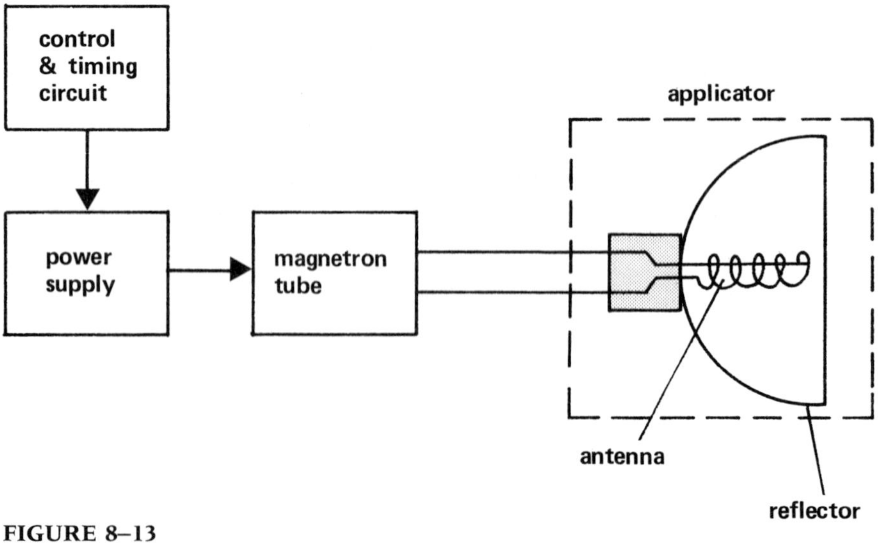

FIGURE 8–13

A schematic diagram of microwave diathermy components. (Adapted from Ward,[7] p 232.)

frequencies shows that for an average thickness of subcutaneous fat, more heat occurs in the subcutaneous tissues (outer 2.1 cm) because of reflection at the fat-muscle interface using the higher frequency. Furthermore, in theory, the depth of penetration is better at the lower frequency.[30] Time to achieve a maximum level of heating with diathermy was found to be 20 minutes, with a drop observed after 30 minutes.[31] Worden and co-workers[32] have demonstrated a significant increase in blood flow from MWD, especially toward the end of the treatment period. Richardson and associates[33] reported that the magnitude of heating played the most significant role in the alteration of blood flow, and this was supported in studies by Leden and colleagues[34] who revealed a significant increase in blood flow when deep muscle temperature was raised to 41°C or more.

Types of Applicators/Electrodes

Over the years, different types of spaced microwave applicators have been developed with the intent of increasing the size of the skin surface area toward which the energy is beamed. One popular applicator is enclosed in a rectangular metallic reflector about 10 cm long and is positioned parallel to the skin surface (type E). When the applicator to skin distance is approximately 3 cm, a tissue temperature increase can be generated over an area of about 150 cm^2.

The heating pattern of the rectangular applicator is oval-shaped providing maximal heat at the center. This microwave applicator is recommended for flat or concave body surfaces. When the applicator is further from the skin, up to about 15 cm away, the area that can be treated increases in size proportionately (inverse square law). However, as the applicator-to-skin distance increases, the wattage output must also be increased. There is another, smaller, rectangular reflector referred to as type C.

Another spaced MW applicator design in clinical use is the hemispheric antenna (type A or B). This electrode is designed to provide a circular heating pattern with an area of minimal energy radiation from its center. The size of this area varies according to the diameter of the metallic reflector that houses the applicator. There will be a strong area of radiation output toward the periphery.

A direct-contact applicator is now commercially available (Fig. 8–14).*† The applicator allows the treatment to be applied at lower forward power levels with minimal stray radiation. The device can be purchased as a new system or can be adapted to an existing MWD generator. A dual power meter on the device displays the forward power as well as the net power delivered to the patient.

An investigation of E field mapping of various MWD applicators by Witters and Kantor[35] provides information to users concerning radiation

* TAG MED: Medical Electronics Corporation of America, Boulder, CO 80301.

† ELMED INC: 60 West Fay Avenue, Addison, IL 60101.

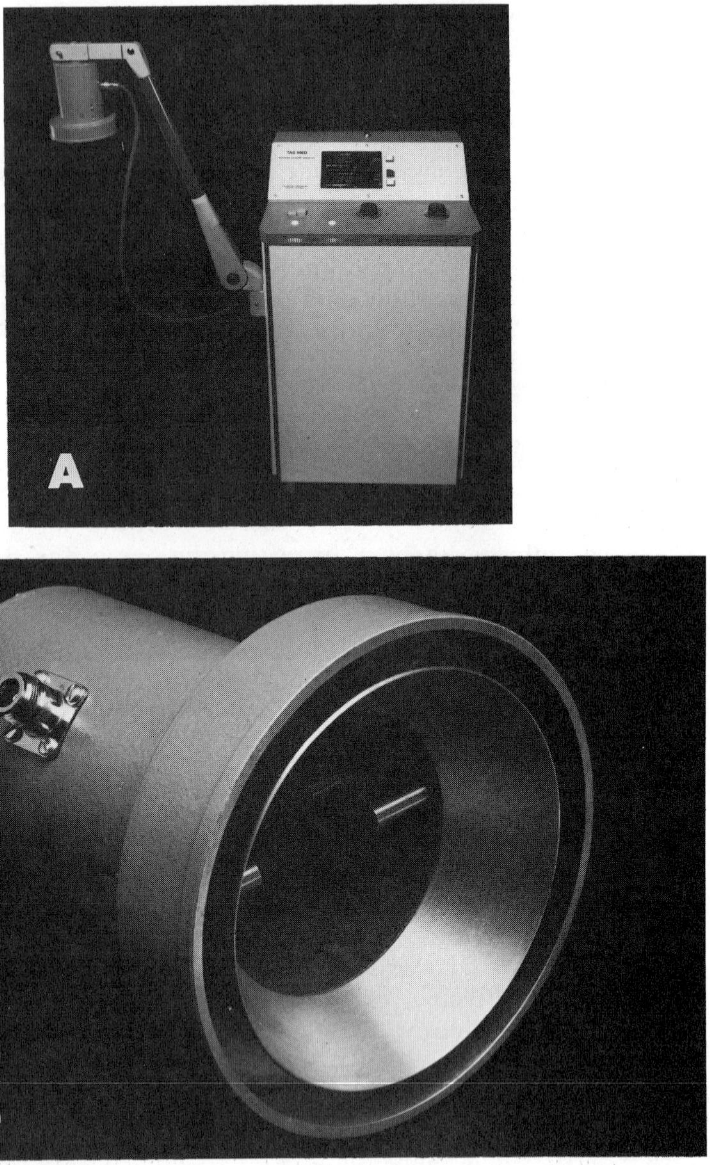

FIGURE 8–14

Microwave diathermy. *A*, 2450 MHz microwave diathermy unit. *B*, Direct-contact applicator. (From Tag Med Co, with permission.)

leakage and applicator efficiency. Their experiment included types B, C, and E applicators; a direct-contact applicator; and one prototype model (a direct-contact applicator with a choke around the center aperture to reduce leakage). In comparing the thermal effectiveness of the applicators, the direct-contact applicators were found to be far superior to types B, C, and E. Furthermore, the radiation leakage around the direct-contact applicators was within the recommended FDA's 10 mW/cm^2 at a distance of 5 cm from the applicator. The leakage for types C and E were variable about the applicator but, as with type B, exceeded the recommended minimum leakage. Lehmann and associates,[36] using phantom models, also found that direct-contact MWD applicators produced much less stray radiation than the type C and E applicators.

Direct-contact applicators that operate at frequencies of 915 MHz and 2450 MHz have been evaluated by Witters and Kantor,[35,37] using a planar phantom model. They found that the specific absorption rate (SAR) remains more constant using the 2450 MHz applicator than using the 915 MHz spaced 1 cm from the phantom; however, the depth of penetration is less for the higher frequency than for the lower (1.3 cm for the 2450 MHz and 1.9 cm for the 915 MHz). More power was required and leakage was considerably higher, when comparing the 915 MHz applicator at 1 cm distance from the phantom with application directly on the phantom. An external choke with a 2.5 cm absorbing material was added to the small direct-contact 915 MHz applicator, which reduced the leakage below the 10 mW/cm^2 measured 5 cm from the applicator. Depth of penetration desired should be a criterion in deciding which frequency to use.

CONSIDERATIONS FOR APPLYING SWD/MWD

Because it is clinically impractical to measure the quantity of electromagnetic energy actually transferred from a SWD/MWD device to the tissues of the body without invasive temperature probes, therapists must use the patient's subjective heat sensation response as a guide for dosage. A significant problem often encountered with those who do not have normal heat sensation is the difficulty they may have in making reliable verbal responses about what they feel. Individuals with cutaneous (sensory) nerve deficit should be tested for pain and temperature sensation prior to beginning treatment.

In evaluating the patient, the therapist should determine whether the stage of the condition to be treated is acute, subacute, or chronic. Having identified the stage of the condition, the extent of involvement (that is, volume of involved tissue) should be determined. This will allow selection of a SWD/MWD device with electrodes that are appropriate for delivering energy to the involved area.

The evaluation should also establish whether there are any bony prominences, metal implants, shrapnel, or surface metal in the area to be treated. Direct application of diathermy over bony prominences or metal may result in tissue destruction. Following the evaluation, the patient should be positioned comfortably for treatment. Clothing, dressings, and bandaging should be removed from the body surface to be treated.

Therapists should always keep in mind that the extent of biologic reactions elicited by SWD/MWD depends on the tissue temperature reached at the end of treatment. Since the therapeutic range for increasing tissue temperature is between 40°C and 45°C, it is imperative that the therapist knows how intensely, how long, and how frequently the treatment should be applied, based on the stage of the condition. According to Thom,[38] the therapeutic effect of a lower dose (intensity) administered over a somewhat longer period of time is better than that of a more intense dose given over a shorter time.

Heat dosage, or the amount of thermal energy delivered to the tissues per unit time, is very important when specific treatment outcomes are desired. Lehmann's definitions of mild and vigorous heating[3] discussed in Chapter 5 may be used in conjunction with the reproducible doses described by Schliephake[39] for SWD application. This dosage scheme may also be used for MWD application:

Dose I, lowest—just below the point of any sensation of heat (acute inflammatory process).
Dose II, low—mild heat sensation, barely felt (subacute resolving inflammatory process).
Dose III, medium—moderate but pleasant heat sensation (subacute resolving inflammatory process).
Dose IV, heavy—vigorous heating that produces a sensation that is well tolerated (chronic conditions). The pain threshold may be reached, but the output is immediately lowered to just below maximum toleration.

Acute conditions like soft tissue trauma should be treated with either dose I or II, with treatment periods of 2 to 5 minutes daily for 2 weeks. The acute condition will not require the deep-tissue temperature rise that results from longer, more intense applications (vigorous heating). Chronic conditions (for instance, contracture) call for either dose III or IV and longer treatment periods of 5 to 30 minutes. The frequency of treatment will vary from once daily to 2 to 3 times weekly, for 1 to 4 weeks.

When SWD devices without deep field efficient circuitry are used for treatment, capacitive air-spaced applicators may be used for heating superficial and subcutaneous structures as well as the outer layers of superficial muscle. When the SWD device has deep field circuitry, deep-tissue heating may be achieved. Capacitive applicators are useful in treating two symmetrical body surfaces.

Remember that the electrical properties of tissues are much higher than they are for air. Thus, use electrodes that are larger than the body part (such as a limb) to be treated, so that field lines bend toward the part and spreading of the field in minimized. It is also very important for the therapist to assess the relative thickness of the patient's subcutaneous fat layer before capacitive electrodes are used.

Inductive (magnetic field) SWD applicators include the minode, monode, diplode, and cable. Generally, these applicators provide more uniform heating of superficial and deep musculature without as much risk of overheating skin and subcutaneous fat. Cable turns should never be allowed to touch one another and should be insulated from the patient with terrycloth toweling of appropriate thickness.

Because of the size of microwave applicators, the use of MWD is more appropriate when smaller body areas or smaller tissue volumes require deep heating. The spaced conventional MW applicators and the direct-contact applicators have been described earlier in this chapter. Recent research has singled out direct-contact applicators as being more effective and safer than the older, spaced applicators. The modern design contact applicators require either direct skin contact or slight spacing within 1 cm of the skin. Generally direct-contact applicators have uniform heating patterns.

For vigorous heating effects, the forward power of the direct-contact applicator should be 50 watts, with an average intensity of approximately 500 mW/cm^2. A comfortable feeling of warmth by the patient is the best available guide for adjusting the dosage of either SWD or MWD.

CLINICAL APPLICATIONS OF DIATHERMY

All of the desired outcomes of treatment with shortwave and microwave diathermy mentioned earlier are based on the elevation of tissue temperature. This section will discuss the clinical conditions for which diathermy has been documented to be effective in achieving these treatment outcomes. The depth of heating achieved with diathermy is more than that which occurs in superficial heating agents but less than that which occurs in ultrasound—with one exception. When a 434 MHz microwave is used in oncology, the depth of heating has been reported to be as much as 10 cm.[40]

Treatment Indications

All of the common indications for thermotherapy are also indications for treatment with diathermy. In fibrous muscular or joint capsular contractures, heating the shortened tissues may enhance collagen extensibility[41] prior to stretching done manually or with automated mechanical (such as continuous passive motion) devices or functional electrical muscle stimulation devices. Either SWD or MWD may be used, since both are able to heat down to the superficial musculature. When contracted structures are deep to heavy layers of soft tissues, microwave will not significantly heat the target tissues.[13]

Muscle guarding and pain, which occur as a result of injury to tendons and joint structures, degenerative joint disease, bursitis, sacroiliac strains, and ankylosing spondylitis, may be relieved by diathermy applications to the muscles that are in spasm (Fig. 8–15).[13]

Joint structures may be selectively heated by shortwave diathermy when the joint is covered by a thin layer of soft tissue (such as the elbow). Vigorous heating of a synovial joint should only be done in chronic disease conditions such as contracture or the burned-out stage of rheumatoid arthritis. The purpose of such treatment is to improve joint range of motion by decreasing stiffness and improving resiliency of contracted soft tissues. In the subacute stage of traumatic arthritis, shortwave diathermy may be beneficial in joints with a thin soft tissue cover to improve blood circulation and thereby to aid in the resolution of edema and hemorrhage. This concept

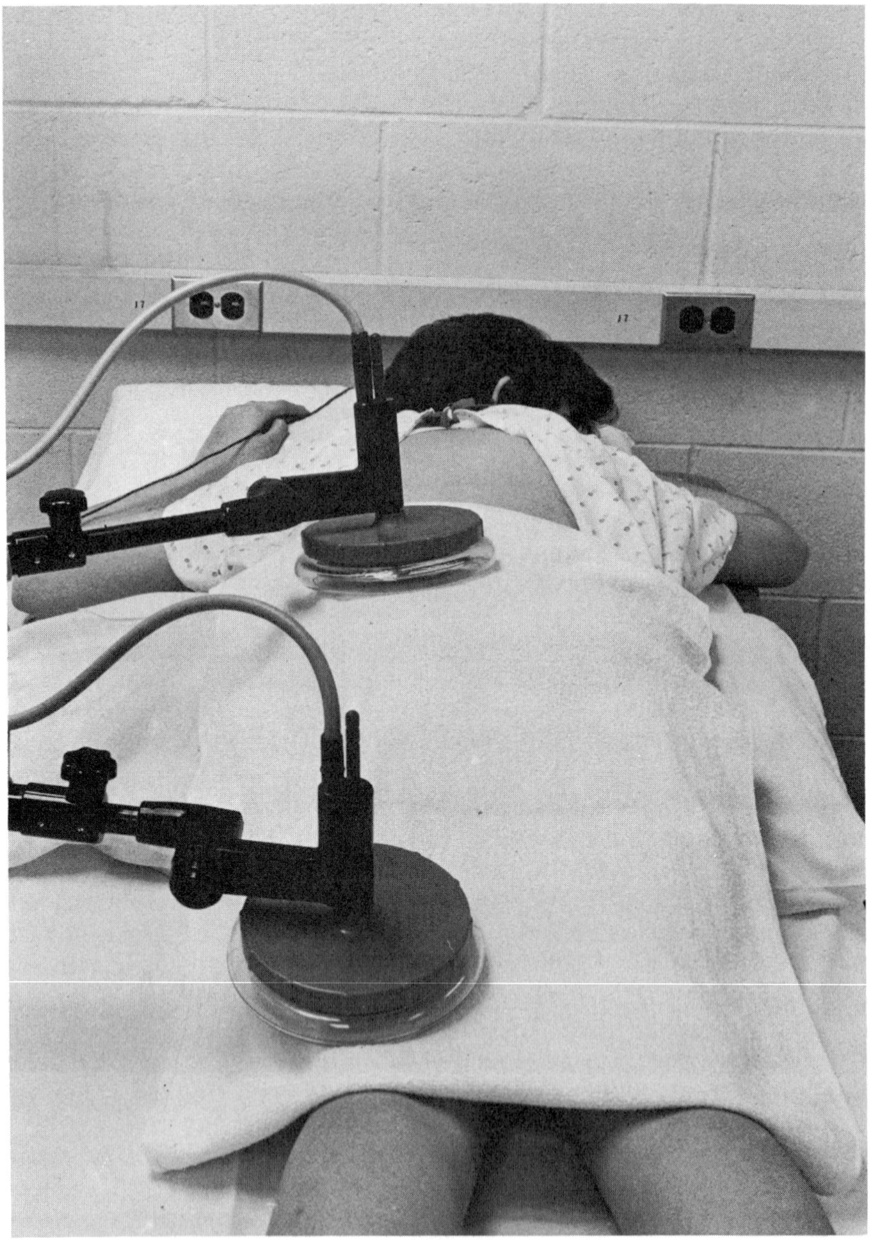

FIGURE 8–15

Capacitive shortwave diathermy using air-spaced plates. Electrode is positioned to give mild heat to musculature of left low back and posterior thigh. Toweling is to absorb perspiration and drape patient.

may also apply to subacute or chronic epicondylitis, for which mild heating from diathermy may assist in reabsorption of inflammatory exudates.

Mild heating from SWD may be used in recurring inflammatory conditions to improve blood flow and facilitate diffusion of oxygen and metabolite clearance.[13] Lehmann[13,42] advocates the use of SWD to induce mild heating (that which produces a mild physiologic response) in the latter stages of traumatic arthritis, chronic pelvic inflammatory disease, epicondylitis, degenerative joint disease, ankylosing spondylitis, and other chronic arthritic conditions.

Reflex or consensual heating of a body part (such as an extremity) is achieved by applying the source of heat proximal to the site of vascular occlusion. If this approach is used in peripheral arterial insufficiency, it avoids the potential for overheating tissues that are poorly vasculated and are therefore incapable of adequately dissipating direct applications of heat. It is not known whether improved deep collateral circulation occurs with this method, in addition to the reflex dilation of skin blood vessels that is evoked.[19]

Shortwave techniques may be used for selective heating of pelvic organs in chronic inflammatory pelvic diseases. According to Lehmann,[13] this treatment produces a significant increase in vascularity and blood flow with the result that cardiac output is increased in the female. As a result of the improved vascularity, antibiotic levels to inflamed tissues may be enhanced.

Allberry[43] and Barnett[44] have reported very successful results with shortwave diathermy therapy, in enhancing the drying up of blisters from herpes zoster and in alleviating the associated pain. Both reports emphasized the importance of applying the mild heating within a few days of the onset of rash, or on the first day if possible. Treatment consists of daily 20-minute applications at the level of the involved dorsal root ganglia until pain is decreased or the scabs fall off.

Many scientific attempts have been made to demonstrate the efficacy of pulsed shortwave diathermy for therapeutic purposes. Some studies[45,46] have shown that the benefits of heat produced in deep tissues with pulsed and continuous SWD have similar therapeutic value. In one of these, Pasila and associates[46] compared two pulsating SWD machines with a placebo in the treatment of 300 ankle and foot sprains. In measurements of strength, joint range of movement, swelling, impairment of gait, and function of disability, they found little significant difference between the placebo group and those treated with pulsed SWD.

Wilson,[47,48] on the other hand, has demonstrated that pulsating SWD reduced pain and disability in several acute ankle sprains significantly better than did continuous wave SWD treatment. The results of this study are shaded by the fact that lower frequencies were used for the pulsed shortwave diathermy than for the continuous shortwave diathermy.

Other claims related to pulsed diathermy have been published, especially those done with animal models.[49–53] Pulsed electromagnetic energy to nerve-damaged rats resulted in quicker regeneration as well as earlier wound healing compared with results from a control group, according to

Wilson and associates.[49] They also noted considerably more scarring and fibrosis around the nerve suture site for the control group. There is insufficient evidence at present that pulsed diathermy has therapeutic nonthermal benefits.[17]

Hyperthermia in Oncology

Hyperthermia induced by diathermy for treatment of cancer is undergoing clinical investigation at present. Moderate elevation of tissue temperature surrounding a tumor may accelerate the rate of growth of the tumor[54] and cause metastasis. At higher temperatures, malignant cells are thermolabile, and they are killed when exposed to temperatures above 42°C.[54] SWD and MWD are effective in treating certain human neoplasms (with hyperthermia), either as single agents or synergistically with ionizing radiation.[55–57] Several investigators[40,58–59] have successfully used the microwave frequency of 433.92 MHz in oncologic hyperthermia studies because of its ability to penetrate fat and muscle and heat at depths of 10 cm.[40,59–60]

Unfortunately, treatment of cancer with microwave or shortwave diathermy is not without iatrogenic side effects that may be manifested as blistering of skin, fat layer burns, and tumor necrosis.[55] The prevention of complications such as these require coordinated health team care and careful planning in selecting diathermy for treatment of the cancer patient. Because physical therapists are familiar with shortwave and microwave diathermy, they may be valuable resources to oncologists who perform hyperthermia therapy.

HAZARDS OF SHORTWAVE AND MICROWAVE DIATHERMY

The literature cites numerous potential hazards of non-ionizing radiation, that is, SWD or MWD. Hazards may result from high levels of unintended exposures to tissues or materials inside the patient's body, adjacent to the patient, or adjacent to the therapist applying the treatment.

Treatment Precautions and Contraindications

Foremost among the potential hazards to be considered for both SWD and MWD are *internal and externally worn metallic objects and electromedical devices.* Neither SWD nor MWD should be applied over surgical metal implants or tissues containing other foreign metallic objects, because focusing of field lines causes excessive charge accumulation on the surface of the metal and raises its surface temperature, resulting in transfer of excessive heat that may burn adjacent tissues.[7,13,17] Women with metallic intrauterine devices should not receive SWD or MWD to the lumbar, pelvic, or abdominal areas.[61–62] Likewise, externally worn metallic items (jewelry and zippers, for instance) should be removed and placed outside the electromagnetic field during SWD or MWD treatment.[24] Metal objects within the immediate treatment area (such as metal in the treatment table, chairs, or swivel stools) should be removed.

In addition to biologic hazards, electromagnetic interference (EMI) may cause disturbances in the function of electromedical or other devices. Wristwatches, other radio-frequency (RF) devices, diagnostic medical equipment (that is, electroencephalographs, electrocardiographs, and electromyographs), cardiac pacemakers, percutaneous electrical nerve/muscle stimulators, electrophrenic pacers, and cerebellar and urinary bladder stimulators[13,63,64] may malfunction when either SWD or MWD is applied in their immediate vicinity. Unpleasant paresthesias or burning sensations may occur beneath percutaneous electrodes that connect the device to the patient, whether the device is in operation or not. Therefore, therapists should avoid directing electromagnetic fields over or near externally worn or implanted electronic devices, their lead wires, or their electrodes.

A prime concern regarding EMI is that diathermy devices (SW more than MW) transmit high-frequency, high-voltage electric and magnetic field energy into and in the vicinity of the patient. The EMI may cause a cardiac pacemaker to stop pacing, revert to a prefixed rate, or to pace rapidly and erratically, if the pacemaker wearer comes within 4.5 meters of a SW device in operation.[7] Secondary to the induced malfunction, the patient's cardiac rhythm may revert to asystole or ventricular fibrillation. Improvements in pacemaker engineering and design have reduced its susceptibility to electromagnetic fields and have even eliminated this problem in some pacemakers.[64] However, it behooves the therapist to place adequate warning signs outside the area where diathermy treatments are being given and to select another nonelectromagnetic thermal agent to treat the patient who is equipped with a cardiac pacemaker.

Specific tissues or anatomic structures that may be adversely affected by SWD or MWD include high–fluid volume areas (such as the eyes and fluid-filled joints); testes; space-occupying lesions; ischemic, hemorrhagic, malignant, and acutely inflamed tissues; as well as sensory-impaired skin.

Areas of the body that contain *a high fluid volume, such as the eye,*[25,42,65–70] *a joint effusion,*[13,72] *moist wound dressings or moist clothing,*[13] *or accumulations of excessive perspiration*[24] will also focus field lines, because of the higher dielectric constant and conductivity of isolated body fluids in comparison to surrounding tissues. The same focusing effect applies to blood vessels that run through adipose tissue. The potential for overheating of the fluids in each case from charge accumulation at the fluid-tissue interface may result in thermal necrosis of adjacent tissues. Terrycloth toweling used with all SWD applicators absorbs surface perspiration, and wide spacing between skin and air-spaced applicators helps to minimize the risk of excessive heating of surface moisture.

When moisture is present in copious amounts, such as occurs in moist wounds or wounds packed with moist dressings, diathermy should not be applied in a manner that would allow energy absorption and selective heating of the moisture.

The high fluid volume of the eye makes it susceptible to selective absorption of unintended or accidental doses of energy from either SWD[65] or MWD.[66] Daily[66,67] and Richardson and co-workers[68,69] have demonstrated that cataracts can develop in the eyes of experimental animals exposed to microwaves. Consequently, exposure of the eye to MWD should be avoided, even though no human studies have reported cataract development or other damage due to diathermy exposure. If SWD is to be applied to the maxillary sinuses of a person wearing contact lenses, the lenses should be removed before treatment to avoid a concentration of field energy that could cause excessive heating of the ciliary body.[70]

The synovial joint that has accumulated an excess of fluid from effusion may also pose a hazard if the temperature of the fluid is raised a few degrees. Intra-articular temperature of normal synovial joints ranges between 30°C and 31°C.[71] Harris and McCroskery[72,73] have demonstrated in vitro that an increase of 5°C produced a fourfold increase in enzymatic lysis of human cartilage by rheumatoid synovial collagenase. Feibel and Fast[74] point out that the intra-articular temperature in knees with rheumatoid arthritis is about 36.5°C and that this increased temperature may accelerate destruction of cartilage. Based on this knowledge, therapists should use caution when considering whether mild, vigorous, or no heating from diathermy is appropriate for the patient who has an inflamed joint condition.

Lehmann and associates[42] suggest that exacerbation of acutely inflamed, fluid-filled joint cavities may occur as a result of selective heating by vigorous treatment using SWD or MWD when the joint is covered by a thin soft tissue layer.

Vigorous heating should be avoided in *acute inflammatory processes* because of the potential for causing tissue necrosis by imposing an inflammatory reaction on an existing acute inflammatory process.[42] Likewise, vigorous heating of tissue adjacent to a space-occupying lesion, such as a protruded nucleus pulposus, may exacerbate symptoms by increasing swelling and congestion of tissue surrounding the disc lesion.[13,42]

In Chapter 5, it was pointed out that a local application of heat from any source to *ischemic tissue* is hazardous, because the compromised blood flow may not meet the increased metabolic demand placed on the tissues by the thermal energy buildup.[75] Lehmann and colleagues[13] have indicated that the time-rate of change of temperature for vascularized tissues treated with SWD should range between 0.8°C and 2.7°C per minute, achieving a critical temperature of 44°C within 10 minutes. This would correspond to absorbed power densities of 50 to 170 W/kg.

To avoid rapid temperature increase in tissues with compromised blood flow, the power density and time-rate of temperature increase should be adjusted to avoid possible tissue necrosis. An alternative method using SWD that avoids potential damage to tissues with arterial insufficiency is to apply the treatment proximal to the area of occluded circulation. This may evoke a consensual increase in distal blood flow owing to reflex vasodilation in the involved area.[76,77] The magnitude of the consensual effect is dependent upon the size of the local area heated. The greater the area heated, the greater the consensual response.[75]

Since an increase in tissue temperature increases blood flow owing to dilation of arterioles, neither SWD nor MWD should be used to treat individuals who are *predisposed to hemorrhage,* such as patients with hemophilia, since the increase in blood flow secondary to the induced vasodilation would potentiate the tendency to bleed.[17,42]

Individuals with *pain and temperature sensory deficits* may be unable to appreciate thermal changes applied to their skin. Since dosage depends on the patient's ability to determine when heat sensation is just comfortably warm, only mild to moderate doses (based on the therapist's knowledge of previous output settings) should be applied in these situations. The patient's condition and the equipment should be checked frequently by the therapist.

Animal studies have demonstrated deleterious effects of MWD on gonad structure and function.[78–80] While the *testicles* and ovaries in humans are generally considered to be sensitive to temperature rise, the testicles (because of their superficial location) are more susceptible to stray radiation than are the ovaries. Therefore, unnecessary exposure of the testes to SWD and MWD should be avoided.[81]

Diathermy should not be applied to the *low back, abdominal, or pelvic regions of pregnant women,* because of the possibility of causing thermal damage to the fetus.[82] Studies on the effect of SWD and MWD on fetal and embryonic growth and development have demonstrated that anomalies occurred in rat fetuses exposed to 27.12 MHz diathermy[83] and that inhibition of growth and development occurred in chick embryos exposed to 2450 MHz microwaves.[84] In both studies, the observed effects were attributed to hyperthermia. Similar effects induced by MWD and SWD on human subjects have not been documented. Case study reports by Rubin and Erdman[85] indicate that MWD exposures of 2450 MHz at 100 W output were given to four women being treated for chronic pelvic inflammatory disease. All four women were either already pregnant or became pregnant during the time of the treatment session, and none experienced any interference with ovulation, conception, or pregnancy. Daels[86] reported no adverse effects in a 1-year followup study of children whose mothers received MWD treatments during pregnancy.

Although exposure of pregnant laboratory animals to MWD[87] and SWD[83] does cause fetal abnormalities, it is not known whether the fetus in the human can be reached with significant microwave radiation at clinically used intensities. Despite the possibility that amniotic fluid may selectively absorb microwave or shortwave energy, there are no clinical reports in the literature to substantiate whether selective heating of the pregnant uterus does or does not occur during exposure. Based on the finding that temperatures of 39.8°C or more are damaging to the human fetus,[88] Lehmann[13] advises that MWD may be hazardous if administered in a way that would allow "a significant amount of energy" to reach the pregnant uterus, and that SWD should not be administered with vaginal electrodes to pregnant women for the same reason.

When diathermy has been *applied to the lumbosacral region* in menstruating females clinical reports have indicated that *an increase* in *menstrual flow* occurred.[13] The low back area of a female may be treated during the menstrual period, but women should be forewarned that their menstrual flow may increase temporarily following treatment.

With respect to the effect of diathermy on bone, it must be emphasized that because of the reflection properties of MWD it should be applied with *caution over bony prominences* to avoid burning of tissues overlying the bone.[89] In addition, one study states that there is a *potential for disturbing bone growth* in children when SWD creates a significant rise in temperature of the epiphyses.[40]

Animal studies have demonstrated that SWD may either enhance[90] or inhibit[91] bone growth. Therefore, therapists applying SWD to children should be aware that bone is not effectively heated when covered by an adequate thickness of soft tissue[13] and that a disturbance in bone growth will occur only at intensities that produce pain.[13] However, the size of the SWD applicator relative to the size of the child may prevent the device from being applied in a way that avoids superficial bone growth centers.

Concern that the therapist who operates diathermy equipment may receive unintended, hazardous exposure of EM energy is not supported by published reports. Mosely and Davison[92] measured the radiation exposure to physical therapists who use MWD and concluded that exposure is not harmful if reasonable care is taken. Unintended exposure will not occur as long as the therapist is 1 meter away from the treatment surface of an operating MWD applicator.[92] A similar study by Stuchly and colleagues[93] concurs that overexposure to the therapist from shortwave diathermy is possible when the distance between the therapist and the applicator is 20 cm or less.

Other materials and objects that may be hazardous during application of SWD include *certain synthetic substances* such as nylon, foam rubber, and plastics. Objects like pillows, pillow cases, treatment tables, sandbag coverings, and clothing often contain these materials, which are nonconductive. However, it has been reported that a pillow being used by a patient receiving an SWD treatment was charred at areas of contact with or directly adjacent to the induction power cables of an SWD unit.[94] Therapists should avoid potential fire hazards such as this by correct placement of equipment and by keeping cables and electrodes well away from synthetic materials.

SUMMARY

Either shortwave or microwave diathermy may be used to produce a rise in tissue temperature within the therapeutically desirable thermal range of 40°C to 45°C. The depth of penetration and extent of temperature rise depends on wave frequency, the electrical properties of the tissue(s) receiving the EM energy and the type of diathermy applicator used. With these factors in mind, the physical therapist must select the appropriate SWD/MWD applicator that produces a selective thermal increase in the target tissues. Either mild or vigorous heating may be produced. Mild heating is usually desired in acute musculoskeletal conditions, whereas vigorous heating may be needed in chronic conditions.[95]

Subcutaneous tissue and muscle at a depth of 3.0 cm may be selectively heated either by direct-contact MW at 915 MHZ or with deep-field–efficient SW circuitry using capacitive plates at 27.12 MHz. Superficial musculature is selectively heated by SW induction coil applicators at 27.12 MHz.

Prior to applying diathermy, it is imperative that the therapist gather information on the status of the patient's circulatory condition to avoid the risk of accidental tissue burning. It is equally important that the therapist take all precautionary measures mentioned earlier to avoid any unnecessary or unwanted exposure to either the patient or therapist.

REFERENCES

1. D'Arsonval, A: *Sur les effects physiologiques de l'état variable et des courants alternatifs.* Bulletin de la Societe Internationale des Electriciens, April, 1892.
2. D'Arsonval, A: *Action physiologique des courants alternatifs a grande frequence.* Archives d'Electricite Medicale 6:133, 1877.
3. Lehmann, JF, et al: *Comparison of relative heating patterns produced in tissues by exposure to microwave energy at frequencies of 2450 and 900 megacycles.* Arch Phys Med Rehabil 46:307, 1965.
4. Lehmann, JF, et al: *Modification of heating patterns produced by microwaves at the frequencies of 2456 and 900 mc by physiologic factors in the human.* Arch Phys Med Rehabil 46:307, 1965.
5. DeLateur, BJ, et al: *Muscle heating in human subjects with 915 MHz microwave contact applicator.* Arch Phys Med Rehabil 51:147, 1970.
6. Bueche, F: *Principles of Physics.* McGraw-Hill, New York, 1965.
7. Ward, AR: *Electricity Fields and Waves in Therapy.* Science Press, NSW, Australia, 1980.
8. Schwan, HP and Piersol, GM: *The absorption of electromagnetic energy in body tissues. Part I.* Am J Phys Med 33:371, 1954.
9. Schwan, HP and Piersol, GM: *The absorption of electromagnetic energy in body tissues. Part II.* Am J Phys Med 34:425, 1955.
10. Schwan, HP: *Electrical properties of tissues and cells.* Adv Biol Med Phys 5:147, 1957.
11. Lehmann, JF, DeLateur, BJ, and Stonebridge, JB: *Selective muscle heating by shortwave diathermy with a helical coil.* Arch Phys Med Rehabil 50:117, 1969.
12. Guy, AW, Lehmann, JF, and Stonebridge, JB: *Therapeutic applications of electromagnetic power.* Proc Institute of Electrical and Electronic Engineers 62:55, 1974.
13. Lehmann, JF: *Therapeutic Heat and Cold,* ed 3. Williams & Wilkins, Baltimore, 1982.
14. Guy, AW: *Analyses of electromagnetic fields induced in biological tissues by thermographic studies on equivalent phantom models.* IEEE Trans Microwave Theory Tech, Vol MTT-19:205, 1971.
15. Guy, AW: *Electromagnetic fields and selective heating patterns due to a rectangular aperature source in direct contact with bilayered biological tissue.* IEEE Trans Microwave Theory Tech, Vol MTT-19:214, 1971.
16. Johnson, CC and Guy, AW: *Nonionizing electromagnetic wave effects in biological materials and systems.* Proc Institute of Electrical and Electronic Engineers 66:692, 1972.
17. Lehmann, JF, et al: *Review of evidence for indications, techniques of application, contraindications, hazards and clinical effectiveness for shortwave diathermy.* DHEW/FDA HFA-510, 5600 Fischers Lane, Rockville, MD 20852, 1974.
18. Millard, JB: *Effect of high frequency currents and infra-red rays on the circulation of the lower limb in man.* Ann Phys Med 6:45, 1961.
19. McNiven, DR and Wyper, DJ: *Microwave therapy and muscle blood flow in man.* J Microwave Power 11:168, 1976.
20. Harris, R: *Effect of shortwave diathermy on radio-sodium clearance from the knee joint in the normal and in rheumatoid arthritis.* Phys Med Rehabil 42:241, 1961.

21. Herrick, JF, Jelatis, DG, and Lee, GM: *Dielectric properties of tissues important in microwave diathermy.* Fed Proc 9:60, 1950.

22. Herrick, JF and Krusen, FH: *Certain physiologic and pathologic effects of microwaves.* Electrical Engineers 72:239, 1953.

23. Saito, M and Schwan, HP: *The time constants of pearl-chain formation: Biological effects of microwave radiation.* Proc Fourth Ann Triservice Conf Biol Effects of Microwave Radiation 1:85, Plenum Press, New York, 1961.

24. Griffin, JE and Karselis, TC: *Principles of Instrumentation.* In Griffin, JE and Karselis, TC: *Physical Agents for Physical Therapists,* ed 2. Charles C Thomas, Springfield, IL, 1982.

25. Shortwave Diathermy Units, Health Devices, 175, June, 1979.

26. Engel, JP, et al: *The effects of microwaves on bone and bone marrow and adjacent tissues.* Arch Phys Med Rehabil 31:453, 1950.

27. Hall, EL: *Diathermy generators.* Arch Phys Med Rehabil 33:28, 1952.

28. Pätzold, J: *Physical laws regarding distribution of energy for various high frequency methods applied in heat therapy.* Ultrasonics Bio Med 2:58, 1956.

29. Guy, AW and Lehmann, JF: *On the determination of an optimum microwave diathermy frequency for a direct contact applicator.* Institute of Electrical and Electronic Engineers Trans Biomed Eng 13:76, 1966.

30. Kantor, G and Witters, DM: *The performance of a new 915 MHz direct contact applicator with reduced leakage—a detailed analysis.* HHS Publication (FDA) S3-8199, April, 1983.

31. Rae, JW, Herrick, JF, Wakim, KG, and Krusen, FH: *A comparative study of the temperature produced by MWD and SWD.* Arch Phys Med Rehabil 30:199, 1949.

32. Worden, RE, et al: *The heating effects of microwaves with and without ischemia.* Arch Phys Med Rehabil 29:751, 1948.

33. Richardson, AW, et al: *The relationship between deep tissue temperature and blood flow during electromagnetic irradiation.* Arch Phys Med Rehabil 31:19, 1950.

34. Leden, UM, et al: *Preliminary studies on the heating and/or effects of microwaves-''radar.''* Br J Phys Med 10:177, 1947.

35. Witters, DM and Kantor, G: *An evaluation of microwave diathermy applicators using free space electric field mapping.* Phys Med Biol 26:1099, 1981.

36. Lehmann, JF, et al: *Microwave therapy: stray radiation, safety and effectiveness.* Arch Phys Med Rehabil 60:578, 1979.

37. Kantor, G: *Evaluation and survey of microwave and radio frequency applicators.* J Microwave Power (2) 16:135, 1981.

38. Thom, H: *Introduction to Shortwave and Microwave Therapy,* ed 3. Charles C Thomas, Springfield, IL, 1966.

39. Schliephake, E: *Carrying out treatment.* In Thom, H: *Introduction to Shortwave and Microwave Therapy,* ed 3. Charles C Thomas, Springfield, IL, 1966.

40. Paliwal, BR, et al: *Heating patterns produced by 434 MHz erbotherm UHF69.* Radiology 135:511, 1980.

41. Warren, CG, Lehmann, JF, and Koblanski, JN: *Heat and stretch procedures: An evaluation using rat tail tendon.* Arch Phys Med Rehabil 57:122, 1976.

42. Lehmann, JF, Warren, CG, and Scham, SM: *Therapeutic heat and cold.* Clin Orthop 99:207, 1974.

43. Allberry, J: *Shortwave diathermy for herpes zoster.* Physiotherapy 60:386, 1974.

44. Barnett, M: *SWD for herpes zoster.* Physiotherapy 61:217, 1975.

45. Silverman, DR and Pendleton, L: *A comparison of the effects of continuous and pulsed shortwave diathermy on peripheral circulation.* Arch Phys Med 49:429, 1968.

46. Pasila, M, Visuri, T, and Sundholm, A: *Pulsating shortwave diathermy: value in treatment of recent ankle and foot sprains.* Arch Phys Med Rehabil 59:383, 1978.

47. Wilson, DH: *Treatment of soft-tissue injuries by pulsed electrical energy.* Br Med J 2:269, 1972.

48. Wilson, DH: *Comparison of shortwave diathermy and pulsed electromagnetic energy in treatment of soft-tissue injuries.* Physiotherapy 60:309, 1974.

49. Wilson, DH, et al: *The effects of pulsed electromagnetic energy on peripheral nerve regeneration.* Ann NY Acad Sci 238:575, 1975.

50. Nadasdi, M: *Inhibition of experimental arthritis by athermic pulsating shortwaves in rats.* Orthopedics 2:105, 1960.

51. Fenn, JE: *Effect of pulsed electromagnetic energy (diapulse) on experimental hematomas.* Can Med Assoc J 100:251, 1969.
52. Cameron, BM: *Experimental acceleration of wound healing.* Am J Ortho 3:336, 1961.
53. King, DR, Hathaways, JW, and Reynolds, DC: *The effect of pulsed shortwaves on alveolar healing.* The Journal—District of Columbia Dental Society, 43:15, 1968.
54. Overgaard, J: *Effects of hyperthermia on malignant cells in vivo: A review and hypothesis.* Cancer 39:2637, 1977.
55. Luk, KH, et al: *The use of 2450 megahertz of microwave in cancer therapy.* Phys Ther 59:405, 1979.
56. Antich, PP, et al: *Selective heating of cancerous tumors at 27.12 MHz.* IEEE Trans Microwave Theory Tech 26:569, 1978.
57. Kim, JH, et al: *Local tumor hyperthermia in combination with radiation therapy.* Cancer 40:161, 1977.
58. Petrowicz, O, et al: *Experimental studies on the use of microwaves for the localized heat treatment of the prostate.* J Microwave Power 14(2):167, 1979.
59. Hornback, NB, et al: *Radiation and microwave therapy in the treatment of advanced cancer.* Radiology 130:459, 1979.
60. Holt, JAG: *The use of V.H.F. radiowaves in cancer therapy.* Australas Radiol 19:1975.
61. Sandler, B: *Heat and the U.U.C.D.* Br Med J 25:458, 1973.
62. Nielsen, NC, et al: *Heat induction in copper-bearing IUD's during shortwave diathermy.* Acta Obstet Gynecol Scand 58:495, 1979.
63. Jones, SL: *Electromagnetic field interference and cardiac pacemakers.* Phys Ther 56:1013, 1976.
64. Smyth, H: *The pacemaker patient and the electromagnetic environment.* JAMA 227:1412, 1974.
65. Konarska, I and Michniewicz, L: *Shortwave therapy of diseases of the anterior portion of the eye.* Klin Oczna 25:185, 1955.
66. Daily, L, et al: *The effects of microwave diathermy on the eye.* Am J Ophthalmol 33:1241, 1950.
67. Daily, L Jr, et al: *Influence of microwaves on certain enzyme systems in the eye.* Am J Ophthalmol 34:1301, 1951.
68. Richardson, AW, Duane, TH, and Haines, HM: *Experimental lenticular opacities produced by microwave irradiation.* Arch Phys Med 29:765, 1948.
69. Richardson, AW, et al: *The role of energy, pupillary diameter and alloxan diabetes in the production of ocular damage by microwave irradiations.* Am J Ophthalmol 35:993, 1952.
70. Scott, BO: *Effect of contact lenses on shortwave field distribution.* Br J Ophthalmol 40:696, 1956.
71. Hollander, JL, et al: *Joint temperature measurement in evaluation of antiarthritic agents.* J Clin Invest 30:701, 1951.
72. Harris, ED Jr and McCroskery, PA: *Influence of temperature and fibril stability on degradation of cartilage collagen by rheumatoid synovial collagenase.* N Engl J Med 290:1, 1974.
73. Harris, ED (ed): *Rheumatoid Arthritis.* MEDCOM Press, New York, 1974.
74. Feibel, H and Fast, H: *Deepheating of joints: A reconsideration.* Arch Phys Med Rehabil 57:513, 1976.
75. Fischer, C and Solomon, S: *Physiological responses to heat and cold.* In Licht, S (ed): *Therapeutic Heat and Cold.* Elizabeth Licht, New Haven, 1958.
76. Abramson, DI: *Physiologic basis for the use of physical agents in peripheral vascular disorders.* Arch Phys Med Rehabil 46:216, 1965.
77. Wise, CS: *The effect of diathermy on blood blow.* Arch Phys Med Rehabil 29:17, 1948.
78. Ely, TS, et al: *Heating characteristics of laboratory animals exposed to ten centimeter microwaves.* US Navy Med Res Inst (Res Rep Proj NM 001-156.13.02) IEEE Tran Biomed Eng 11:123, 1964.
79. Gorodetskaya, SF: *The effect of centimeter radio waves on mouse fertility.* Fiziol Zh 9:394, 1963.
80. Imig, CJ and Free, JR: *Testicular degeneration as a result of microwave irradiation.* Proc Soc Exp Biol Med 69:382, 1948.
81. Van Demark, WR and Free, JR: *Temperature effects.* In Johnson, AD, et al (eds): *The Testis,* Vol 3. Academic Press, New York, 1973.

82. Smith, DW, Clarren, SK, and Harvey, MAS: *Hyperthermia as a possible teratogenic agent.* J Pediatr 92:878, 1978.

83. Dietzel, F: *Effects of non-ionizing electromagnetic radiation on the development and intrauterine implantation of the rat.* In Tyler, AE (ed): *Biological Effects of Nonionizing Radiation.* Ann NY Acad Sci 247:367, 1975.

84. Van Ummersen, CA: *The effect of 2450 mc radiation on the development of the chick embryo.* In Peyton, MF (ed): *Biological Effects of Microwave Radiation,* Vol 1. Plenum Press, New York, 1961.

85. Rubin, A and Erdman, WJ: *Microwave exposure of the human female pelvis during early pregnancy and prior to conception.* Am J Phys Med 38:219, 1959.

86. Daels, J: *Microwave heating of the uterine wall during parturition.* J Microwave Power 11:166, 1976.

87. Rugh, R, et al: *Are microwaves teratogenic?* In Czerski, P, et al (eds): *Biological Effects and Health Hazards of Microwave Radiation.* Polish Med Pub, Warsaw, 1974.

88. Harvey, MAS, McRorie, MM, and Smith, DW: *Suggested limits of exposure in the hot tub and sauna for the pregnant woman.* Canadian Medical Association Journal 125:50, 1981.

89. Lehmann, JF: *Diathermy.* In Krusen, FH (ed): *Handbook of Physical Medicine and Rehabilitation.* WB Saunders, Philadelphia, 1966.

90. Doyle, JR and Smart, BW: *Stimulation of bone growth by shortwave diathermy.* J Bone Joint Surg 45-A:15, 1963.

91. Hutchinson, WJ and Burdeaux, BD: *The effects of shortwave diathermy on bone repair.* J Bone Joint Surg 33-A:155, 1951.

92. Mosely, H and Davison, M: *Exposure of physiotherapists to microwave radiation during microwave diathermy treatment.* Clinical Physics and Physiological Measurement No 3, 2:217, 1981.

93. Stuchly, MA, et al: *Exposure to the operator and patient during shortwave diathermy treatments.* Health Physics 42:341, 1982.

94. Progress Report American Physical Therapy Association, June, 1980.

95. Kloth, LC, Morrison, M, and Ferguson, B: *Therapeutic microwave and shortwave diathermy—a review of thermal effectiveness, safe use, and state-of-the-art—1984.* Center for Devices and Radiological Health, DHHS, FDA 85-8237, December, 1984.

CHAPTER 9

LOW-POWER LASER: ITS APPLICATIONS IN PHYSICAL THERAPY

LAURENCE M. SEITZ, M.S., R.P.T., AND
JOSEPH A. KLEINKORT, M.A., P.T.

Laser is an acronym for *l*ight *a*mplification by *s*timulated *e*mission of *r*adiation.[1] Radiation is the process by which energy is propagated through space.[2] The common characteristics of all forms of radiant energy are as follows: (1) They are produced by applying electrical and other forces to various forms of matter; (2) they all may be transmitted without the support of a sensible medium; and (3) their velocity of travel is equal in a vacuum but varies with different media. Their direction of propagation is normally a straight line; they undergo reflection, deflection, and absorption by the media. They are designated collectively as electromagnetic radiations. A laser is generally used as a source or generator of radiation.[3] Low-power laser is utilized in physical rehabilitation for pain control and soft tissue healing.

The objectives of this chapter are to (1) establish a basic understanding of the physical principles of therapeutic laser; (2) delineate the differences between low- and high-power laser as therapeutic modalities; (3) present the clinical application of laser in physical therapy for wound healing and pain management; and (4) discuss the contraindications, precautions, and guidelines for the safe and effective use of laser in physical therapy.

BACKGROUND

One must understand how laser is produced and what makes it unique from other forms of light before its use as a therapeutic agent is to be discussed. Einstein[4,5] proposed the concept of stimulated emission as it related to the atom and its component parts. Einstein reasoned that a stimulus can cause the electron configuration of an atom to be momentarily rearranged. In returning to its original configuration, surplus energy will be released in the form of a photon, the basic unit of light. This massless particle, in turn, can release a photon from every pre-excited atom or molecule with which it collides. A chain reaction is initiated and the stimulated emission of radiation occurs.[4]

Beginning in 1953, an interest in stimulated emission reappeared with the advent of microwave amplification.[5,6] Microwave radiations are wavelengths that possess optical properties; that is, they can be refracted, diffracted, and reflected and can be focused by suitable lenses.[2] With the development of masers (*m*icrowave *a*mplifiers by the *s*timulated *e*mission of *r*adiation), speculation arose concerning the possibility of extending this principle into amplification and generation in the region of visible radiation.

Schawlow and Townes presented the feasibility of producing stimulated emission in the microwave wavelength area near the optical regions of the spectrum.[7] Their paper, considered to be the impetus for the initial discoveries of all types of lasers, turned out to be surprisingly accurate in predicting the size, wavelength range, and output power for typical gas lasers having moderate input power excitation requirements.[8] (However, it did not propose the use of a gas discharge for excitation of atomic components.[9])

Two years later, Maiman successfully produced the first working model of the ruby laser.[6] Javan, Bennett, and Herriott discovered the helium-neon (HeNe) laser in the fall of 1960.[6] The discovery of visible red laser output at 632.8 nanometers (nm) by White and Rigden occurred in early 1962.[10] This work generated interest in other possible applications for the laser that were in the infrared, nonvisible emission, range.[9]

PHYSICAL PRINCIPLES

When a photon, or energy particle of light, is directed at an atom, it may be absorbed, reflected, or transmitted. If the particle is reflected or transmitted, no light energy change occurs. However, if the photon is absorbed, energy in the orbital electrons is increased. One or more electrons undergo a positional change from an inner orbit to a more outer orbit. The affected atom will have gained energy and is then said to be "excited."[9]

Excited atoms are unstable and will seek their ground state in random fashion, after a short time without further external stimulation. This phenomenon produces spontaneous emission of light. This process, if allowed to reach its end, will prevent the energy transfer level necessary for laser radiation. If, however, a photon of appropriate energy strikes an atom while it is maintained in an excited state, the atom is immediately stimulated to emit its excess energy and make its transition to the ground state. This process is called stimulated emission. The emitted photon is an amplification of stimulating radiation[9] (Fig. 9–1). Laser is electromagnetic energy that is within the visible and infrared regions of the electromagnetic spectrum (Fig. 9–2).

In a laser, when electrons are stimulated by an external power source at a rapid rate, resultant photons are aligned in a reflecting chamber. When they hit a semipermeable silver resonating mirror, the photons are reflected back to a reflecting mirror. The back-and-forth reflection of photons be-

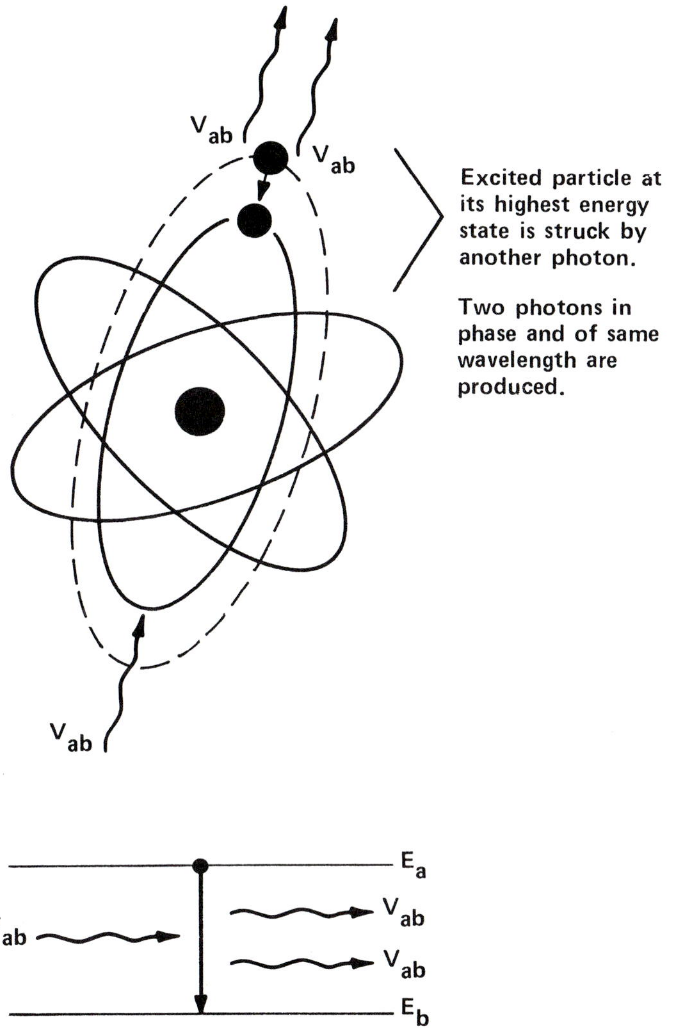

FIGURE 9–1

The principle of stimulated emission. Two photons are emitted from orbit when another photon strikes. E_a, E_b = electrons; V_{ab} = energy of photons.

tween the two mirrors through the laser medium further amplifies the light (Fig. 9–3). This process continues as more and more photons are stimulated, until the chamber cannot contain the energy level. Photons are then ejected through the semipermeable mirror and out a fiber optic cable. The fiber optic is a thread-like filament composed of glass that guides the stimulated photons by directing them to the surface to be treated. As photons pass through the cylindrical stylus, some of the excited atoms in the reflecting chamber begin to revert back to their ground state. This previously mentioned process of spontaneous emission creates a lower intensity of emitted photons to the tissue. Another type of laser uses a diode in the applicator tip rather than a fiber optic.

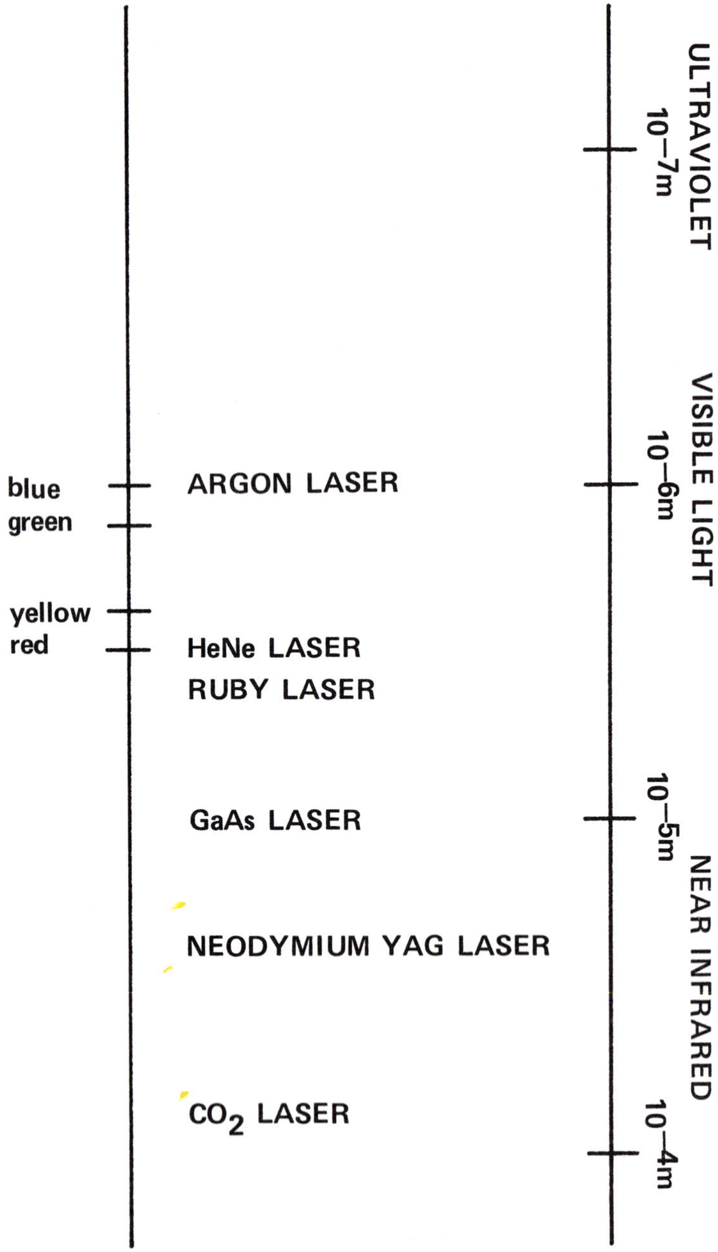

FIGURE 9–2

The visible light and infrared portions of the electromagnetic spectrum (EMS). Some different types of lasers are placed in their approximate location on the EMS.

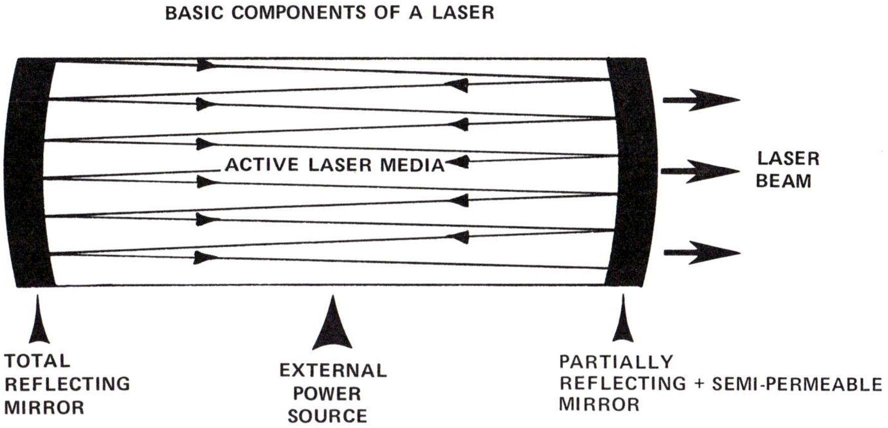

FIGURE 9–3
Basic components of laser.

Basic Components of Laser

There are three properties of the laser that distinguish it from incandescent and fluorescent light sources: coherence, monochromaticity, and a collimated beam.

The property of *coherence* denotes several things. All of the photons of light emitted from individual gas molecules are of the same wavelength. The individual light waves are locked in step with one another. Having the same phase, waves are said to be temporally coherent. Last, they are all traveling in the same direction; this is called *spatial coherence* (Fig. 9–4).

When light is spatially coherent, it can be focused to a very small spot by a lens. Sunlight is spatially coherent and should never be looked at directly. Since light from a laser is similarly coherent, possible damage to the eyes can occur if that light is focused by the lens of the eye onto a small retinal spot.[11]

Monochromaticity refers to the specificity of light in a single, defined wavelength, which gives it added purity not found in most light sources. If this specificity is in the visible spectrum, it is of a single color. For example, helium-neon (HeNe) produces a red light. A laser is one of the few light sources that produces a specific wavelength. The shorter the wavelength, the greater the purity of the light. HeNe has a 632.8 nm wavelength. Gallium arsenide (GaAs) has a wavelength of 910 nm.

The laser beam is well *collimated.* There is minimal divergence or moving apart of the photons.

Power is the rate at which energy is being produced and is measured in watts (joules/sec) or as a lower power such as milliwatt (mW) or 10^{-3} watts (W). If the laser produces one pulse per second, its average power, the amount of energy transferred in 1 second, would be 0.001 joule/1 sec = 0.001 W or 1 mW. When the average power of a laser is 1 mW or lower,

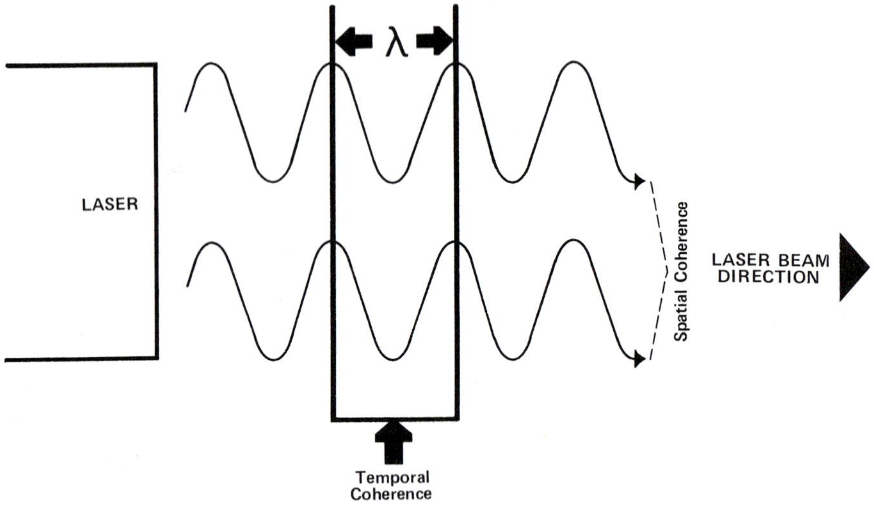

FIGURE 9–4

Coherence—The laser is highly coherent in temporal and spatial planes.

it is called a low-power or "cold" laser.[11] Sometimes it may be referred to as a low-energy or soft laser, as well.

Dosage is equal to the total energy delivered. Therefore, it is equal to the average power multiplied by the time. When using a HeNe laser such as the Dynatron 1120, in a chopped or pulsed mode, its average power would be 0.45 mW.

Power density describes the concentration of power in a particular area. It is determined by power divided by area. Therefore, a 1-mW laser source distributed over a 1-cm^2 area has a power density of 1 milliwatt per square centimeter (1 mW/cm^2).

When the laser is focused on the epidermis, the amount of energy absorbed is proportional to the absorption quality of the tissue. Human epidermis absorbs approximately 99 percent of the laser radiation.[12] Laser energy absorption is greater with darker or pigmented tissues. As tissues are not homogenous, the quality of each structure produces a varying absorption of laser energy. The physiologic variability of the effect on the tissue also depends upon wavelength, energy, and exposure time. This will be elaborated on throughout the chapter.

Classification of Laser

Laser can be classified as high-power or low-power (cold). At present, the most common image of laser radiation and its biologic effects is associated with damaging changes to cells and tissues through its thermal effects. This concept probably originated and was exaggerated by science fiction literature and movies. With the advent of the surgical laser, controlled heating and cutting have become more realistically associated with the device.

The different intensities of lasers are represented by different wavelengths. Tissue responses produced by a high-intensity laser are directly linked to intensity and include five effects: (1) elevation of tissue temperature, (2) dehydration of tissue, (3) coagulation of protein, (4) thermolysis, and (5) evaporation.

The magnitude of thermal reactions produced by high-intensity lasers depends on (1) the absorption, reflection, and transmission of the tissues at the laser wavelength; (2) the power density of the laser beam; (3) the speed of incision or time of exposure; (4) the volume and the velocity of blood flow of local blood vessels; and (5) the degree of tension at the area of incision when cutting is used.[12] Table 9–1 indicates some of the medical uses of high-intensity lasers.

The use of a laser under 1 mW (a "cold" laser) will cause only a nonthermal response. Total optical illumination in this case is limited to less than 1 mW at total peak power or to less than 0.5 mW in a pulsed mode. At this low milliwattage the bright red, in the case of the HeNe laser beam, does not even warm the tissues. Tissue temperature has been measured by Seitz and Kleinkort (unpublished data) using liquid crystal thermography in conjunction with the use of the laser. Photographs taken before, during, and after the application of laser stimulation, at the point of dysfunction, have not demonstrated any indication of change in heat production or thermal variability. However, when laser stimulation was applied at distant acupuncture sites or auricular points, a decrease in temperature (indicating a decrease in inflammation) was demonstrated by thermograms. This is thought to be related to a reflexogenic or autonomic nervous system response. This was hypothesized originally in auricular medicine by Nogier.[13] Interested readers may consult his work for further detail.

Since low-power laser is postulated to stimulate the biologic field around the cell, tissue, and organ, it may be called a biostimulation instrument.[11] This point is further noted in the section of this chapter on Theoretical Considerations. Low-energy laser systems have been used experimentally and clinically to stimulate wound and fracture healing and to

TABLE 9–1
Some Medical Uses of High-Intensity Laser

Laser	Spectrum	Most Frequent Use
CO_2	Invisible	Epithelial dysplasias Surgery: tumor destruction
Argon (skin)	Blue-green	Superficial vascular lesion such as removal of tattoos
Argon (eye)	Blue-green	Diabetic retinopathy
YAG	Invisible	Surgical incision

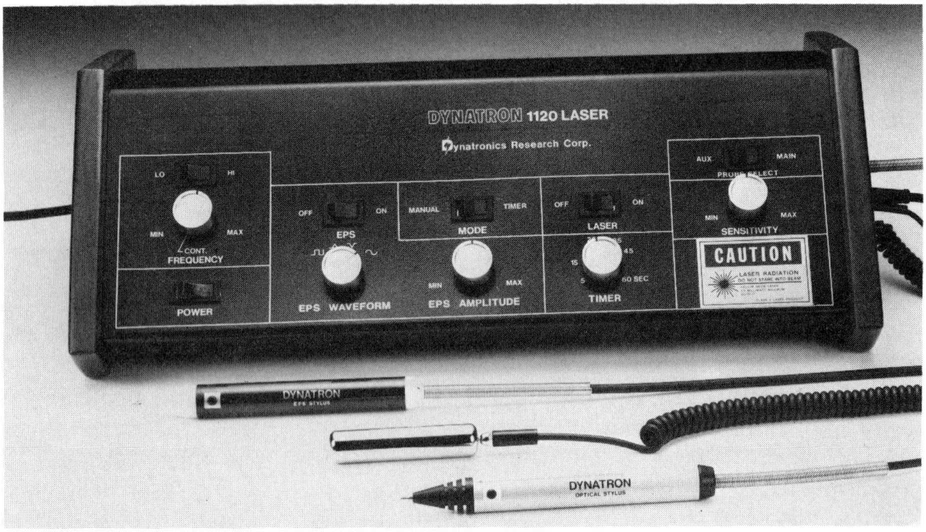

OPERATION OF LASER

Dynatron 1120

1. —Turn power switch on.
   —Turn laser switch on.
   —Select probe switch to main.
   —Select mode switch to timer.
   —Adjust timer to 20 seconds for pain and 30 seconds for tissue healing.
   —Frequency switch should be set on continuous.
   (Note: If the patient is unable to tolerate continuous frequency owing to strength, then you may select a frequency of 2 to 200 Hz. This adjusts the frequency of the pulse of light.)
   —To turn the laser light on, press the button on the wand, and the preadjusted time will maintain the laser for the amount of time set.

2. —To determine low-resistance points in tissue, have the patient hold the inactive electrode in one hand and scan with the laser wand in the other. The only adjustment for this is power on. Then the sensitivity knob may be adjusted depending on the conductance of the tissue. Moist tissue requires minimum sensitivity and dry tissue requires maximum sensitivity.

3. —If low-output (50-500 μa) A.C. stimulation is required, either with laser stimulation or separate, it can be added with adjustment of the EPS section. Turn EPS knob on, adjust the wave form desired: square, positive spike, negative spike, or sine. Then adjust amplitude: minimum is 50 μa and a maximum is 500 μa. This stimulation may be administered either with the main probe or auxiliary probe.

FIGURE 9–5
Dynatron 0.9 mw HeNe laser. (Courtesy of Dynatronics, Salt Lake City, UT.)

obtain analgesic effects. The low-energy systems used include helium-neon and gallium arsenide.

Helium-Neon (HeNe) Laser

Helium-neon laser is produced by a tube with atoms of these two gases (Fig. 9–5). The helium gas is elevated from the ground state to one of two excited states by electrical excitation. These states are a direct result of either stimulated or spontaneous emission. The atoms of the gas are in a vacuum chamber and are stimulated with a special light called a flash gun. The excited levels of the helium atom very closely approximate ground state levels of the neon atom. When an excited helium atom collides with a ground state neon atom, the energy produced is transferred to the latter, and the helium reverts to the ground state.

The wavelength of helium-neon laser is 632.8 nm (within the red band of visible light). It is directed toward the tissue in a pulsed or continuous mode via a fiber optic.[5] The helium-neon depth penetration is up to 0.8 mm directly and from 10 to 15 mm indirectly. Direct penetration refers to the characteristic properties of laser that have not been altered. In indirect penetration, the light is transmitted into the deeper tissues through hyperscopic absorption properties of the surrounding tissue. Once this occurs, the coherent and collimated properties of laser are altered. Therefore, the difference between the two depths is due to the dispersion of light in tissue.

Gallium Arsenide (GaAs) Laser

The first "semiconductor" laser, used in 1962, was the gallium arsenide laser. This laser is housed in a diode (Fig. 9–6). A diode is an electrical component that allows electric current to pass in one direction through the device, offering high electrical resistance in the reverse direction. Using GaAs, upon which has been deposited a thin coating of zinc, a junction diode may be formed. This design allows the current to flow more readily in the direction from the zinc to the GaAs. The laser reaction occurs in this junction region. The energy is delivered in the pulsed mode.

One further difference between the two low-powered lasers is that the indirect depth of tissue penetration of the GaAs output is 5 cm, compared with that of the HeNe laser, which is 10 to 15 mm. GaAs, at a wavelength of 910 nm, is within the infrared or invisible spectrum.

BIOPHYSICAL EFFECTS OF LASER

The investigation into the biologic and physical effects of cold laser radiation is still in its early stages. Some of the preliminary proposed physiologic effects attributed to low-power laser energy include an acceleration in collagen synthesis, an increase in vascularization of healing tissue, a de-

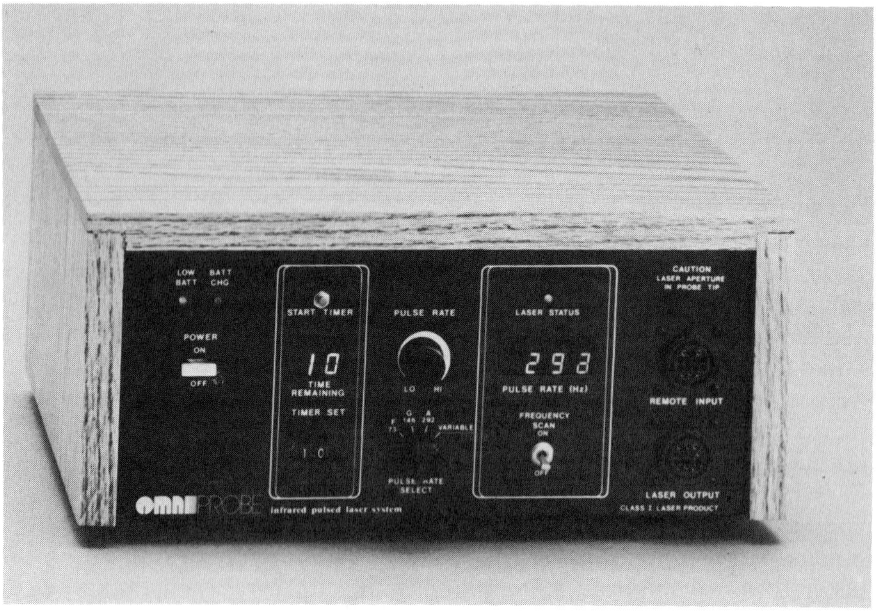

OPERATION OF LASER

Omni Infrared

1. —Turn power switch on.
   —Adjust desired frequency:
      —73 Hz for acute pain or early wound healing.
      —146 Hz for subacute pain or routine wound healing.
      —300 to 1200 Hz for chronic pain or long-term wounds.
         (Note: The authors have found 1000 Hz to be a more effective frequency in the majority of the chronic pain patients.)

2. —Set timer for the desired number of minutes and then press the timer button. The red "laser" light will then come on, indicating that laser is being produced. Since this laser is set at 904 nm, it is is in the infrared range and cannot be seen. The only way to determine if the laser is on is by the red status laser light. You also can determine if the laser is operating by listening for a high-pitched whine from the laser applicator.
   —Frequency scan switch when on will automatically cause the frequency to scan 20% below and above the adjusted setting.
   —The pulse knob is used on variable mode to adjust the frequency from 300 to 1200 Hz.

FIGURE 9–6

Omniprobe 0.9 mw GaAs infrared laser. (Courtesy of Physiotechnology, Inc., Topeka, KS.)

crease in micro-organisms, and pain reduction. Much of the work reported to date is empirical observations, which can serve as a foundation for the design of well-controlled laboratory and clinical studies on the bioeffects of laser irradiation.

Mester,[14] in a reported study of 100 healed clinical cases, showed some of the changes that take place in wound healing when low-power laser was applied. He found that there was a marked increase in collagen formation, as viewed through the electron microscope. He also noted an increase of vasodilation and accelerated DNA synthesis. Castro[15] has shown, however, that after 2 weeks of daily radiation, the collagen synthesis ceases. In the continuation of laser biostimulation, Gamaleya reported on various Russian studies that resulted in (1) the healing of skin grafts in rabbits, (2) regeneration of burns in the skins of rats and mucous membranes of the tongues of mice, (3) the uniting of fractured bones in dogs, (4) the healing of bone defects in rabbits, and (5) bone growth after HeNe laser irradiation.[16]

Yew, Wong, and Chan[17] studied whether there is really an increase of intercellular matrix in the eye, and if so, what is the mechanism of such an increase. Earlier in 1976, the investigators studied the effect of low-dose laser on the histochemical pattern of increases in the para-aminosalicylic acid (PAS)–positive intracellular matrix of mucopolysaccharides located between the pigment epithelium and cells of the retina, following treatment. Their results indicated an increase in the intercellular matrix surrounding the outer segments of the visual cells of the retina. They also noted that the response appeared to be dose dependent; that is, the longer the exposure, the greater the increase. At the same time, an increase in labeled uridine uptake of the pigment epithelium was recorded, indicating a possible increase of RNA production. Such a study may shed some light on the possible use of low-power laser whenever an increase of intercellular matrix would benefit the healing process.

Kovacs, Mester, and Gorog[18] used a HeNe laser of 5 mW power output on the ear chamber of rabbits. They investigated the development of blood vessels that sprouted from the central artery of the ear chamber. Observation was performed using a high-power microscope. According to the results, the development of blood circulation in the growing tissue was significantly increased by laser radiation. The important implication is that low-power laser can assist vascularization after surgery or implantation. Therefore, the laser could accelerate the time of postoperative healing when applied at 5 mW.

Lethal photosensitization of micro-organisms with light of 632.8 nm from a continuous wave gas laser was observed by Macmillan, Maxwell, and Chichester.[19] Eleven strains were examined for their susceptibility to death by irradiation using 21 to 30 mW of light. Washed cells of seven species were rapidly killed when irradiated aerobically in aqueous solutions to toluidine blue. Therefore, an endogenous photosensitizer was not acting at 632.8 nm. None were killed if not suspended in this solution. Although this study used, in theory, a low-dose laser, the power ranges that were used placed it out of the low range and into the high range of power.

Haina and associates[20] reported on stimulation of wound healing by laser light. Their investigations showed that, when using a HeNe laser as a stimulant, the formation of granulation tissues in rats and the epidermal regeneration from thermal defects in guinea pigs were significant. Five series of experiments with applied energy densities of 0.5 joule/cm^2, 1.5 joule/cm^2, 4.0 joule/cm^2, 10 joule/cm^2, and 20 joule/cm^2 were performed at a power density of 50 mW/cm^2. Time was altered at each application but no specific parameters were indicated. They concluded that the beneficial effects of laser therapy in the treatment of slow healing wounds in humans may also be due to promotion of granulation and epithelialization.

Kana and associates[21] undertook a study to determine whether laser radiation of low-power density would affect the healing of open skin wounds in rats. The wounds were irradiated daily with a HeNe laser or argon laser (514.5 nm). The closure of skin defects was practically complete in all animals within eighteen days of treatment. Between the third and 12th postoperative days, the rate of wound closure was significantly accelerated in wounds subjected to a HeNe irradiation of 4 joule/cm^2 daily. No significant acceleration of wound closure was observed after the use of the argon laser. The conclusion is that collagen production in wounds can be increased significantly by HeNe light and not by argon.

In two separate studies, Fine and associates and Goldman and associates[12] studied the effects of laser irradiation on the skin. Using the ruby laser, a lesion was produced on the skin of a pigmented hamster. There was a small central area of less-intense damage similar to a second-degree burn that went on to vesiculate. When a white animal was irradiated, only a mild superficial lesion was produced. However, in the absence of pigmentation, energy was transferred to a deeper level, and the damage produced was much greater.

In a later experiment, Goldman[12] irradiated the skin of a normal white human volunteer with an unfocused 100-joule ruby laser beam. An area of instantaneous, mild erythema was produced that was insensitive to touch. This area persisted for 4 days, at which time a biopsy was performed. Pathologic diagnosis on the excised tissue was "consistent with carcinoma in situ of the skin."

Theoretical Considerations

The Soviet scientist Guravich proposed a theory of the biologic field in which connections between tissues and organs in the intact organism are not limited to the effects of various humors and nervous control mechanisms.[16] Humors are the extracellular fluids of the body (such as blood and lymph).[22] The theory purports that a biologic field exists around every cell, tissue, and organ. Normalizing influences of high structural levels (such as the organism and organ) are exerted on lower levels (such as the tissues and cells).

In the biologic field, a vibratory system exists that responds with maximum amplitude under the action of harmonic force. This phenomenon, called resonance, occurs when the frequency of the applied force is the same as a natural frequency of the vibrating body. Guravich postulated that the resonance of the vibratory bodies is the same as the low-power laser.

In 1923, Guravich discovered mitogenetic radiation.[16] This finding described the weak ultraviolet radiation emitted by the dividing cell during mitosis. The radiation, in turn, stimulated the division of other cells. The significance of this discovery was that mitogenetic division would occur through the equal resonance substitution produced by the low-power laser.

Soviet actinotherapy, as part of physiotherapy, uses light rays of varying wavelengths to evoke a reaction in the organism in a way that produces equal resonance between the organism and the low-power laser. Thus, the applied light sources can attempt to approach the energy characteristics of the organisms' metabolic processes.

According to Inyshin and Chekurov, migration of light energy travels to the organisms' zones of conductance in those conditions that are at present in disharmony and not in the normal or equal resonance of the HeNe laser radiation. Once the laser radiation enters the different parts of the cell that participate in the transmission of wavelengths, a change in the cells' energy level occurs. What results is a restoration of reversal of the organism to its normal physiologic state.[18]

Under very specific conditions, low-power laser systems can produce an inhibition of the stimulation effect within the local cellular area, a general systemic effect, or both. This condition occurs in conjunction with Arndt's law. The law states that "weak stimuli excite physiologic activity, moderately strong ones favor it, strong ones retard it, and very strong ones arrest it."[23] Therefore, this law implies that a minimal amount of therapeutic application of the laser for biostimulation purposes is most conducive to increasing physiologic activity. Hence, a reciprocal relationship exists between the application of laser and the physiologic outcome.

INDICATIONS AND CLINICAL APPLICATION

The indications for the therapeutic use of cold or low-intensity laser can be separated into categories of tissue healing and pain management (acute or chronic).

Tissue Healing

The effectiveness of the laser in wound healing can be most dramatic, and the application techniques are simple. There are basically two different techniques: gridding the wound and surrounding the wound.

To grid a wound, the clinician should imagine a grid or screen over the wound with 1 to 1½ cm^2 open squares. Irradiation of each of these squares should take place for 20 seconds with the HeNe laser and 10 seconds with the use of the GaAs type. If indicated for cleansing and debridement, the whirlpool should be introduced before laser application. One daily application of whirlpool is sufficient and more than this should be discouraged, because the granulation of new tissue may be disrupted. This, in turn, can disturb and retard the time of wound healing. If there is eschar present or the wound is unusually large, one may choose to surround the healthy tissue on the periphery of the wound. Stimulation is then applied every 2 cm^2 for 30 seconds using the HeNe laser and 20 seconds using the GaAs. If the wound is closing from the outside, sterile saline or hydrogen peroxide can be poured into the wound. This fluid is then stimulated for 1 to 2 minutes with the laser. The evidence of effectiveness is based upon the clinical protocol adopted by Seitz and Kleinkort (unpublished data).

Stimulation for wound healing every other day at a frequency of 80 Hz using either the gridding or the surrounding technique is recommended. After approximately 10 to 15 treatments, the therapist may note a drop-off in the rate of healing. When this occurs, treatment should be halted temporarily for 5 days. Finally, treatment shall be reinitiated but at a lower frequency, such as 20 to 40 Hz, and continued until the wound closes.

A specific time course for wound healing has not been clearly defined. Healing time is extremely variable, owing to the specific etiology of a wound, the age and skin color of the patient, and the pre-existing physical condition of the healing site. In general, a wound that is directly related to a poor circulatory bed, such as a diabetic or stasis ulcer, will respond the slowest, whereas a decubitus ulcer will respond quicker. The fastest-healing wound is one that has been caused by surgical intervention or some form of dermatologic eruption. Examples are amputation, open reduction with internal fixation with an orthopedic appliance, herpes simplex, episiotomy incisions, opened acne blemishes, cauterized skin ulcers, and dental surgery.

Following trauma, when the laser was applied immediately to an area where a hematoma might be expected to form, the hematoma usually did not appear. When the laser was applied to a traumatic edema, such as a sprained ankle, a decrease in edema was seen.

The application of laser to a herpes simplex lesion of the mouth also immediately decreased the pain, and resolution of the lesion took place within a day or two.

In the case of tissue healing, if the healing process appears to be slowing down, the therapist should reduce the laser treatment. For such a case, one accomplishes this reduction by lowering the power, which can be achieved by turning a dial. If this approach is ineffective, the patient's weekly sessions should be curbed from three to two times.

PAIN MANAGEMENT

In acute pain management, the application techniques are straightforward. After the area of pain is localized, the laser is applied for 20 seconds with the GaAs laser or 30 seconds with the HeNe unit. The GaAs laser is usually set at a frequency of 73 Hz, and the HeNe is best used in the continuous setting.

CASE STUDY NO. 1

A.F., an 87-year-old Caucasian male, was referred for wound closure at the greater trochanter of the right femur. The patient was a resident of a local nursing home. He had suffered a left cerebral vascular accident 7 months prior to his laser treatment. The patient was mildly confused but very eager to walk again.

The patient was referred to physical therapy in New Jersey by a general surgeon who had been debriding the decubitus ulcer while maintaining the wound free of infection.

The decubitus had been ulcerated for 6 months, without healing, prior to his initial visit to physical therapy. According to family members, the ulcer had enlarged during the 6 months.

The patient was treated for 6 weeks, for a total of 12 treatments, only twice weekly owing to travel constraints. Upon evaluation, the patient had normal and appropriate sensory findings. Range of motion and manual muscle testing at the hip joint were within normal limits.

The patient's ulcer was irrigated with hydrogen peroxide, a mild antiseptic solution. Then, using the grid technique, the wound was irradiated. This procedure continued for approximately 30 minutes, owing to the size of the ulcer. The stimulation occurred over a 2 cm^2 area at a power of 80 Hz for 30 seconds. The initial dimensions were 6.25 cm wide by 2.54 cm deep by 1.27 cm long. At the completion of 6 weeks, the wound was almost totally closed. This procedure was used because it was within the previously selected timeframe and was part of the protocol that had always been successful.

The patient has since begun gait training with no further indication of skin ulcerations.

The use of trigger points or other such body points in conjunction with the painful site can be included when treating the acute patient.

When the laser was applied immediately to an area where a hematoma might form, to a traumatic edema, or to an oral herpes simplex lesion, the pain usually associated with the inflammation was interrupted. The elimination of the anticipated pain, which can be a part of the acute inflammatory process, was managed by the laser. This approach implies an important point for physical therapy intervention. The application of laser, in a specific time period, can assist in the resolution of a pathologic process.

Laser has been used successfully to reduce pain in the chronic state. Many different protocols are used, including direct stimulation over the site of dysfunction or stimulation of associated acupuncture, trigger, or auricular points. Some of the more commonly treated dysfunctions will be discussed in this section.

In the treatment of the patient with pain, different responses have been noted with each laser. The GaAs laser produces a more immediate response than the delayed one of the HeNe laser. This delay can be as long as two or three treatments. Aside from the faster times response to stimulation, the GaAs laser seems to be more effective in acute injuries, whereas the HeNe unit appears to have a latency period for pain relief. Often the patient begins to respond only after two or three treatments. However, once the response occurs, a rather dramatic pain reduction has been noted. In most circumstances, the patient should require no more than 8 to 12 treatments. If no response is forthcoming after four to five sessions, the use of laser is discontinued.

BACK DYSFUNCTION. In pain conditions associated with the vertebral column, four cases when laser may be of benefit have been identified. These include nerve inflammation, muscle guarding spasm, osteophytosis, and facet inflammation.

When there is an inflammatory nerve root without known anatomic impingement, the laser will be directed toward the affected neural foramen. If spasms of the paravertebral musculature are present, a second stimulation site 1 inch lateral from the first stimulated point is added. This second point is stimulated for 30 seconds with HeNe and for 20 seconds with the GaAs. If there is a facet inflammation stimulation should be as close to the site as possible. Equally, with osteophytosis, stimulation should occur as close to the osteophyte as possible.

Numerous patients have been treated who gained range of motion and had a decrease of pain from laser stimulation for osteophytosis. Results have been better in the cervical spine than in the lumbar spine.

For compression fractures of the spine, the technique of surrounding the affected vertebrae is used. This technique has been sufficient for reducing pain, increasing motion, and promoting healing time.

BURSITIS. In the case of trochanteric bursitis, the following approach should be considered. Because this condition is an inflammatory pain syndrome, continuous laser is used. The patient is scheduled for eight to 10 treatments every other day. The patient should notice pain relief by the third to fourth treatment or the laser is discontinued. The area to treat is located by palpating the trochanter. An imaginary grid is formed just distal to the trochanter, about the size of a half dollar. The area is marked in 1 cm^2 sizes. The continuous laser stimulates each of these 1 cm^2 segments within the area distal to the trochanter and tender to palpation for 30 seconds. Usually, after eight to 10 treatments, pain reduction and return to full range of motion will be maximal.

HEADACHE. In the area of headache management, there are as many treatment techniques as there are headaches. In general, laser may be more effective in those patients who are not suffering from a severe episode when examined. The most general and overall effective technique for a variety of headache patients is the corona technique first described by Caspers.[10] This technique is especially effective in the migraine patient. A circumferential technique with the laser is used around the entire head.

ARTHRITIS. Clinical results with laser application to inflammatory joint conditions have proved to be very beneficial. Osteoarthritis and rheumatoid arthritis do well when only one or two joints require radiation. The only exceptions to this observation are in the hand, foot, cervical, and lumbar areas. The typical treatment of a joint is to approach it on all sides. The only time that circumferential exposure appears to be unproductive is when one treats multiple joints in the foot or hand. In this case, irradiation both medially and laterally are sufficient. The times remain the same as previously mentioned.

Goldman and associates[24] undertook a study using 30 people with classic or definite rheumatoid arthritis. They were classified by American Rheumatism Association criteria, 26 having classic and 4 having definite rheumatoid arthritis. There were 25 women and 5 men who ranged in age from 22 to 73 years. Twenty-one patients noted improvement of both their metacarpal phalangeal joints and proximal interphalangeal joints of both hands during laser therapy. Twenty-seven patients noted improvement of their proximal interphalangeal joints, and 26 noted improvement of their metacarpal phalangeal joints during therapy. The improvement was in both hand function and hand activity. The changes were usually bilateral, although more improvement in grip strength and tip pinch, and less erythema and pain were noted on the side treated with laser. Activity levels related to duration of morning stiffness and motion restricted by joint heat, erythema, tenderness, pain, and swelling.

TRIGGER POINTS. Snyder-Mackler and Bork[25] undertook a double-blind study to determine the effect of cold laser on musculoskeletal trigger points. They defined a trigger point as a site that elicits referred pain on deep palpation and demonstrates lowered skin resistance in comparison to surrounding tissue. Thirty patients with musculoskeletal pain were included in the study. Trigger points were treated for three successive treatments. They noted that the patients who received the cold laser treatment demonstrated a significant increase in skin resistance when compared with the control. The difference was $p < 0.05$. They concluded that the results indicated that the increases in skin resistance associated with the resolution of trigger points may be elicited by using cold laser therapy.

OTHER TECHNIQUES OF STIMULATION. Although there are many different protocols that may be used in the application of laser to the chronic pain patient, the simplest is the direct application to the site of physiologic dysfunction. An additional therapeutic approach for pain management with laser may be associated with the stimulation of motor points, trigger points, acupuncture points, auricular points, and meridian balancing techniques. A detailed description of these techniques is beyond the scope of this chapter, but some suggested protocols are outlined in Table 9–2.

PRECAUTIONS AND CONTRAINDICATIONS

Research and safety criteria are necessary for any new therapeutic agent. Investigations on the safety of laser continue in Europe, Russia, and the United States.

Lasers below 1 mW are classified by the Food and Drug Administration (FDA) as a class III medical device. The low-power laser, at the time of this

TABLE 9–2

Suggested Protocol for Laser Application of Trigger Points and Acupuncture Points

Condition	Laser Characteristics	Time	Area
Tendinitis, bursitis	HeNe (cont.) or infrared (1000 pps) (GaAs)	30 sec per pt (HeNe) 20 sec per pt (infrared)	Local area of inflammation 5–10 placements to both areas of inflammation
TMJ syndrome	Same as above Same as above	Same as above	TMJ joint only
TMJ/MPD	Same as above Same as above	Same as above	TMJ joint + St. 6, 7, SI 19, & tai yang.
Cervical or lumbar nerve root radiculopathy	Same as above Same as above	Same as above	At root site 3–4 angles to root, then peripheral points in UE or LE (i.e., B67, 54 [LE]). LI4, H 2.5 (UE).
Arthritis—limit to 1 or 2 joints	Same as above Same as above	Same as above	Bathe joint 10–12 points per large joint; 4–6 per small joint.

Note: There are man, other placements that can be used. This is just an example of what may be done with various diagnoses. Often the use of auricular points are used to augment the treatment.

CASE STUDY NO. 2

K.J. is a 28-year-old Caucasian woman with a 3-year history of severe pain radiating along the distal medial aspect of the upper arm through the medial epicondylar region down the volar aspect of the right forearm. A surgical exploration and median nerve entrapment release were performed.

Postoperatively, she developed a very painful keloid scar at the incision located from the midmedial aspect of the upper arm to the midvolar aspect of the forearm.

Physical therapy evaluation revealed a 20-degree limitation in elbow extension. The scar could not be palpated because of excruciating pain. She presented with painful, contractured forearm flexor muscles. This resulted in a 20-degree wrist flexion contracture.

Treatment was initiated 8 months after surgery. The patient received laser treatments including scar tissue points, web space acupuncture points of the hand, acupuncture large intestine meridian points 4, 10, 11, 12, and multiple auricular points. This was the clinical procedure used based upon previously successful treatments. An appropriate mobilization and exercise program was also initiated to the right upper extremity. She was seen for a total of 10 treatments over a 1-month period. The stimulation occurred over a 2 cm area at a power of 80 Hz for 20 seconds over the keloid surface. The initial dimensions were 1.1 cm wide by 11 cms long. At the conclusion of her treatment time, she was totally asymptomatic of pain and had regained the loss of range of motion in the elbow and wrist. Her scar tissue coloration had turned from a purple-red to nearly normal tissue coloration. The height and breadth of the scar tissue decreased markedly.

writing, is still considered an investigational device and the user should have an investigational device exemption (IDE) under the abbreviated requirements of section 812.2(b)a of the FDA regulations prior to therapeutic intervention with laser. The FDA is concerned not only with safety but also with therapeutic efficacy. The FDA's Center for Devices and Radiological Health now regulates the manufacture and sale of laser products in the United States (US Department of Health, Education and Welfare, 1979). This regulation requires the manufacturer to classify the laser product.

The basic concept of the classification schemes of ANSI, AGGIH, WHO, IEC, and FDA is as follows:

Class I laser products are essentially safe and are typically enclosed systems that do not emit hazardous levels.

Class II laser products are limited to visible lasers that are safe for momentary viewing but should not be stared into continuously unless the exposure limits (ELs) and the dazzle of the brilliant visible light source would normally preclude staring into the source.[12]

Low-power lasers are class II or I laser devices. This means that they are considered an insignificant risk to humans unless held close to the cornea of the eye.

The safety of these devices can further be evaluated by the American National Safety Institute Standard 2-136.1. A review of the maximal permissible emission value of the lasers under 1 mW shows a good margin of safety.[26]

Safety standards for laser aid considerably in hazard analysis and controls. The most prominent standard was first produced in 1973 and has since been revised: American National Standards Institute (ANSI, 1976), Safe Use of Lasers.

A new edition of the ANSI standard was approved in 1980. Several other organizations have followed suit with safety standards that are comparable: the American Conference of Governmental Industrial Hygienists (ACGIH, 1976), the World Health Organization (WHO), and the International Electrotechnical Commission (IEC).

There are some contraindications to which the clinician should adhere. One should refrain from use of laser in the pregnant female. Laser is not used over the unclosed fontanels of children. The use of laser near cancerous lesions should be avoided. Laser should not be radiated directly into the cornea.

Ophthalmologic research has shown that in rabbits, laser levels of 25 mW producing retinal lesions in the continuous wave HeNe laser mode. These lesions were obtained after 2.5 seconds with a rise of temperature at the lesion site of 7.8°C. However, no lesions were present with the use of the 2 or 5 mW lasers.[27]

Lappin[28] has measured ocular damage thresholds for the helium-neon laser in the rhesus monkey. Exposure time of radiation was 2 msec to 10 seconds with peak power of 50 mW. Mean values of the visible damage threshold for power versus time were determined for each eye in the macula and in the extramacula. Approximately 500 exposures were made to determine mean damage threshold levels in 70 eyes for the macula and an extramacula area between the optic disc and the macula. The macula was found to have a lower damage threshold than the extramacula area, the ratio of thresholds decreasing as exposure time is increased. The macula-extramacula threshold ratio varied from about 2:1 at 5 msec to 1.3:1 at 1 second.

Ham and associates studied the retinal burn thresholds for the HeNe laser in the rhesus monkey.[29] They concluded that the data indicated the threshold power for irreversible burn damage in the monkey is about 7 mW at the cornea for the worst case of accidental exposure to HeNe lasers. For this exposure the whole beam entered the eye and was focused on a minimal spot size. Available data indicate that the human retina is less susceptible to thermal damage than is that of the monkey or the rabbit. Until more reliable data are available, the total power of the HeNe laser entering the human eye should be limited to 1 mW or less. This recommendation is based solely upon the irreversible thermal damage to the retina.

CLOSING REMARKS

The use of cold laser by the physical therapist has become a controversial but important area of clinical discussion. Its potentially wide applicability in wound healing and pain modulation adds a new agent for physical therapists. One must fully understand that the low-power laser, at this time, is felt to be a clinical tool for therapeutic purposes and not an instrument of destruction.

There have been numerous articles dating back to the 1960s pertaining to laser application, principally in medicine and surgery. However, only in the past decade have purposeful investigation and clinical testing persisted to assess the efficacy of this modality for use in rehabilitation. Although the actual physiologic mechanisms of therapeutic laser are incompletely understood, there is little doubt that it has a definite role in the profession of rehabilitation.

With every scientific discovery, there is frequently a certain amount of trepidation. The use of the low-power laser as a tool of healing and analgesia is certain to be accompanied by numerous fears. Low-power laser may likely be recognized as an extremely valuable device in the future. The fact that the physical therapist can now investigate with a modality that is aseptic, pain free, and noninjurious to tissues, and that may promote rapid return to functional recovery may create a whole new dimension to the field of rehabilitation.

REFERENCES

1. Kleinkort, JA and Foley, RA: *Laser acupuncture: Its use in physical therapy.* American Journal of Acupuncture 12:51, 1984.
2. Watkins, AL: *A Manual of Electrotherapy.* Lea & Febiger, Philadelphia, 1968, pp 12–15, 24–26, 197–199.
3. Bloom, AL: *Gas Lasers.* John Wiley & Sons, New York, 1971, pp 1–24.
4. Calder, N: *Einstein's Universe.* Greenwich House, New York, 1982, pp 29–30.
5. Goldman, L: *Biomedical Aspects of the Laser.* Springer-Verlag, New York, 1967, pp 1–7.
6. Lengyell, BA: *Lasers-Generation of Lightly Stimulated Emission.* John Wiley & Sons, New York, 1962, pp 1–15, 22–23, 83–99.
7. Kroetlinger, M: *On the use of laser in acupuncture.* International Journal of Acupuncture and Electrotherapy Research 5:297, 1980.
8. Kovacs, L: *Experimental investigation of photostimulation effect of low energy HeNe laser radiation.* In *Laser in Basic Biomedical Research (IV).* Plenum, New York, 1977.
9. Litwin, MS and Glew, DH: *The biological effects of laser radiation.* JAMA 187:842, 1964.
10. Caspers, K: *Laser Stimulation Therapy.* Physikalishe Medizin and Rehabilitation 18:426, 1977.
11. Dynatronics: *Dynatron 1120 Operators Manual.* Dynatronics, Salt Lake City, UT, 1983.
12. Goldman, L: *Basic reactions in tissue.* In Goldman, L (ed): *The Biomedical Laser: Technology and Clinical Applications.* Springer-Verlag, New York, 1981, pp 6–9.
13. Nogier, PFM: *Treatise on Auriculotherapy.* Maisonneuve, Sainte-Ruffine, France, 1972.
14. Mester, E: *Neu Utersuehungen Under Die Wirkung Der Laserstrahlung Aug Die Wundhelung.* A Exp Clin 89:212, 1980.
15. Castro, D: Personal communication, March 1983.
16. Gamaleya, NF: *Laser biomedical research in Tae-USSR.* In Wolbarsht, ML (ed): *Laser Applications in Medicine and Biology.* Plenum, New York, 1977.
17. Yew, DT, Ling Wong, SL, and Chan, Y: *Stimulating effect of the low dose laser—A new hypothesis.* Acta Anat 112:131, 1982.
18. Kovacs, IB, Mester, E, and Gorog, P: *Laser-induced stimulation of the vascularization of the healing wound: An ear chamber experiment.* Experientia 4:341, 1974.

19. MacMillan, JD, Maxwell, WA, and Chichester, CO: *Lethal photosensitization of microorganisms with light from a continuous-wave gas laser.* Photochem Photobiol 5:555, 1966.
20. Haina, D, et al: *Animal experiments on light-induced wound healing.* In *Laser in Basic Biomedical Research (IV).* Plenum, New York, 1977, pp 221–223.
21. Kana, JS, et al: *Effect of low-power density laser radiation of healing of open skin wounds in rats.* Arch Surg 116:3, 1981.
22. *Stedman's Medical Dictionary.* Williams & Wilkins, Baltimore, 1977.
23. Lehninger, AL: *Biochemistry.* Worth Publishers, New York, 1975, p 995.
24. Goldman, JA, et al: *Laser therapy of rheumatoid arthritis.* Lasers in Surgery and Medicine 1:1, 1980.
25. Snyder-Mackler, L and Bork, C: *The effect of cold laser on musculoskeletal trigger points: A double blind study.* Poster-Presentation, National Convention, American Physical Therapy Association, Las Vegas, 1984.
26. Moore, W: *Biological aspects of laser radiation. A review of hazards.* US Government Printing Office (DHEW Monograph), Rockville, MD, 1969.
27. Kohtiao, A, et al: *Temperature rise and photocoagulation of rabbit retinas exposed to the CW laser.* Am J Ophthalmol 62:3, 1966.
28. Lappin, PW: *Ocular damage thresholds for the helium-neon laser.* Arch Environ Health 20:2, 1970.
29. Ham, WT, et al: *Retinal burn thresholds for the helium-neon laser in the rhesus monkey.* Arch Ophthalmol 84:6, 1970.

PART 3

CLINICAL DECISION MAKING

CHAPTER 10

CLINICAL EVALUATION OF THERMAL AGENTS

MARY P. WATKINS, M.S., P.T.

Evaluation of the effectiveness and efficiency of therapeutic intervention is an essential function of every health care professional. Participation of each individual in this process can vary from critical reading of the medical and scientific literature to conducting sophisticated research projects. In order to participate at all, health professionals must have an understanding of the existing problems and questions about current practice and have the ability to incorporate into practice those therapeutic advances that have been demonstrated to be effective by sound critical analysis. Acquisition of such understanding and ability depends upon a working knowledge of the aims, uses, and limitations of clinical investigation.

This book presents a comprehensive review of the physical and physiologic mechanisms that serve as the basis for the characteristics of energy delivered by and the potential applications of thermal agents. For example, from the physical sciences, we have gained knowledge of heat transfer mechanisms. From the biologic sciences, we have gained information on the responses of cells, tissues, and organs to thermal agents. In vitro laboratory studies include the influence of temperature changes on the viscoelastic properties of collagen and changes in ion fluxes across cell membranes when temperature is altered. Animal studies, in vivo, have examined such changes as blood flow, muscle spindle activity, synaptic transmission, and induction and resolution of inflammation and edema. These kinds of information are useful for establishing a rationale for employing thermal agents in the treatment of patients. Throughout this book, current instrumentation and techniques are also described, which demonstrate clinical application of heat, cold, and laser. In many instances, however, the therapeutic effects of these modalities are based on anecdotal reports or on empirical evidence of success in amelioration of patient problems.

The number of formal clinical studies that document the effects of treatment procedures is very limited. To illustrate, a review of the journal *Physical Therapy* reveals that from 1973 to 1984, 30 articles related to the subject of thermal agents were published. Of these, 15 could be classified as clinical research articles, but only four presented data obtained from patient samples. Findings based on normal subjects may assist in understanding physiologic responses to therapeutic applications. Such studies, however, do not answer the important questions regarding clinical efficacy. Clinical research efforts must be expanded to accomplish the goal of providing patient care of high quality in an economically sound manner. Three essential approaches toward this goal are to (1) determine the appropriateness of current techniques, (2) develop new methods tested by scientific inquiry, and (3) discard methods that do not stand up to such scrutiny.

The purpose of this chapter is to examine selected elements of the research process applicable to the clinical evaluation of thermal agents. General principles, samples of methodology and instrumentation are presented to highlight the uses and limitations of the clinical research process. Examples of research questions, concerning the application of thermal agents identified throughout this book, will be used.

GENERAL PRINCIPLES OF CLINICAL RESEARCH

Planning and Preparation

The basic process of conceiving, planning, and preparing to conduct research can be described in several well-defined steps. These preliminary steps are

1. Definition of the research question
2. Collection of the relevant information
3. Statement of a hypothesis or the specific aims of the research activity
4. Selection and development of the method of study

This process applies to all types of research design and involves careful planning, including the recognition of the problems that potentially can invalidate the outcome of a study. Several general principles or process guidelines can be defined to ensure well-planned and well-executed clinical research projects.[1,2]

THE RESEARCH QUESTION. The research question or problem must be specific and delimited, identifying the research variables precisely. The first potential failure in the research process is posing a question that is diffuse or broad, containing confounding elements that make it impossible to derive a useful answer. For example, *What is the effect of cold on edema?* The two key elements of a research question can be identified here: (1) the independent variable, *cold,* which the investigator will control, manipulate, or apply; and (2) the dependent variable, *edema,* which will be observed or measured to determine the effect of applying the modality. The question, however, is unmanageable. Many confounding elements, or extraneous variables, have not been taken into account. What kind of cold is being questioned? How often will it be applied? In what setting? On what category of patient? Will age of the patients or the duration of illness or injury affect the outcome? What specific outcome is relevant—range of motion, limb circumference, limb volume, or functional abilities? These kinds of questions must be addressed and resolved during the process of defining the research question.

COLLECTION OF THE RELEVANT INFORMATION. Background information must be carefully accumulated and analyzed. Clinical observation and experience are valuable sources of background information; indeed, the question at hand is often derived from some clinical event. Although clinically derived knowledge is important, it is never thorough enough to substitute for a critical review of the current medical and scientific literature. As the investigator defines the problem to be studied and formulates the specific elements of the research project, several pertinent pieces of information should be incorporated, or at least considered. Regarding the illustrative question of cold and edema, the literature search would include both laboratory and clinical studies. From animal studies, the investigator will learn the mechanisms of edema formation and, as discussed in Chapter 4, that the intensity and duration of cold application may influence the tissue response, possibly adversely. This knowledge should lead to careful consideration of the method of cold application to be used. From clinical studies, there is evidence that the application of cold may control swelling. In at least one study, however, compression wraps were also part of the treatment. This problem suggests a more definitive series of questions than did the first, vaguely stated one. In general, the investigator needs to know if his or her question has been studied, how it has been studied, what has not been studied, and what constitutes the scientific rationale for the proposed study. This information is useful and necessary to solidify the importance of the current problem and to develop an appropriate approach to the research question.

At this point, the investigator should be able to pose an important, clinically relevant, sensible research question. Taking the initially stated global question, for example, a more refined question may be asked: *Is cold or cold plus intermittent compression more effective in reducing edema following ankle sprains in college athletes?*

Then the question can be transposed into a working or research hypothesis.

HYPOTHESIS OR SPECIFIC AIMS. Most research questions can, and should, be transposed into hypotheses. Certainly, if the study compares two treatment methods, a prediction of the outcome can be made on the basis of the available background information. A hypothesis must be stated to clearly identify the independent and dependent variables to be studied and proposes a relationship between the two. This statement can be made in two ways: nondirectional or directional.

A statement of difference declares that the application of the independent variable will result in a change in the dependent variable. If the investigator predicts a change but not the direction of that change, the statement can be referred to as a *nondirectional hypothesis*. For example, "There will be a difference in the amount of residual ankle edema when sprains are treated with cold alone, compared with cold plus intermittent compression." A *directional hypothesis* predicts not only a difference but also the direction of that difference: "The application of cold plus intermittent compression will be more effective in reducing edema following ankle sprains than the application of cold alone."

There is a third form of hypothetical statement, the *null hypothesis*, which is a statement of *no difference* and is used in the application of procedures to determine the statistical significance of research data.

In studies of a descriptive or correlational nature, when the purpose is to describe a particular phenomenon, a predictive hypothesis may not be appropriate or necessary. In this case, a clear statement of the *specific aims* of the study should be made.

METHOD. In order to answer the question or test the hypothesis, a method of study must be carefully selected and specifically described. The purpose of this major task is to make certain that (1) all extraneous variables (those factors, other than the independent variable, which could affect the outcome) are controlled for or eliminated; and (2) the kind and use of the measurement tools are appropriate.

An explicit written description of the method must be prepared and must include the following details: (1) The specific conditions of the study are stated (such as the age, sex, and health status of subjects and the setting in which the study is to be conducted). (2) The testing instruments and their application are specifically defined to answer: what test, when used, how used, and by whom? (3) The procedure for applying the independent variable is defined in order to outline, using our example, such details as: what type of cold? how frequently administered? how will the subject be positioned? and, what kind of supervision or monitoring? (4) Statistical procedures or other techniques that will be used to analyze the data are outlined. Throughout this written protocol, "operational definitions" will be stated: the *meaning* of cold and the *meaning* of edema should become clear.

At this point in preparing to conduct a research study, the investigator must analyze the proposed method to ensure that the design is correct and meets certain necessary criteria. This process may require consultation with other investigators and clinicians, as well as a pretrial pilot study. Three important criteria should be met: reliability, validity, and objectivity.

Reliability is synonymous with dependability, stability, consistency, predictability, and accuracy. If the same set of objects is measured again and again with the same or comparable instruments, under the same conditions, will the results be the same? There are statistical techniques to estimate the degree of reliability of a testing situation.[3,4] (These techniques in many cases simply serve to confirm the investigator's good common sense.)

Validity refers to the soundness, logic, and appropriateness of the study design.[5] The *internal* validity of a study depends upon the extent to which the method controls those extraneous factors that interfere with the true relationship between the stated independent and dependent variables. Is the investigator measuring what he or she thinks is being measured? What factors, in addition to the application of cold alone or cold and compression, are important: weight bearing, elevation of the limb, anti-inflammatory medication? *External* validity refers to the extent to which the results can be generalized to other subjects, settings, or conditions. How representative are the findings to the "outside" world? Will cold gel packs have the same effect as the application of chipped ice? Will the response of an athlete, anxious to return to competition, be the same as the response of a sedentary executive?

Objectivity means the extent to which the testing situation and the measurement tools control for the biggest kind of extraneous variable: the biases, subjective impressions, and "feelings" of the investigators and subjects.

Implementation and Dissemination of Results

At this point in the process, the investigator has a carefully considered and prepared protocol. This is the guide that must be strictly followed during every phase of carrying out the study. When data collection is complete and the results are analyzed according to plan, the investigator has one more responsibility: to share the results with professional colleagues. The results of clinical studies may also be useful to the engineers and manufacturers who are responsible for the design, construction, and safety of therapeutic devices.

Two general considerations should be uppermost as the final report is being prepared. First, the information must be accurate and detailed enough so that the reader or listener can identify the question asked, assess the appropriateness of the method, replicate the study, and evaluate the strength and veracity of the conclusions.

The primary goal of any research is to improve or increase the body of knowledge in the relevant clinical or scientific arena. This can best be done by gathering and disseminating sound, reliable, accurate information.

TYPES OF CLINICAL RESEARCH

Some types of research are more rigorous than others, but all carefully planned and executed projects that follow the aforementioned principles will make a contribution to the existing body of knowledge. An understanding of the purposes and limitations of research approaches will permit appropriate interpretation and analysis of information in the proper perspective. The research designs discussed here are those that seem most applicable to the clinical evaluation of thermal agents. Real and hypothetical examples will be cited.

The Single-Case Study

Many will argue that the report of a single case does not fit the criteria for research. On the other hand, the description of a single case can provide useful information, particularly if questions exist about the applicability of a known method of treatment in an unusual circumstance or to elucidate a new approach to an old clinical problem. An innovative case report may be a stimulus for the author and others to investigate a topic in greater depth.

A report by Wing[6] illustrates that a well-planned, well-documented single case will contain several elements of the research process. The question asked was "What is the effect of phonophoretically driven hydrocortisone on the range of motion (ROM) of the temporomandibular joint (TMJ) and pain level in a patient with TMJ dysfunction?" Supportive rationale was provided in the introductory paragraph. The methods for assessment of ROM and pain were presented and were conducted before and after treatment. The specific treatment protocol was described. The conclusion was stated clearly and appropriately: phonophoresis with hydrocortisone "was influential in reducing pain and increasing range of motion in this case." This statement, as written, acknowledges the most distinct disadvantage of the single-case study, which is the inability to generalize the result to a broader population. There is an inherent lack of control over extraneous variables such as the effect of the passage of time, the patient's attitude toward treatment or, in this case, the patient's desire to eat more heartily.

Single-Group Design

The same problems of lack of control and inability to generalize results exist in the single-group pretest, post-test design, whereby a number of subjects are tested before and after the application of a specific treatment regimen. Quillen and Rouillier[7] presented such a single-group study. The purpose of their project was to evaluate the effect of rapid pulsed pneumatic compression in conjuction with cold on acute grade I sprains. Their conclusion, based primarily on edema reduction as measured by volumetric displacement, was that this form of compression was effective. A comparison of the pretreatment and post-treatment volumetric measurements was presented to support their conclusion. There can be more confidence in the effectiveness of treatment when the same or similar results are obtained in a group of individuals, in contrast to the single case.

The important questions, however, remain unanswered. Is the change in measurement caused by the treatment alone, or do other factors (such as time, bed rest, medication, or daily activities) contribute to the outcome?

Is this group of patients different in some way from other patients with a similar clinical problem?

Campbell and Stanley[5] categorize these kinds of studies as "pre-experimental." The implication is that more rigor and control are needed to increase the value of the findings.

Comparative Research Designs

Several approaches to comparative research have been described and used to study clinical questions. The common factor among them is that at least two carefully defined circumstances are compared. The choice of the approach to a specific clinical research problem must be based (1) on the nature and content of the question to be studied; and (2) on a number of pragmatic details (such as the availability of subjects; the support and cooperation of patients, their families, and other health care personnel whose intervention may have an effect on the study; and whether withholding treatment from some subjects is ethically sound).

GROUP STUDIES. Two "traditional" methods for comparison are the two-group pretest, post-test design and the two-group post-test–only design.[5] Both require a rigorous control of patient selection and group assignment. Both will test the effect of a treatment scheme imposed on one group but not the second. The difference between these two designs is that to use a pretest determination, there must be a common pre-existing condition that can be measured and remeasured after the experimental period. For example, the question "Is cold or cold plus intermittent compression more effective in reducing edema following ankle sprains?" presupposes that edema is present and measurable prior to administering the two treatment regimens. Measured pretreatment edema becomes one criterion for patient selection, and a change in that edema becomes a determination of effectiveness. In contrast, the post-test–only design applies when the condition to be measured (the dependent variable) does not exist prior to treatment. If the question were "Does the application of cold packs prevent edema following arthroscopic meniscectomy?" the preoperative condition would not necessarily include edema, and, therefore, a pretreatment measurement would be irrelevant and noncontributory to answering the research question.

Both of these traditional experimental designs customarily require the most rigorous control of subject selection and assignment to treatment or control groups. The designs, for example, by classic definition require that subjects for study be drawn randomly from some defined, existing population. This requirement assumes that such a population is available to the investigator at the time a study sample is to be selected. In the case of studying the effect of cold on edema in college athletes, the investigator could hope that a huge number of athletes will suffer ankle sprains at 4 P.M. on a particular Wednesday afternoon. Of course, such an event is unrealistic. Furthermore, if that should happen and if the study sample could be randomly drawn from that number, would the investigator have adequate work force, equipment, and facilities to conduct the evaluations and treatments outlined in the research protocol, in a timely manner? It is highly unlikely and suggests one of the serious practical problems in performing traditional experimental research in the real clinical world.

Traditional designs can and are employed in the clinical setting, despite such problems, although compromises are usually made. Deriving the study sample is often done by the method of sequential assignment. In a two-group comparative study requiring 10 patients per group, for example, 20 slips of paper (10 with the number 1 and 10 with the number 2 written on them) can be placed in a hat and drawn out one by one. The order of the drawn numbers becomes the method of assigning the eligible patients as they appear to either group 1 or group 2.

A second kind of adaptation or compromise can be made when the investigator believes that certain characteristics of subjects must be controlled by the process of group assignment. A common variable in clinical studies is the age of the subjects. In this case, an investigator who believes that healing time or functional recovery or any element of the dependent variable may be affected by age may choose to match the subjects in pairs according to age and assign them to different groups.

TIME SERIES DESIGNS. Research questions about treatment effectiveness and efficiency focus on the patient and on the management of the patient's problem in the clinic. In the clinical setting, practical issues such as time, numbers of patients with specific disorders, space, and at times, ethical considerations make it difficult to conduct two- or multigroup studies with random samples. Procedures for conducting research have been described that may apply when the clinic is the "laboratory," the clinician is the "investigator," and the patient who has been referred for treatment is the "subject." Of particular relevance in this clinical setting is that the time series designs presented here can be applied to a *single subject* as well as to groups of subjects. As the name "time series" implies, these methods of evaluation are based on serial assessment of the dependent variable over time. Depending upon the question, this may mean repeated measures over a period of hours, days, or weeks. The most important factor is that decisions about the measured variable are based not on a single assessment but on a series of assessments.[8–10]

The simplest time series model is the *simple baseline design* (A-B), in which A is a period of baseline measurement and B is a period of measurement while treatment is being administered. In this and in all time series designs, the baseline period continues until the measured values are stable over repeated measures.[10] Figure 10–1 *(top)* represents a hypothetical example of the use of the A-B design to investigate the effect of ultrasound on range of motion of the shoulder in a patient with "frozen shoulder." The results of this study would be less than convincing because there is no way to be sure that some confounding variable is not responsible for the effect during phase B.

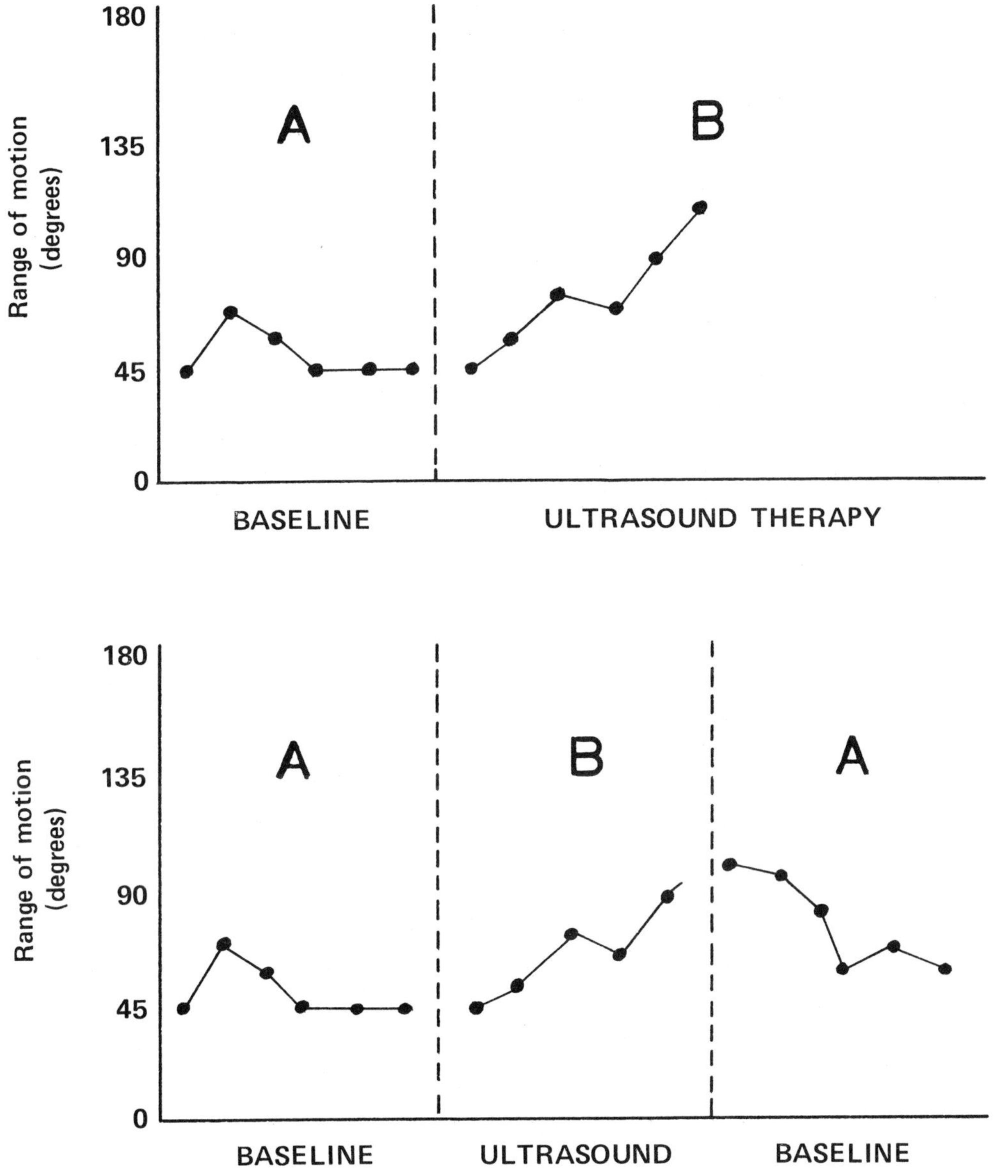

FIGURE 10-1
Hypothetical record representing the time series designs.

The investigator may have more confidence in the effect of treatment during phase B, if the treatment can be withdrawn for a period of time while baseline measurements are made again. If, during the second baseline period, the treatment effect is reversed toward the original baseline, while all other activities or aspects of management of the patient are unchanged, the evidence is strengthened that the treatment administered during phase

B was responsible for the change in measurement values. The A-B-A, or even an A-B-A-B, time design can be used to evaluate treatment of those conditions in which a return to baseline values might be expected, such as the chronic inflammatory states of rheumatoid joints or limitations of motion secondary to long-term changes in joint structure (Fig. 10–1, *bottom*). These designs will not work when return to baseline is not expected. For example, when a patient is treated following a temporary period of immobilization and resumes normal activity, a return of limited motion or weakness should not happen. In this case, the A-B-A designs are inappropriate.

A variation of time series research is the *multiple-baseline design*, whereby more than one measurement is obtained and evaluated. Two or more baseline measures can be derived in several ways: (1) within a single subject, studying multiple joints or limbs or muscle groups; (2) across subjects, whereby the same method is applied to several subjects over a staggered time course; or (3) across settings, whereby a single subject is studied in different treatment settings introduced sequentially.[2,9]

SEQUENTIAL MEDICAL TRIALS. The sequential medical trials model is a comparative experimental system in which the results of each *pair* of observations, as they are obtained, determine if the experiment must continue in order to reach a definitive answer or if the experiment is to be terminated.[2,11–13] It is based on alternative treatments randomly administered to individual subjects or to paired subjects. Subjects are admitted to the study until a decision is made about which of the two treatments is superior. That decision is determined by the sequential plan, chosen in advance, based on the selected probability of obtaining a statistically significant result.

Formulas and calculations for these determinations have been presented by Bross[11] and Armitage.[12] Using the Bross model at a significance level of 0.05, for example, a grid is constructed. This grid with a hypothetical set of data is illustrated in Figure 10–2. When a preference for one treatment over the other is made for each pair of observations, and X is placed in the direction (vertical or horizontal) of that preference. As soon as the path of X's crosses one of the bold lines, indicating a decision in favor of one of the two treatments (or in favor of neither, if the central portion lines are crossed), the study is terminated. In order for the X's to progress, a clear decision within each pair must be made: "preference" for one or the other treatment must be achieved in each pair. If there is no "preference" (that is, if neither achieves or if both achieve the selected goal for success), then no X is recorded for that pair. This represents a potential fault with the design in that data are lost from the total evaluation of the comparison, unless the investigator reports this occurrence separately.

The essential requirements for employing the sequential medical trials model include those that apply to all research designs: the alternative treatments and the measurement procedure must be specifically defined, and the criteria for subjects to be included in the study must be established in advance. Two other important requirements must be fulfilled. First, observations are made in pairs, one for each treatment. If the comparison

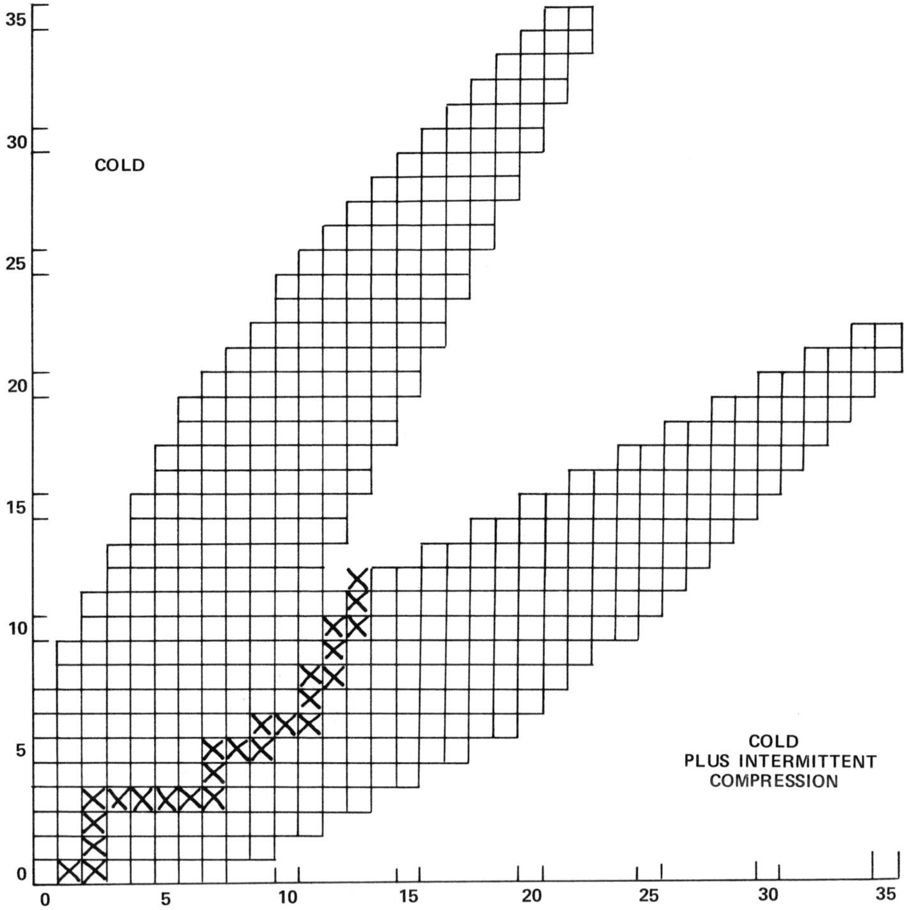

FIGURE 10-2

Sequential medical trials grid with significance level of $p \leq 0.05$. Data are *hypothetical,* comparing cold alone and cold plus intermittent compression in the treatment of ankle sprains.

is between pairs of subjects, successive subjects eligible to participate become a pair, and the assignment of the two treatments to each of the pair is random. If the comparison is between two treatments in the same subject (within-subject comparison), the order of presentation or administration of each of the treatments is random. Second, because the decision to place the X's is based on a preference (that is, treatment A or B or neither is "better"), the criterion or definition of "better" must be specified. For example, if the dependent variable is passive range of motion, what value will indicate "better:" an increase of 15 degrees over the initial value; some percentage of the initial value; or a value relative to a normal value, perhaps of the uninvolved extremity?

Using the sample question "Is cold or cold plus intermittent compression more effective in reducing edema following ankle sprains in college athletes?" this research model can be illustrated. The investigator will define "ankle sprain," perhaps limiting the sample to grade 2 sprains, and will determine the exact methods of applying the two treatments. The management of all subjects should be the same in all respects, except for the application of intermittent compression in one group. The number of treatments and treatment days should be specified. The daily activities of the subjects during the experimental period should be specified, to control for such variables as weight bearing on the involved ankle. The criterion measure should be defined, perhaps a 50 percent reduction in foot and ankle edema measured volumetrically on the fourth day postinjury.

Hypothetically, 50 athletes suffered grade 2 ankle sprains during an academic year. The effect of the two treatments was determined on each pair and recorded on the grid (Fig. 10–2). With the 25th pair, the central bold line was crossed, thereby indicating that neither method was "superior." In 13 pairs, cold plus intermittent compression resulted in a 50 percent reduction in edema on the fourth day and, in 12 pairs, cold alone resulted in achieving that criterion measure. Furthermore, the opposite member of each pair had *not* achieved the criterion measure. It can be noted that with the results obtained from the 20th pair, cold alone would not be found superior. However, at that point, it was not known if cold plus compression would be determined to be superior or, as happened, if neither could be considered significantly better.

The efficiency of a sequential medical trial is a major advantage for the clinical investigator. Patients who meet the defined criteria are admitted to the study as they appear. This process is easily adapted to the clinical setting where the on-going clinical service cannot be disrupted in a major way and where it is unlikely that a large number of patients are available at any one time to be randomly assigned to treatment groups. The recording of results on each pair is immediate and on-going until the selected level of significance is attained. This process means three things: (1) Data analysis is simple; (2) the study is terminated as soon as a "preference" is determined; and (3) when there is a clear demonstration of "superiority," the impact on clinical decision making can be immediate.

The major argument against sequential trials is that an answer may be obtained after a small number of observations or may require a relatively large number: in the Bross model, 20 pairs to reach the central "no difference" area or 58 pairs to reach either favorable choice.[2] This issue of frequency or numbers is of concern in interpretation of the role of chance and traditional statistical significance.[14]

This design, however, is certainly more rigorous than the single-case study or single-group design. It is economical and practical as a research approach in the setting of a busy clinical practice.

As an example, Light and co-workers[15] have employed this model to compare two methods of stretching in patients with chronic knee flexion contractures.

The approaches to research presented here are not all inclusive, but rather were selected to exemplify the kind of options and some of the constraints that must be considered in the plan to answer any question about the value of a therapeutic regimen.

INSTRUMENTATION FOR CLINICAL EVALUATION

Clinical evaluation of thermal agents depends upon the use of measurement techniques that will provide accurate documentation of therapeutic effectiveness. Selecting appropriate measuring tools must be based on (1) the therapeutic aims of treatment; (2) the reliability, validity, and objectivity of the measurement procedures; and (3) the value of the evaluation to the advancement of knowledge and practice of the clinician. Throughout this book, a number of clinical signs and symptoms have been discussed repeatedly: pain, edema, limitation of motion, and interference with normal muscular function. Each problem means something special to the patient and should be of major concern to the clinical investigator. Appropriate evaluation procedures, therefore, should be those that will accurately document changes in these clinical conditions.

Many clinical characteristics are measurable in *quantitative* terms (for example, temperature, limb volume, muscle force, range of motion, and recovery time). Some values are *qualitative* in nature (for example, pain assessment and manual muscle test grades). The importance of this distinction is that the approach to statistical analysis of data depends on an understanding of the measurement values.[2]

The following discussion will be limited to a review of the instrumentation that is currently available to the clinician or that is economically feasible to acquire and useful for measurement of the clinical problems enumerated above.

Pain Scales

The presence of pain for many patients is a most debilitating problem; therefore, pain relief becomes a priority in clinical management. For this reason alone, the evaluation of pain is important. The comprehensiveness of the evaluation may also provide information about the causes of pain.

The complexities of the pain experience include not only the sensation itself but also the impact of the patient's past experience, emotional state, and cultural attitudes on the interpretation of the quality and magnitude of the symptom. Herein lies one of the difficulties, for both the patient and the clinical investigator, in determining pain levels and changes in the pain state.

Newton has discussed the evaluation of pain and described current rating scales in Chapter 2. Of these tools, it appears that the McGill Pain Questionnaire has been most thoroughly scrutinized for establishing validity and reliability.

When pain scales are used to generate research data, every possible caution must be taken. For example, Melzack[16] points out a potential problem with the reliability of administering the McGill Questionnaire when patients make errors in filling out the questionnaire by themselves. He suggests that the instructions be read aloud and that the researcher or assistant may need to work with patients to aid their comprehension of the words presented for selection. Of course, the ability of the researcher or assistant to interact with a patient without bias is another potential source of variability.

When a pain assessment scale is used to evaluate the effects of thermal agents (or any other physical therapy procedure), the investigator must take into account other aspects of the patient's management. Of particular importance is the administration of analgesics and anti-inflammatory drugs, which will undoubtedly influence the pain state. Cooperation between the patient, physician, and physical therapy investigator is mandatory during a clinical trial. Clinical judgment will determine the reasonable course to follow in such a case. Occasionally, stopping or withholding medication may be possible. If not, as is likely, medication administration may be regulated to ensure that no new medication is introduced and that the dosage schedule remains constant during the trial. At the very least, a record of drug intake should be maintained, as it will be if the patients are hospitalized. Control and compliance[17,18] of outpatients is more difficult, but every attempt should be made to document the extent of this important extraneous variable.

The presence and magnitude of pain often accompanies or results in other physiologic changes. Concurrent muscle spasm or muscle guarding may interfere with range of motion. Pain may be the limiting factor in the patient's performance of daily activities. The converse may also occur if, for example, the patient has no pain at rest but, because of muscle tightness, has pain on motion. Many times, therefore, other measures of clinical effectiveness may be and should be obtained conjointly with the assessment of pain.

Range of Motion

Techniques of goniometry are well known to physical therapists. When these techniques are used accurately, they provide quantitative data about limitation in joint range of motion.

Common methods have been described[19,20] and are used as guides throughout the United States. Reliability of these methods has been evaluated.[21,22] The data on reliability deserve particular attention when the investigator plans to use goniometry as a dependent measure in clinical studies. Accurate goniometry requires skill and consistent performance of the examiner. These attributes may be assessed by determining intra-rater reliability on repeated trials. Knowledge of intra-rater variability for specific measurements may be used to establish criteria for a change in patient status. Based on Boone's data, for example, a change of greater than 5 degrees in the upper extremity and 6 degrees in the lower extremity must occur to state an improvement or a decline in range of motion. Because of the documented differences between testers, the performance of each examiner should be evaluated before a clinical trial and it appears necessary to use only one examiner in a given study.

In addition to establishing reliability, the responsibility of the clinical investigator is to select and define a specific protocol for goniometric measurement. The protocol should include such details as the type of goniometer, placement landmarks, patient position, and patient participation. The last consideration may seriously affect the validity of testing. The choice is whether to measure passive, active-assisted, or active range of motion. The results may be quite different depending upon muscle guarding, spasm, segmental reflex interactions, or the patient's ability to follow instructions.

Volumetric and Girth Measurements

The presence of edema is a common problem in several of the clinical conditions for which thermal agents are employed and may be a major cause of pain, limitation of motion, and decreased functional ability. Reduction of swelling, therefore, becomes another important therapeutic goal. Two relatively inexpensive and efficient methods for obtaining quantitative data about limb edema are volumetric measurement and girth measurement.

Volume of an entire limb or a distal limb segment can be estimated using a water displacement system,[23,24] in which the part to be evaluated is submerged in a water tank with an outflow spout from which the water displaced by the limb is collected in a graduated cylinder. The indicator of limb volume is the quantity of displaced water, measured in milliliters. The accuracy of this method depends upon (1) the initial level of water in the tank relative to the outflow spout; (2) the position of the limb in the tank, particularly depth of submersion; and (3) the state of relaxation of the patient's limb. Tanks made of clear material such as Lucite (Volumeters Unlimited, 524 Double View Drive, P.O. Box 146, Idyllwild, CA) are probably best to permit the examiner to observe the position of the limb within the tank (Fig. 10–3).

As previously mentioned, this method of volmetric measurement is appropriate when the swelling is distally located (that is, hand and wrist or foot and ankle), or when swelling involves a large area from distal to proximal. If swelling is limited to a more proximal site (that is, knee, thigh, or upper arm), this measurement method may not be sensitive enough to detect a change in such a delimited location, because the entire limb must be immersed.

In this case of limited proximal or localized swelling, girth (or circumferential) limb measurements may be more appropriate. The only equipment required is a measuring tape; one made of flexible steel is probably preferred over one of cloth or plastic, which may change in length over time by stretching. Because examiner skill is required in placing and reading the tape, intra-rater reliability should be evaluated prior to using this procedure for clinical evaluation. Limb posture and relaxation of the part to be measured may be confounding variables; therefore, careful instructions to the patient seem necessary.

Evaluation of Muscle Performance

Muscle strength may not be of primary concern during the acute stage of injury or illness; however, ultimately, restoration of normal muscle perfor-

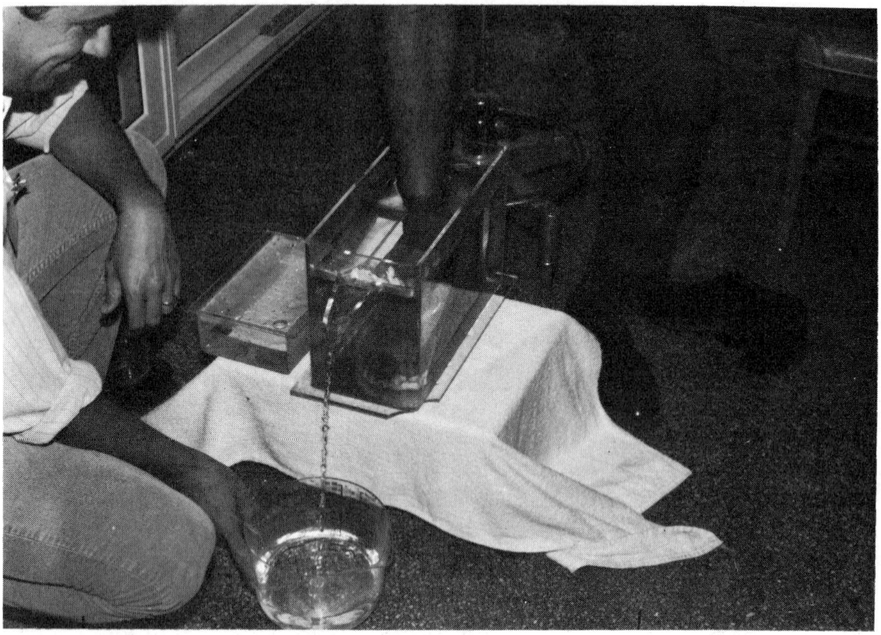

FIGURE 10-3

Foot and ankle volume is being measured using a volumeter.

mance is usually found on any list of long-term therapeutic goals. The direct effects of cold on muscle strength have been discussed in Chapter 4. In addition, skeletal muscle performance may be altered secondary to the demonstrated effects of thermal agents on nerve conduction velocity, muscle spindle activity, and synaptic transmission. For these reasons, muscle strength may be an important dependent variable in evaluating the long-term effects of applying thermal agents.

If so, the investigator must make a series of decisions in selecting the appropriate test instrument. The first problems to solve are the *operational definitions* of strength and the selection of criteria for determining whether strength is improving or declining. None of the currently used terms (such as force, tension, work, and power) are synonymous, although all can be used to describe a quality of being "strong" or "weak." Criteria for improvement or decline should be based on knowledge of the reliability or reproducibility of the selected test procedure. The second important consideration must be both the local and the systemic conditions of the patients who will be studied. For example, testing procedures that require patients to generate high levels of force may be impractical and inappropriate in the presence of acute inflammation or serious debilitation secondary to prolonged bed rest. A third factor relates to the nature of the research question. If it is one in which the muscle testing should be correlated with functional activity, a determination of the functional requirements of the muscles to be tested will have to be made. Then, the investigator can select a test condition, such as isometric or dynamic, at low or high speed, that most closely relates to those functional requirements.

There is an imposing array of testing instruments for the measurement of muscle strength. Only three of the choices will be mentioned to illustrate the available spectrum: the manual muscle test, the cable tensiometer, and the isokinetic dynamometer. These instruments represent the diversity of kinds of information which can be obtained under the category of "strength" testing.

The manual muscle test[25] was developed by Lovett and Merrill in 1912 and, since that time, has periodically fallen in and out of favor without careful analysis of the attendant reasons. One of the criticisms has been that it is not an "objective test." The objectivity of this test very definitely depends on the skill and precision of the examiner and on the adherence to strict rules for grading. Under sensible, controlled conditions, the reliability of the manual muscle test was assessed[26] and, based on the demonstrated reliability of the testing procedures, this test was effectively employed during the polio era.

The qualitative ranking of muscle strength can be used to determine change, particularly in muscles that cannot move through the complete arc of motion against gravity or an externally applied resistance. In fact, there may be no other measure in common usage to assess muscle strength in this circumstance.

The arguments against the manual muscle test become more appropriate when the variable of the examiner's manual resistance is introduced, as in the range of grades above "fair" (50 percent). Not only is the examiner's resistance part of the determination, but also the grade of "normal" (100 percent) may be interpreted to mean full recovery and normal function, which is not necessarily so. For example, Watkins and colleagues[27] documented deficits in isokinetic torque production in the so-called uninvolved thigh musculature of patients with hemiparesis whose manual muscle test grades for quadriceps and hamstrings muscles were graded "normal."

When the muscles under study are able to develop higher levels of force, the quantitative measures of that force can, and should, be employed.

The cable tensiometer measures *isometric* tension.[1] The recorded values are pounds or kilograms of force. A calibrated length of cable is placed within a fixed cable or chain system, which is attached to the subject's limb and against which the muscle or muscle group exerts force. The force, translated through the calibrated cable, is recorded using a tensiometer attached to that cable. The advantage of this instrument is that with the versatility of hardware attachments, the subject and tensiometer can be aligned to test a muscle at several points within the arc of motion.

The capability of testing *dynamic* muscular performance requiring motion through an arc of motion is no longer limited to weightlifting and values such as the 10-repetition maximum of DeLorme and Watkins,[28] although this method may continue to be used if it suits the needs and criteria of a particular research question.

The concept of isokinetic exercise and the introduction of isokinetic dynamometers[29] interfaced with recording devices (such as the Cybex II, Lumex Corporation, Cybex Division, Ronkonkoma, NY) have expanded the choices of instrumentation for clinical measurement of "strength." With isokinetic exercise devices, which are based on the force-velocity principle, speed of motion can be preselected and the instrument will prevent acceleration beyond that preset speed. Several measures of muscular performance, such as peak torque and joint angle at peak torque, can be obtained from the torque curves generated by the patient's attempts to accelerate. Assessment of performance over a range of speeds which may more closely simulate functional requirements is an advantage of these systems.[30]

Assessment of muscular performance can make an important contribution to the evaluation of long-term effects of thermal agents. There is, however, one final caution: all of these procedures designed to measure muscle strength depend on the *voluntary* participation and cooperation of the patients. Apprehension, motivation, inattention, and the ability to follow instructions are factors that may interfere with the validity of these measures.

Functional Tests

Eventually, in the course of therapeutic intervention, the question of effectiveness and efficiency of treatment procedures becomes: "How well does the patient function in carrying out the physical activities relevant to the patient's lifestyle?" In considering the efficacy of thermal agents and any comparison of specific modalities, the question may be: "How quickly does the patient return to his or her optimal level of function?" In this case, the measure is "recovery time." "Function," "recovery," and "time to recovery" then can become dependent variables in clinical studies. Again, the first necessary step is to define operationally those terms in a manner relevant to the specific research question.

The performance of functional tasks can be documented qualitatively or quantitatively as appropriate. The system of noting whether a patient can perform a given activity independently, with an assistive device, or not at all can be translated into a qualitative rating scale for research purposes.

A number of quantitative measures are available or could be created. These are timed tests of functional performance in which the dependent variable is the time (usually in seconds) it takes to accomplish a defined task. An objective and standardized test of hand function by Jebsen[31] is an example of such a measure of upper extremity function, including such items as writing a short sentence and stacking checkers. The time required to walk a fixed distance or climb a set of standard stairs[32] are other examples of timed tests.

Temporal and spatial characteristics of gait may also be quantitatively and reliably measured.[33,34] The basic implements of the method described by Boenig[33] are a mat or paper strip secured to the floor, inked tapes on the shoes of the subject, and a stop watch. Using this method, the data obtained include step length, stride length, step width, foot angle, and cadence. Using more sophisticated instrumentation such as the computerized gait mat described by Wall and associates,[34] additional data can be collected—namely, stance time, double support time, and velocity of walking.

All of the preceding examples of clinical instrumentation can be employed by physical therapy clinicians for both the assessment of individual patients who are referred for treatment and, with careful planning and organization, the evaluation of therapeutic effectiveness or efficiency of thermal agents.

Related Evaluative Procedures

The practitioner and clinical investigator should be aware of other instruments relevant to the evaluation of thermal agents. Some have been cited elsewhere in this book. These measurements do not directly document *clinical* progress or outcomes. However, the information they provide may be correlated with signs and symptoms that limit function. These techniques may be useful to draw attention to and further elucidate the underlying

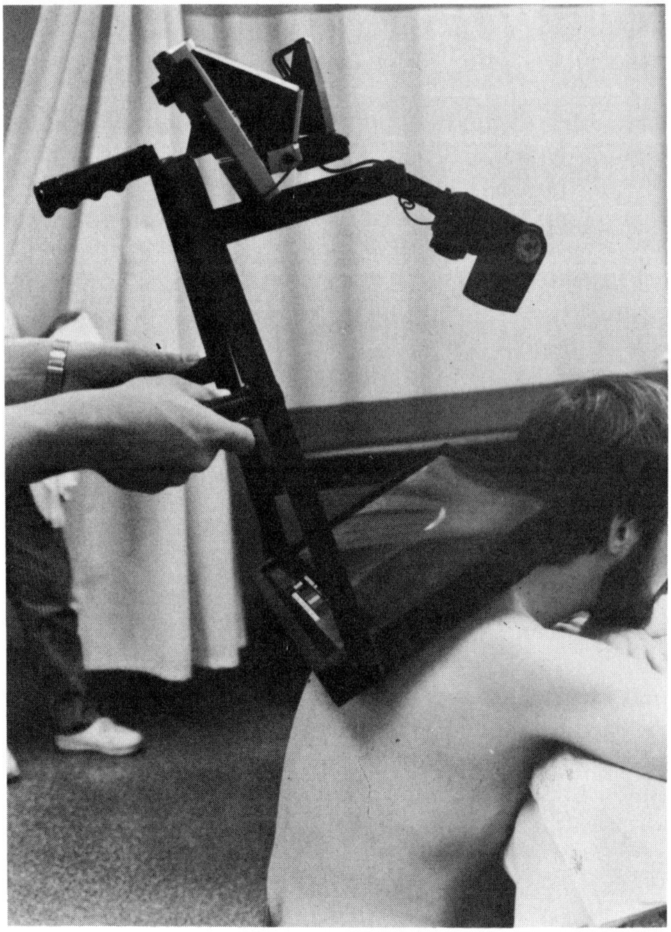

FIGURE 10-4
The cervical area is being examined using liquid crystal thermography.

mechanisms of pathology or to document the nature and extent of a patient's problem. Because of the "distance" between these techniques and the functional status of patients, only one, thermography, will be defined, and others will be listed (with references) for the reader's information.

Clinical *thermography* is a method of detecting and recording infrared radiation specifically from the body surface. One of the available systems is liquid-crystal contact thermography, which uses selected cholesteric esters embedded in elastomeric sheets. The configuration of crystals allows calibration of color responses to specific temperature ranges.[35] These sheets are placed in contact with the area to be assessed. As the colors are displayed through a clear plastic frame, they are photographed to record the colored thermogram (Fig. 10–4).

Thermography is based on the principles that infrared rays are radiated from any object having a temperature above absolute zero[36] and that superficial blood flow contributes to surface temperature.[37] Variations of detected emissions over a given area may represent autonomic or metabolic reactions to pathologic conditions.

The reported applications of this instrumentation include detection of spinal root compression,[35] observation of pain,[38] and evaluation of low back pain.[39]

The accuracy of thermography will be influenced by several factors including room temperature, ambient infrared radiation, materials (for instance, oils and powder) on the skin surface, and pressure.[40] Obviously, thermography could not be used to evaluate the immediate effects of a thermal agent, because the surface temperature will simply reflect the temperature of the applied agent. It may be more useful during initial assessment to delineate the specific area to be treated.

Effects of thermal agents on blood flow and blood volume have been discussed in Chapters 4 through 8. Techniques to ascertain assessment of these functions include the Doppler ultrasound flowmeter,[41,42] plethysmography,[42,43] and ^{133}Xe washout studies.[43] Electromyography and nerve conduction velocity studies[44] have been cited elsewhere (see Chapters 4, 5, and 7) and may continue to provide insight regarding neuromuscular responses to thermal agents.

SUMMARY

This chapter has identified the need and selected methods for conducting clinical studies to evaluate the effectiveness and efficiency of applying thermal agents for ameliorating conditions of pain, swelling, limited motion, and functional limitation. Such evaluation cannot be done by informal opinions of practitioners whose private experiences are not tested in a well-organized manner. It must be done through sound, systematic research, most properly conducted in the clinical setting where the physical therapist and associates become the investigators and the patients referred for treatment become the subjects of study.

The success of this kind of clinical research depends on multiple collaborations. Coordination and cooperation among physical therapists, physicians, other allied health professionals, and most certainly the patients is important to ensure adequate control of extraneous variables. Consultation with a biostatistician during the process of establishing the appropriate research design will facilitate proper application of data analysis procedures. In the case of thermal agent evaluation, the accuracy of energies delivered should be determined by the appropriate biomedical or electrical engineer. In summary, it is foolhardy to expect that clinical research can or should be done by a single individual.

The data derived from this kind of collaborative clinical investigation will contribute to the professional body of knowledge about therapeutic intervention and will enhance the process of clinical decision making to the benefit of both the practitioner and the patient.

REFERENCES

1. Currier, DP: *Elements of Research in Physical Therapy.* Williams & Wilkins, Baltimore, 1979.
2. Payton, O: *Research: The Validation of Clinical Practice.* FA Davis, Philadelphia, 1979.
3. Colton, T: *Statistics in Medicine.* Little, Brown, Boston, 1974, p 39.
4. Fleiss, JL and Shrout, PE: *The effects of measurement errors on some multivariate procedures.* Am J Public Health 67:1188, 1977.
5. Campbell, DT and Stanley, JC: *Experimental and Quasi-Experimental Designs for Research.* Rand McNally College Publishing Co, Chicago, 1963.
6. Wing, M: *Phonophoresis with hydrocortisone in the treatment of temporomandibular joint dysfunction.* Phys Ther 62:32, 1982.
7. Quillen, WS and Rouillier, LH: *Initial management of acute ankle sprains with rapid pulsed pneumatic compression with cold.* Journal of Orthopedic and Sports Physical Therapy 4:39, 1982.
8. Barlow, DH and Hersen, M: *Single-case experimental designs.* Arch Gen Psychiatry 29:319, 1973.
9. Martin, JE and Epstein, LH: *Evaluating treatment effectiveness in cerebral palsy.* Phys Ther 56:285, 1976.
10. Wolery, M and Harris, SR: *Interpreting results of single-subject research designs.* Phys Ther 62:445, 1982.
11. Bross, I: *Sequential medical plans.* Biometrics 8:189, 1952.
12. Armitage, P: *Sequential Methods in Medical Research.* John Wiley & Sons, New York, 1971.
13. Gonella, C: *Designs for clinical research.* Phys Ther 53:1276, 1973.
14. Oldham, PD: *Measurement in Medicine.* JB Lippincott, Philadelphia, 1968.
15. Light, KE, et al: *Low-load prolonged stretch vs high-load brief stretch in treating knee contractures.* Phys Ther 64:330, 1984.
16. Melzack, R: *The McGill Pain Questionnaire: Major properties and scoring methods.* Pain 1:277, 1975.
17. Carpenter, J: *Medical recommendations followed or ignored: Factors influencing compliance in arthritis.* Arch Phys Med Rehabil 57:241, 1976.
18. Vincent, P: *Factors influencing patient non-compliance.* Nurs Res 20:509, 1971.
19. Moore, ML; *The measurement of joint motion. Part II: The technic of goniometry.* Phys Ther Rev 29:256, 1949.
20. American Academy of Orthopaedic Surgeons: *Joint Motion: Method of Measuring and Recording.* American Academy of Orthopaedic Surgery, Chicago, 1965.
21. Hellebrandt, FA, et al: *The measurement of joint motion. Part III: Reliability of goniometry.* Phys Ther Rev 29:302, 1949.
22. Boone, DC, et al: *Reliability of goniometric measurement.* Phys Ther 58:1355, 1978.

23. Engler, HS and Sweat, RD: *Volumetric arm measurements: Technique and results.* Am Surg 28:465, 1952.
24. Devore, GL, et al: *Volume measuring of the severely injured hand.* Am J Occup Ther 22:16, 1968.
25. Daniels, L and Worthingham, C: *Muscle Testing: Techniques of Manual Examination.* WB Saunders, Philadelphia, 1980.
26. Lilienfeld, AM, Jacobs, M, and Willis, M: *Study of reproducibility of muscle testing and certain other aspects of muscle scoring.* Phys Ther Rev 34:279, 1954.
27. Watkins, MP, Harris, BA, and Kozlowski, BK: *Isokinetic testing in patients with hemiparesis: A pilot study.* Phys Ther 64:184, 1984.
28. DeLorme, TL and Watkins, AL: *Progressive Resistance Exercise: Technic and Medical Application.* Appleton-Century-Crofts, New York, 1951, p 23.
29. Thistle, HG, et al: *Isokinetic contraction: A new concept of resistive exercise.* Arch Phys Med Rehabil 48:279, 1967.
30. Watkins, MP and Harris, BA: *Evaluation of isokinetic muscle performance.* Clinics in Sports Medicine 2:37, 1983.
31. Jebsen, RH: *An objective and standardized test of hand function.* Arch Phys Med Rehabil 50:311, 1969.
32. Vignos, PJ, Spencer, GE, and Archibald, KC: *Management of progressive muscular dystrophy of childhood.* JAMA 184:103, 1963.
33. Boenig, D: *Evaluation of a clinical method of gait analysis.* Phys Ther 57:795, 1977.
34. Wall, JC, Dhanendran, M, and Klenerman, L: *A method of measuring the temporal/distance factors of gait.* Biomed Eng 11:409, 1976.
35. Pochaczevsky, R, et al: *Thermographic study of extremity dermatomes in the diagnosis of spinal root compression syndromes.* In *Biomedical Thermography.* Alan R Liss, New York, 1982, p 339.
36. Atsumi, K (ed): *Medical Thermography.* University of Tokyo Press, Tokyo, 1973, p 11.
37. Love, TJ: *Thermography as an indicator of blood perfusion.* Proc NY Acad Sci 335:429, 1980.
38. Hobbins, WB: *Thermography and pain.* In Gautherie, M and Albert, E (eds): *Biomedical Thermography.* Alan R Liss, New York, 1982, p 361.
39. Rubal, BJ, Traycoff, RB, and Ewing, KL: *Liquid crystal thermography: A new tool for evaluating low back pain.* Phys Ther 62:1593, 1982.
40. Fujimasa, I, Sakurai, Y, and Atsumi, K: *Some physical and physiological aspects of thermography.* In Atsumi, K (ed): *Medical Thermography.* University of Tokyo Press, Tokyo, 1973, p 31.
41. Guyton, AC: *Textbook of Medical Physiology,* ed 6. WB Saunders, Philadelphia, 1981, p 209.
42. Hirsh, J: *Noninvasive tests for thromboembolic disease.* Hosp Pract (Sept) 1982, p 77.
43. Lassen, NA, Henriksen, O, and Sejrsen, P: *Indicator methods for measurement of organ and tissue blood flow.* Section 2: In Shepherd, JT and Abboud, FM (eds): *Handbook of Physiology, The Cardiovascular System.* American Physiological Society, Bethesda, MD, 1983, p 40.
44. Goodgold, J and Eberstein, A: *Electrodiagnosis of Neuromuscular Diseases,* ed 2. Williams & Wilkins, Baltimore, 1978.

CHAPTER 11

THE APPLICATION OF COLD AND HEAT IN THE TREATMENT OF ATHLETIC INJURIES

WAYNE SMITH, M.ED., P.T., A.T.C.

Kraus has described athletic injuries as "those injuries produced by circumstances inherent in respective athletic performances."[1] These injuries can vary from minor strains and sprains to fractures. The goal in treatment of an injured athlete is to restore the greatest possible degree of function in the shortest period of time. Physical agents, such as cold and heat, can be instrumental in reducing an athlete's recovery time.[2–7] The purposes of this chapter are (1) to review the literature on thermal agents as applied to injured athletes and (2) to suggest guidelines to follow in treating athletic injuries.

COLD

Cold has become an increasingly versatile agent among sports medicine practitioners. It is not only useful in first aid to control hemorrhage and edema, but also to relieve pain and muscle spasm. The use of cold allows passive and active exercises of muscles and joints, and reduces the morbidity immediately following acute injury.[8–11]

Edema

One of the earliest attempts to establish guidelines for application of cold in sports medicine was by Bennett,[12] who advocated the use of cold (8°C) whirlpool baths to control hemorrhage and edema. Bennett believed that this temperature would allow vasoconstriction but avoid the vasodilatation response reported by Lewis.[13–15] Even though there was no formal research undertaken, his article did serve as an impetus for future clinical practice. Therapists and trainers assumed that the properties of cold were effective in treating acute injuries because of their physiologic effects. However, it was only after Hocutt and associates[16] compared cold versus heat that any clinical documentation was formulated. The study assessed patients recovering from ankle sprains. Participants were categorized according to the severity of injury, and according to the use of cryotherapy versus the use of heat therapy (each 15 minutes, one to three times daily, for a minimum of 3 days). Therapy commenced either less than 1 hour, from 1 to 36 hours, or more than 36 hours after traumatic injury. Patients who were treated on the first day of injury with cold (that is, whirlpool baths or ice packs) returned to preinjury activities an average of 8 days sooner than did their counterparts who were treated with heat (that is, warm soaks or heating pads).[16] The significance of the study was threefold: (1) It was the first controlled study of its kind reported in the literature; (2) it attempted to establish parameters with regard to temperature and duration of cold application; and (3) it was found that early cryotherapy allowed patients to return to full activities sooner than did late cryotherapy or early heat treatments.

COLD AND COMPRESSION. Cold has been reported to be effective when combined with other modalities in treating athletic injuries.[17–21] The addition of compression to cold application appears to enhance the effectiveness of treating sprains.[2,16,19,21,22] A basic cause of swelling is a change in capillary filtration pressure. Edema will occur when factors controlling the equilibrium between intra- and extravascular fluids are disturbed. The use of a mechanical intermittent compression device appears to assist in maintaining the homeostasis with respect to osmotic pressures and hydrostatic pressures in the capillary beds. Several clinical studies have sought to evaluate the efficacy of combining cold and intermittent compression in treating ankle sprains. Starkey,[21] using high school athletes, compared the simultaneous use of cold, elevation, and intermittent inflatable compression with that of cold, elevation, and compression wrapping. According to the author of the study, 30 minutes of intermittent compression at a 15-second cycle along with cold and elevation proved to be more effective in edema reduction than were cold, elevation, and compression wrapping. In addition, time lost from practice was reduced with the former regimen by approximately 2 days.[21] Similar results were reported by Quillen and Rouillier,[19] who combined cold and elevation with a rapid pulse pneumatic compression device in the treatment of athletic sprains among college athletes. A protocol of 5 minutes of rapid pneumatic pulse compression (70 to 90 mm Hg) along with a cold wrap placed around the injured joint was used, followed by removal of the cold and a continuation of compression for an additional 15 minutes. Volumetric displacement of the foot and ankle confirmed the significant reduction in edema.[19]

Case number 1 illustrates the use of cold and compression.

COLD AND HIGH-VOLTAGE PULSED GALVANIC STIMULATION. High-voltaged pulsed galvanic stimulation along with ice to reduce effusion has

CASE STUDY NO. 1

A 16-year-old male high school athlete sustained an inversion sprain to his right ankle. He reported to the training room and was seen by the school trainer, complaining of pain on weightbearing. Physical examination of the right ankle revealed no gross deformities, limited range of motion, palpable tenderness distal to the right lateral malleolus, and moderate swelling of the anterolateral aspect of the right foot and ankle complex. Initial treatment consisted of a combination of 30 minutes of cold, intermittent compression (50 mm Hg), and elevation. The patient was given crutches and a compression wrap and instructed in a home program of 20 minutes of ice and elevation for a period of 24 hours. On the second day postinjury, he reported to the trainer, who noted a marked reduction of edema; then a prescribed regimen of cryokinetics was instituted: cold whirlpools (9°C for 15 minutes), followed by range-of-motion exercises and weight-bearing as tolerated. On the fourth day postinjury, swelling and pain appeared stabilized, and the patient was progressed to a program of 15 minutes of alternating cold application and light resistive exercises. The athlete resumed full activities by the ninth day postinjury.

recently become a popular therapy mode (Fig. 11–1). Although research is pending regarding the use of this modality with cold, several preliminary reports have suggested that this combination appears to be effective in the management of postfractures and sprains.[17,18,20] Lamboni and Harris[18] have reported good results in reducing edema using cold, compression, and high-voltage pulsed galvanic current at 30 pulses per second, using negative polarity stimulations for 30-minute periods at 15-second intervals. Smith[20] reported similar results in postfractures using cold packs, elevation, and high-voltage pulsed galvanic stimulation at 60 pulses per second, negative polarity alternating stimulations for 10 seconds per pad. However, it should be pointed out that the aforementioned were the results of clinical observations and in no way was there a comparison of methods involving research principles.

MUSCLE INJURY. Conditions that involve injury at the musculotendinous junction or at the tendon itself can pose a difficult problem for the trainer. The joint must be kept mobile to avoid morbid complications during healing without producing further damage. In an attempt to initiate early motion in these painful conditions, cold has been demonstrated to be effective in relieving pain and allowing passive and active exercising.[10,16,23,24] Grant[8] and Hayden[9] both reported that ice massage of 5 to 7 minutes' duration achieved sufficient anesthesia to permit range of motion and immobilization exercises. Waylonis[25] who later repeated Grant's study under controlled conditions, measured some of the physiologic changes of ice massage—pain stimuli, blood flow, and skin temperature. The author reported that although numbness occurred at 5 minutes of ice application, those who

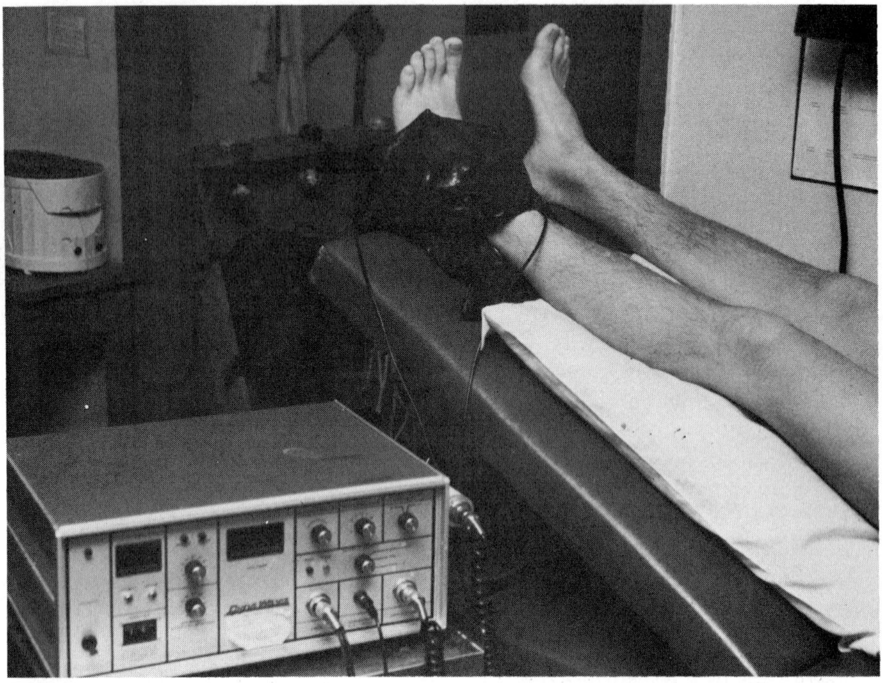

FIGURE 11–1

The use of cold in combination with high-voltage pulsed galvanic stimulation for the acute management of an ankle sprain.

received 10 minutes' application had a greater reduction of temperatures to the deeper tissues.

Prentice[26] used electromyography (EMG) to evaluate the effectiveness of heat and cold, along with some form of stretching for inducing skeletal muscular relaxation, among college athletes suffering from exercise-induced muscle soreness. The study involved a four-way comparison among heat and contract-relax stretching, cold and static stretching, heat and static stretching, and a control group. The findings indicated that those who received a combination of 20 minutes of ice pack followed by static stretching exhibited less EMG activity than did the three other groups. Therefore, the implications for using cold and stretching in such conditions as muscle spasm may have some validity as shown by experimental research. However, Yackzan and associates[27] investigated the efficacy of 15 minutes of ice massage in reducing delayed muscle soreness to determine the optimal time within a stated protocol. Three groups receiving cold were tested: those individuals receiving ice immediately after exercise, those receiving it 24 hours after exercise, and those receiving it 48 hours after exercise were studied. Pain and range of motion were assessed after the patient's undergoing eccentric-based exercises to the elbow flexors. The investigation reported no consistent patterns of significant differences on various comparisons between the treated versus the untreated arms and of the treated arms that were iced at different times. The results of this study failed to dem-

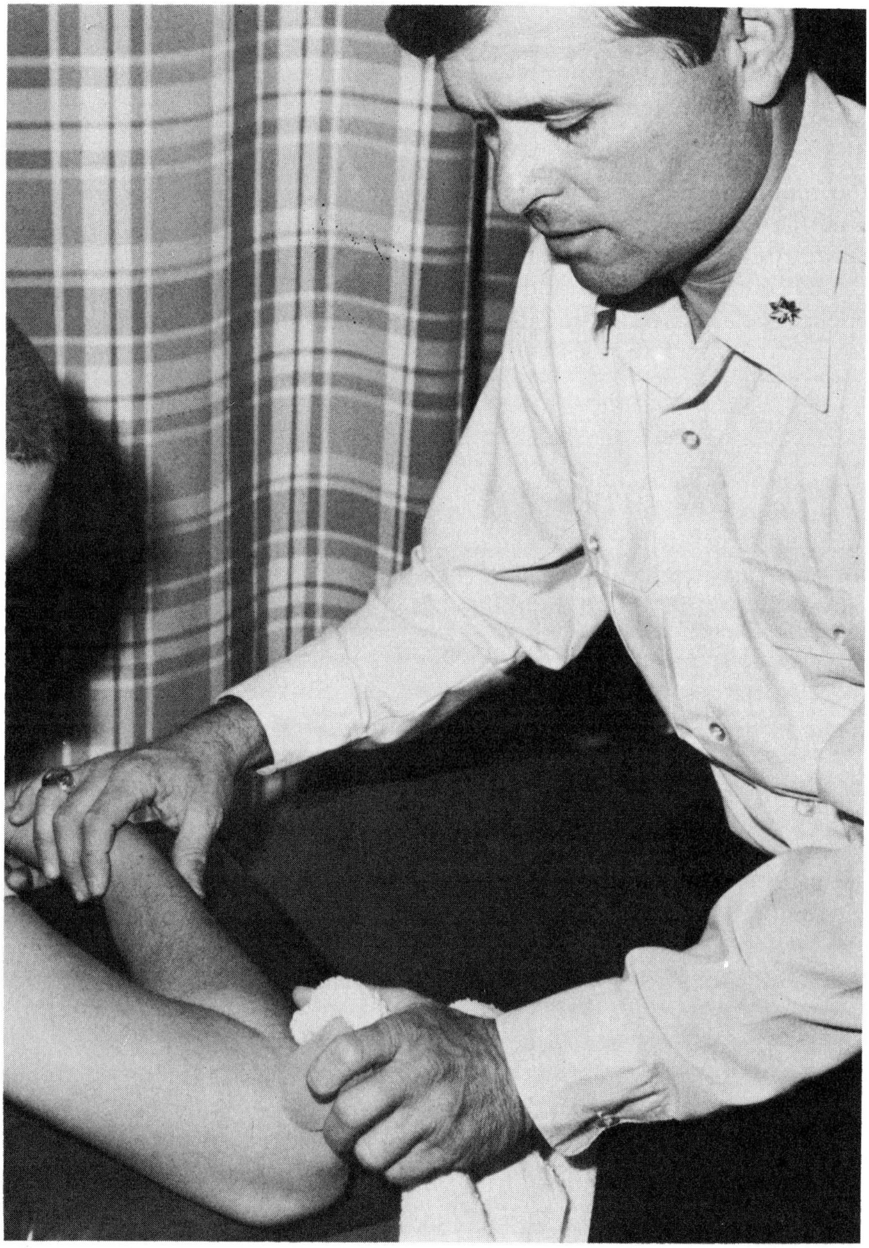

FIGURE 11–2

Cryokinetics in the management of tennis elbow. Ice massage is being applied to the area of the lateral epicondyle to be followed by a slow, gentle stretch to the forearm extensor muscles.

onstrate that cold alone was effective in preventing the occurrence of or in alleviating pain in delayed muscle soreness.

CRYOKINETICS. In the preceding paragraphs, reference was made to the use of cold and exercise. Cryokinetics (cold and exercise) is an essential part of an athlete's rehabilitation program. The key to successful rehabilitation is the use of cold along with graded exercises. Ice is used to numb the affected area; 10 to 12 minutes of application are necessary to achieve the required anesthesia (Fig. 11–2). Unlike the dangers involved when pain-alleviating pharmaceutical agents are injected to enable the patient to perform exercises, the use of cryokinetics has a built-in safety valve. Although the clinical application of cold produces a degree of analgesia, the application is generally not enough to completely anesthetize the involved tissue. If the athlete is experiencing pain during analgesia of the injured part when exercising, it indicates to the practitioner that the patient is exercising too vigorously; this then should be avoided and the patient's activity level should be decreased.

The procedure involving cryokinetics is simple. Cold is initially used to numb the injured part by applying either ice massage, ice packs, immersion baths, or towels soaked in ice water (Fig. 11–3). If the therapist or trainer chooses to use an immersion bath, a technique sometimes employed for injuries of the distal joints, the duration of treatment should not

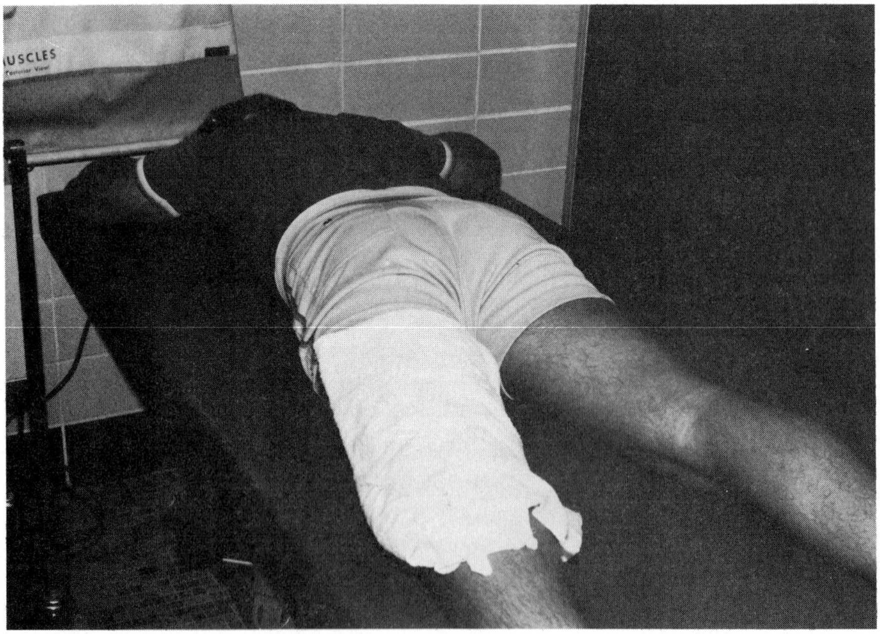

FIGURE 11–3

Towel soaked in ice water is applied along the length of the hamstrings. This will be followed by a hamstring stretch.

TABLE 11-1

Therapeutic Guidelines for the Application of Cold and Heat in the Management of Ankle Sprains

Conditions	Management Phase	Basic Management	Combination Treatment	Objectives of Treatment
Inversion Ankle sprain (grade 2–3)	Phase 1; immediate; 0–72 hours	*Cold* Ice pack 15–30 min Whirlpool 12–20 min (13–21°C) Ice towels 15–30 min	Compression (constant) (intermittent) HVPG stimulation	Reduce swelling and pain
	Phase 2; subacute; 72–96 hours	*Cryokinetics* (cold) 7–10 min ice massage Whirlpool (13–21°C)	Passive/active exercising	Improve mobility Increase blood flow Strengthening
		Heat (edema controlled) Whirlpool × 15–20 min (35.5–38°C) Hot pack × 15–20 min	Same as above Mobilization	Same as above
		Ultrasound (dosage dependent) Continous		Selective heating of joint structures
		Pulse		Tissue repair
		Phonophoresis		Induce medication to injury site
	Phase 3	*Heat* Whirlpool × 12–20 min (37–39°C)	Isokinetic cycle Preprogram jogging	Strengthening Improve blood flow
		Ultrasound (dosage dependent)	Friction massage to fibular collateral ligament	Removal/prevention of adhesions or scarring

TABLE 11–2

Therapeutic Application of Cold and Heat in the Management of Thigh Contusion

Conditions	Management Phase	Basic Management	Combination Treatment	Objectives of Treatment
Thigh Contusion "Charley horse" (grade 2–3)	Immediate; 0–48 hr	*Cold* Ice pack 15–30 min Cool whirlpool (13-21°C) 10 min	Elevation—crutches Compression wrap Rest HVPG stimulation	Control hemorrhaging Reduce muscle spasm and pain
	Subacute; 48–variable	*Cryokinetics* 8–10 min ice massage to injury site	Isometric exercise Passive ROM to tolerance	Improve blood flow Mobility Strengthening
		Ice pack × 12–20 min	Electrical stimulation	Muscle re-education. Reduce congestion
	Phase 3; injury site stabilized or chronic	*Heat* Whirlpool (38–39°C) Hot pack	Isokinetic cycle Preprogram	Strengthening injury site Improve blood flow
		Ultrasound (dosage dependent)	Passive stretching	Softening deeper tissues Clot reabsorption

exceed 12 minutes and the clinician should ensure that the patient has an intact peripheral circulation. Prolonged exposure of cold over an extremity has been reported to result in nerve palsies.[28]

Because use of cold can be a valuable tool in the early management of rehabilitation of the injured athlete, it is important that the therapist or trainer knows what specific effects cold has on the body, when to use this agent, and how it can help in the rehabilitation processes. Tables 11–1, 11–2, and 11–3 provide the reader with a basic guideline for the application of thermal agents in three common sports-related injuries.

HEAT

The effects of heat on circulation, metabolism, and nerves must be taken into account when beginning a new phase of rehabilitation. Heat improves capillary flow and increases the fluid quantity of tissues by speeding the blood flow and dilating the vessels in the involved parts. As a result, metabolism of heated parts is increased, hastening chemical changes and diminishing congestion brought about by the inflammatory process. Heat may reduce muscle spasm by increasing the threshold of sensory endings; hence, it is a pain-relieving modality. To help the therapist decide when it is safe to apply heat to the injured athlete, certain criteria should be met. There should be no increase in swelling of the affected part within the prior 24 hours, and there should be minimal point tenderness with no severe

TABLE 11–3
Application of Cold and Heat Management of Achilles Tendinitis

Conditions	Management Phase	Basic Management	Combination Treatment	Objectives of Treatment
Achilles tendinitis	Swelling and redness present	*Cold* Ice pack 12–30 min Cool whirlpool 10 min (13–21°C)	Crutches ¼″ heel lift; HGV 12–30 min bipolar I	Reduce swelling Pain reduction
	Gradual onset; crepitation, pain present	*Cryokinetics* 8–10 min ice massage	Non-weight-bearing heel cord stretching; temporary orthotic ¼″ heel lift	Increase blood flow Mobility Biomechanical control
	Phase 3; Pain, intermittent—edema not present	*Ultrasound* (dosage dependent) *Heat* Whirlpool × 10–15 min (37–39°C)	Phonophoresis, active exercising and flexibility program; consider permanent orthotic control	Induce medication Increase blood flow Strengthening Biomechanical control if necessary
	Chronic (≥ 3 wk) Intermittent pain with excessive activities	Ultrasound continuous before friction massage; *or* (ice massage, ice pack, or whirlpool)	Friction massage to Achilles tendon	Soften tissues Break up adhesions Reduce irritation after massage

aching of the body part. If heat is applied too soon after an injury, inflammation and extravasation of blood vessels, lymph, and synovial fluid will be aggravated.

Techniques of Heat Application

The way heat is employed is usually predicated on convenience of application, availability of method, and the depth of penetration. In most training rooms, heat is usually administered by either Hydrocollator packs, hydrotherapy, or ultrasound. Hydrotherapy is the most frequently used modality in athletic training. The use of warm whirlpools is indicated in treating postacute sprains, strains, and contusions. When choosing a therapeutic temperature, one must take into account the disadvantages of using whirlpools. The difficulty lies in controlling the therapeutic effects primarily caused by the rapid dissipation of heat radiation, which causes difficulty in maintaining constant tissue temperatures. Studies have shown that topically applied wet heat to raise superficial tissue temperatures is best produced when temperatures between 37°C and 43°C are obtained.[29] Therefore, water should be kept constant at these temperatures using variances that take into account the amount of edema and patient sensitivity. Researchers have found that whirlpool baths at temperatures between 40.5°C and 46.1°C produce up to 25 to 140 ml of increased volume in the extremities.[30] Consequently, whirlpool baths at high temperatures are contraindicated in cases when edema is potentially a problem.

The practice of full body immersion for treating extremities at high temperatures should be avoided. Two serious problems can result from this technique. As blood vessels throughout the body dilate, blood is drawn away from the parts not submerged. The change in blood pressure can result in an athlete's fainting. Second, the dangers also exist of the athlete's suffering from heat exposure, since the body's surface is surrounded by water that is warmer than normal body temperatures. Heat may not be able to dissipate from the body via evaporation or radiation. Special care should be taken by the trainer to avoid full body immersion of an athlete who has just completed vigorous exercising. A proper cool-down is first necessary to dissipate the internal body heat that has resulted from exercise.

The clinical application and guidelines for administration of ultrasound and hot packs have already been discussed in previous chapters. The literature involving control studies using these modalities among the athletic population is "sparse." However, the significance of what is reported can be applied to the population. Ultrasound is commonly used by therapists and trainers as an adjunct in the management of soft tissue injuries.[4,6,31–33] Conditions such as supra- and infrapatellar bursitis appear to respond to ultrasound at low intensities because of the possible mechanical breakdown of large protein molecules that are a major factor in the change of osmotic pressure within the bursa.[7]

The technique of delivering anti-inflammatory drugs via ultrasound (phonophoresis) (Figs. 11–4, 11–5) is becoming increasingly popular

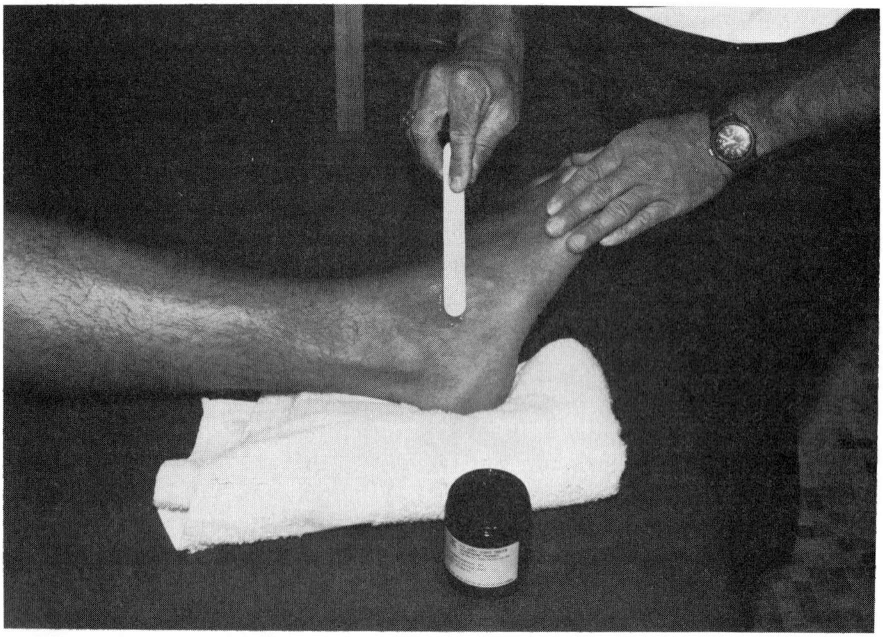

FIGURE 11–4

Massaging a 10 percent solution of hydrocortisone ointment into the skin overlying the sinus tarsus. This will be followed by ultrasound.

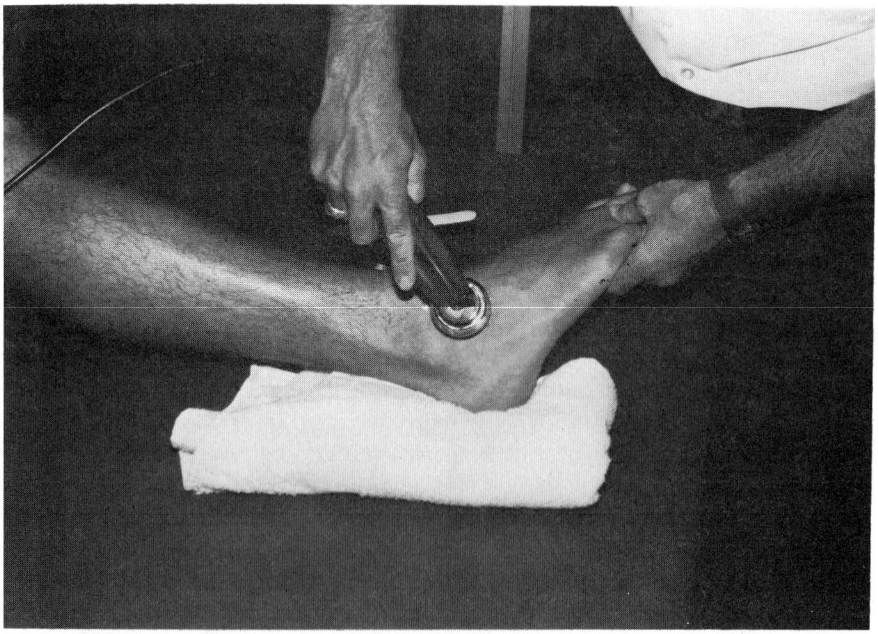

FIGURE 11–5

Phonophoresis (driving in hydrocortisone by ultrasound) to the sinus tarsus in the management of a subacute lateral ankle sprain.

among practitioners. Kleinkort and Wood[32] have demonstrated its effectiveness using hydrocortisone in treating certain types of tendinitis of the elbow and the Achilles tendon. When using this procedure in treating joint and tendon dysfunction, one must take into account the stage of inflammation. After considering the physiologic effects of continuous ultrasound in elevating tissue temperature and increasing the possibility of edema, phonophoresis may have its greatest value in treating subacute and chronic conditions rather than acute conditions. Depth of penetration, which is between 4 and 6 cm, and anatomic positioning are also factors to keep in mind when using phonophoretic treatments. Intensities between 1 and 2 W/cm^2 for a 6-minute duration appear to have the better success in treating musculoskeletal disorders.[33] Conditions such as subdeltoid bursitis may be difficult to treat owing to the excessive amount of tissue the drugs must pass to reach the inflamed area.

Plantar fasciitis, a common occurrence in runners, appears to respond to the therapeutic application of ultrasound. Clark and Stenner[33] studied the effects of ultrasound among patients who were diagnosed for plantar fasciitis. Eight of the 10 patients treated reported they felt improvement after nine applications of 15 to 20 minutes of 1.5 W/cm^2 of continuous ultrasound. Kleinkort and Wood[32] on the other hand reported poor results after six phonophoretic treatments. They postulated that thickened epidermis may have hampered delivery of the hydrocortisone to significant levels. The success of the Clark study may have been attributed to the thermal effects of ultrasound, i.e., blood flow and tissue metabolism.

Ultrasound is often used to facilitate the healing of soft tissue contusions during the post-traumatic period. However, the intensity applied by the therapist must be a consideration. Histologic studies using ultrasound on traumatized tissues (hematomas) indicate that intensities of 1.5 W/cm^2 or greater were needed to effect the healing process.[34] In addition, the same researchers also reported that there were no significant differences between the pulsed and continuous modes, nor between treatment times of 3 and of 7 minutes.

Heat can be of value to the patient when it is used to warm connective tissue that has been scarred following injury or surgery. Strains involving the tearing of either muscle or connective tissue are a common affliction among athletes. The cellular response by the body is to produce fibroblasts, which in turn leads to the production of collagen. Injury and subsequent immobilization can affect movement of tissues, causing joint stiffness. Studies have shown that under heated conditions, the viscous properties of collagenous tissue can become dormant, allowing residual elongation of this tissue when combined with the load. Sapega and co-workers[35] have suggested that prolonged low-intensity stretching at elevated temperatures and maintaining that stretch while the tissues cool can be effective in gaining range of motion. Permanent lengthening of connective tissue is maximized, while the deterioration of tensile strength is minimized.

A treatment plan that utilizes cold and heat is illustrated in case study number 2.

CASE STUDY NO. 2

A 23-year-old female distance runner developed left Achilles peritendinitis while participating in a 6-mile run. She was initially treated with ice and high-voltage pulsed galvanic stimulation and given a ¼-inch heel lift for a period of 72 hours, at which time swelling and pain subsided. However, she continued to have intermittent discomfort 5 days postinjury. Physical examination revealed tightness in the gastrocnemius-soleus muscle complex with mild crepitation within the Achilles tendon. Rehabilitation of the gastrocnemius-soleus muscle tendon unit consisted of gastrocnemius-soleus flexibility exercises and 6 minutes of 1 W/cm^2 of continuous ultrasound to the Achilles tendon, followed by 5 minutes of friction massage to alleviate scar tissue. The patient was able to resume activities 3 weeks after onset of the initial injury.

SUMMARY

The implications for using heat and cold among athletes has been reviewed. Cold appears to be effective in reducing swelling and managing inflammatory processes. It is also an effective modality when combined with exercise. Heat is still a universal treatment for pain after the acute stage of injury. It has many beneficial physiologic effects that the practitioner must take into account when beginning a new phase of rehabilitation.

REFERENCES

1. Kraus, H: *Evaluation and treatment of muscle function in athletic injury.* Am J Surg 98:353, 1959.
2. Esterson, P, Knortz, K, and Wallace, L: *Immediate care of ankle injuries.* Journal of Orthopedic and Sports Physical Therapy 1:46, 1979.
3. Knight, K: *Ice for immediate care of injuries.* Physician and Sports Medicine 10:137, 1982.
4. Millar, A: *Strains of the posterior calf musculature (tennis leg).* Am J Sports Med 7:172, 1979.
5. Moore, RJ: *Uses of cold therapy in the rehabilitation of athletes: Recent advances.* Presented at 19th AMA National Conference on the Medical Aspects of Sports, San Francisco, June 18, 1977.
6. Novich, M: *Physical therapy in treatment of athletic injuries.* Tex State J Med 61:672, 1965.
7. Wise, D: *Physiotherapeutic treatment of athletic injuries to muscle-tendon complex of the leg.* Can Med Assoc J 8:117, 1977.
8. Grant, AE: *Massage with ice (cryokinetics) in the treatment of painful conditions of the musculoskeletal system.* Arch Phys Med Rehabil 45:233, 1964.
9. Hayden, CA: *Cryokinetics in early treatment program.* Am J Phys Ther 44:990, 1964.
10. Knight, K: *Cryostretch for muscle spasm.* Physician and Sports Medicine 4:129, 1980.
11. Moore, RJ, Nicolette, RL, and Behnke, R: *The therapeutic use of cold (cryotherapy) in the care of athletic injuries.* Journal of National Athletic Trainers Association 6:12, 1967.
12. Bennett, D: *Water at 67° to 69°F to control hemorrhage and swelling encountered in athletic injuries.* Journal of National Athletic Trainers Association 1:12, 1961.

13. Aquird, J, et al: *A re-examination of Lewis' cold-induced vasodilation in the finger and the ankle.* Athletic Training 15:248, 1980.
14. Knight, K and Loadere, RB: *Comparison of blood flow in the ankle of uninjured subjects during therapeutic application of heat, cold and exercise.* Medicine and Science in Sport and Exercise 12:217, 1980.
15. Lewis, T: *Observation upon the reaction of the vessels of the human skin to cold.* Heart 15:177, 1930.
16. Hocutt, JE, et al: *Cryotherapy in ankle sprains.* Am J Sports Med 10:316, 1982.
17. Brown, S: *Ankle edema and galvanic muscle stimulation.* Physician and Sports Medicine 9:137, 1981.
18. Lamboni, P and Harris, B: *The use of ice, airsplints, and high voltage galvanic stimulation in effusion reduction.* Athletic Training 18:23, 1983.
19. Quillen, WS and Rouillier, LH: *Initial management of acute ankle sprains with rapid pulsed pneumatic compression and cold.* Journal of Orthopedic and Sports Physical Therapy 4:39, 1982.
20. Smith, W: *High galvanic therapy in the symptomatic management of acute tibial fracture.* Athletic Training 16:59, 1981.
21. Starkey, J: *Treatment of ankle sprains by simultaneous use of intermittent compression and ice packs.* Am J Sports Med 4:142, 1976
22. Cooper, D and Fair, J: *Contrast baths and pressure treatment for ankle sprains.* Physician and Sports Medicine 7:143, 1979.
23. McMaster, W: *Cryotherapy.* Physician and Sports Medicine 10:112, 1982.
24. Smith, C: *Physical management of muscular low back pain in the athlete.* Can Med Assoc J 117:632, 1977.
25. Waylonis, GW: *The physiological effects of ice massage.* Arch Phys Med Rehabil 48:37, 1967.
26. Prentice, WE: *An electromyographic analysis of the effectiveness of heat or cold and stretching for inducing relaxation of injured muscle.* Am J Sports Med 9:133, 1981.
27. Yackzan, L, Adams, C, and Francis, K: *The effects of ice massage on delayed muscle soreness.* Am J Sports Med 12:159, 1984.
28. Drez, D, Faust, DC, and Evans, JP: *Cryotherapy and nerve palsy.* Am J Sports Med 9:256, 1981.
29. Abramson, D, et al: *Comparison of wet and dry heat in raising temperature of tissues.* Arch Phys Med Rehabil 12:654, 1967.
30. Magness, J, Garrett, T, and Erickson, D: *Swelling of the upper extremity during whirlpool baths.* Arch Phys Med Rehabil 5:297, 1970.
31. Blazina, M, et al: *Jumper's knee,* Ortho Clinics of North America, 4:665, 1973.
32. Kleinkort, J and Wood, F: *Phonophoresis with one percent versus 10 percent hydrocortisone.* Phys Ther 55:1321, 1975.
33. Clark, GR and Stenner, L: *Use of therapeutic ultrasound.* Physiotherapy 62:185, 1976.
34. Stratton, SA, Heckmann, R, and Francis, RS: *Therapeutic Ultrasound: Its effects on the integrity of a non penetrating wound.* Journal of Orthopedic and Sports Physical Therapy 5:278, 1984.
35. Sapega, A, et al: *Biophysical factors in range of motion exercise.* Physician and Sports Medicine 9:57, 1981.

CHAPTER 12

THE USE OF HEAT AND COLD IN THE MANAGEMENT OF RHEUMATIC DISEASES

SUSAN L. MICHLOVITZ, M.S., P.T.

A well-planned physical therapy program is an integral part of the comprehensive management of the patient with rheumatic disease. The overall objective of physical therapy is to improve or maintain the patient's level of function.

The physical therapy evaluation serves as a foundation from which a treatment program can be designed. In developing treatment goals, it is important to assess pain (at rest and on activity), range of motion (ROM), muscle strength, posture, gait, and functional status (such as stair climbing, activities of daily living, occupational demands). The component parts of a treatment plan are developed from short- and long-term goals and can include techniques for pain relief, exercises for increasing/maintaining ROM and muscle strength, and cardiovascular conditioning. Assistive and adaptive devices may be required to improve gait and functional activities. An important aspect of treatment, patient education, should include joint protection and energy conservation techniques.

Physical agents including electrical stimulation, heat and cold can be used as an adjunct to provide pain relief prior to exercise or positioning, decrease muscle guarding spasm, improve ROM, or facilitate muscle reeducation. In most cases, it is important to emphasize that the use of a physical agent is only an adjunct in the total treatment plan and may only help reach a short-term goal. Most important to consider is that the patient with arthritis has a chronic disease often associated with exacerbations and remissions and unrelenting pain.

The purposes of this chapter are to (1) discuss the role of thermal agents in the total treatment strategy; (2) review previous work that has used heat or cold agents as an adjunct in the management of arthritis; and (3) suggest guidelines for application of these agents and evaluation of treatment outcome.

GENERAL CONSIDERATIONS

All of the thermal agents have been incorporated at some point in the various treatment regimens for arthritis management. The decision of which agent to use in which situation is not always clear. Certain basic questions come to the forefront. Should a superficial or a deep-heating agent be applied? Is heat or cold the more effective in treating the arthritis patient? Will cold increase stiffness in persons with arthritis? Will deep heat accelerate the destruction of joint structures in the patient with inflammatory arthritis? As will become evident in the forthcoming review and discussion, some of these questions have been partially or fully answered. Others still require further investigation.

The choice of when to apply a thermal agent and which to use is dependent on a number of factors, including some of the following:

1. *Inflammatory versus noninflammatory polyarthritis.* As an example, if the goal of medical treatment of rheumatoid arthritis is to reduce joint inflammation and temperature, it may be best to choose a physical agent that will alter only skin and subcutaneous tissue temperature (such as hot packs or cold packs). These will provide pain relief and relaxation through reflex mechanisms and counterirritation, rather than a deep-heating agent (such as ultrasound or diathermy), which has the potential to increase joint temperature and inflammation. In the case of osteoarthritis, when muscle guarding spasm or joint contracture is present, heating can usually be more aggressive.
2. *Acute versus chronic inflammation.* When a joint is actually inflamed (hot and swollen), heat application may exacerbate symptoms. During this time, cold application and/or electrical stimulation can be effective in reducing pain and inflammation. Cold can also be effective during the chronic stages of rheumatoid arthritis to provide pain relief prior to exercise (see subsequent section on rheumatoid arthritis).
3. *Loss of range of motion.* The origin of the limitation in motion must be delineated. If joint capsular shortening or musculotendinous contracture are limiting mobility, deep heat in combination with a slow, gentle stretch can be more effective than heat or stretch used in isolation. If the patient can tolerate cold application, simultaneous use of cold and slow stretch may produce desired results. This technique should be used with caution, because cold analgesia prior to exercise may mask both pain and potential damage to soft tissue. If the joint space is reduced, then the techniques to increase range of motion will be less successful.
4. *Position for treatment.* The patient should be discouraged from sitting while receiving a thermal agent. This is particularly important to stress with the patient who has inflammatory arthritis. This patient will have a tendency to develop flexion contractures, which will be facilitated with the patient in the seated position. Joints should be positioned so pain is not markedly increased. If one of the goals of treatment is to decrease pain, the therapy administered should not increase pain. A sharp, aggravating pain must be differentiated from a more subdued aching of short duration (less than 2 hours) which can be expected when performing exercise or positioning to maintain or increase ROM.

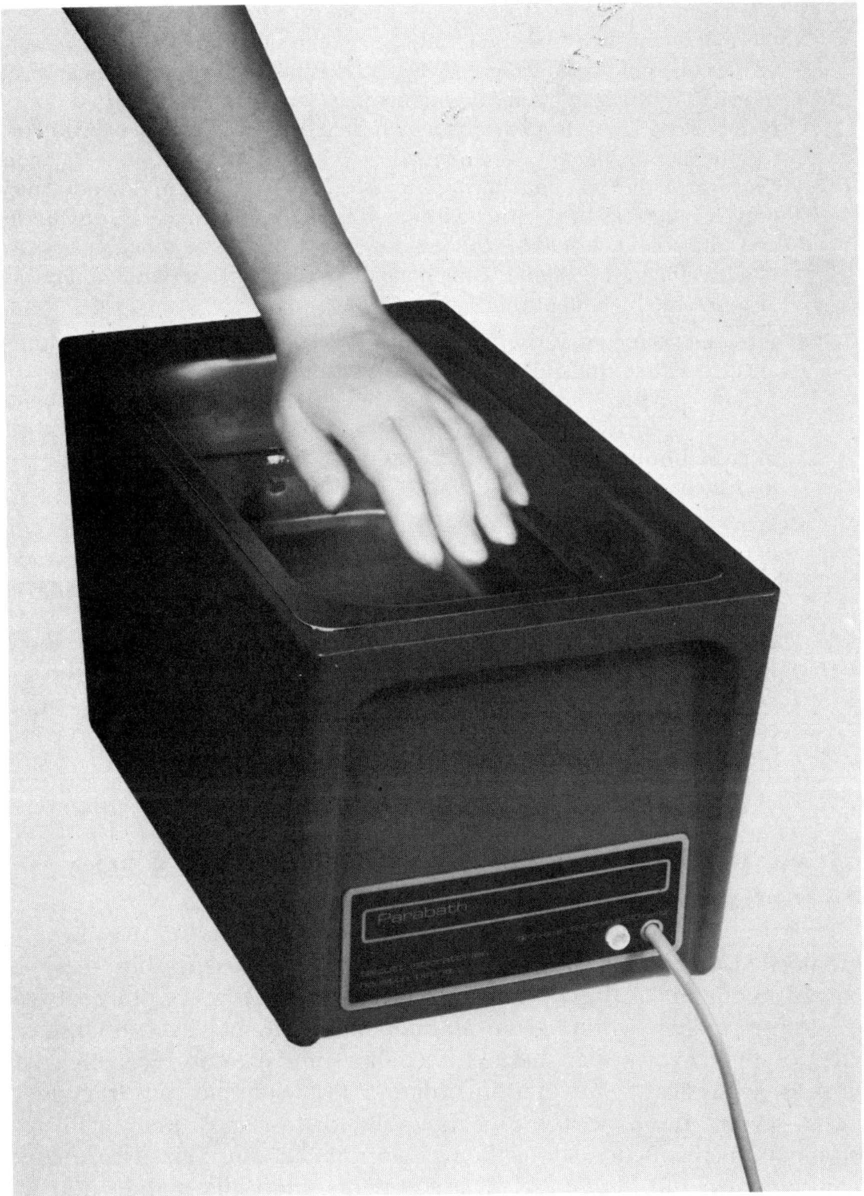

FIGURE 12-1
A home model paraffin unit. (Courtesy of Talcott Laboratories, Houston, PA.)

5. *Number of joints involved.* With multiple joint involvement, the use of some of the thermal agents may be impractical. For example, application of hot packs to more than four joints can be cumbersome. In this instance, hydrotherapy (especially Hubbard tanks and therapeutic pools) can assist in reducing the effects of gravity and stress on painful joints, thus promoting ease of motion. In addition, psychological aspects of pool therapy should not be overlooked.

6. *Clinic versus home care.* If a patient is placed on a home care program, some thermal agents are more practical to use than others. A table-top paraffin unit can be purchased or rented (Fig. 12–1); this is more practical and safe to use than the suggested "home mixtures" that are prepared in a double boiler or crock pot. Hot packs can be heated as needed, but may be difficult for the arthritic patient to handle. Electric heating pads should be avoided because of the potential for falling asleep on the pad and producing a burn. Cold packs can be made from ice chips and a plastic bag. Diathermy and ultrasound should be applied only by or under the *direct* supervision of a qualified professional, which precludes their unsupervised application at home by the patient or a family member.
7. *Precaution/Contraindication.* Some medical conditions and patient appliances preclude the choice of many of the thermal agents; thorough evaluation and good clinical judgment can screen for those cases when a thermal agent can be potentially harmful. These conditions have been discussed in earlier sections of this text, and some will be reiterated later in this chapter.
8. *Preconceived notions.* Many patients with arthritis have experienced periods of unrelenting pain and loss of function. They may have been given useful tips by well-meaning neighbors and friends. Many friends and neighbors have offered a myriad of topical salves and home remedies. It is not uncommon to hear a patient say, "Cold is bad for arthritis." Some people with arthritis favorably respond to heat, some to cold. Often the choice is empirically based. Therefore, patient education regarding the disease process and principles and goals of conservative management can be one of the keys to successful therapeutic intervention.

POLYARTICULAR ARTHRITIS: GUIDELINES FOR MANAGEMENT WITH THERMAL AGENTS

Foremost in the therapist's choice of thermal agent usage should be the goals of treatment of the arthritic patient. Short- and long-term goals can be determined after a completed evaluation of the patients' functional status, extent of joint involvement, and pain. Unlike some patients receiving treatment in a physical rehabilitation program (for example, postfracture or tendon repair), the patient with a rheumatic disease most likely will have chronic problems. Patients must be well educated about their disease, functional abilities, and limitations. These patients, more likely than not, will return for treatment more than once. Patients will be done a disservice if a heat/cold agent is given without providing them with information and instructions about long-term management.

Successful therapeutic management of arthritis is difficult to achieve and assess. The more than 100 rheumatic diseases are not all managed in the same way. For the purpose of discussion in this chapter, two different categories of polyarticular arthritis will be considered: disorders associated with systemic disease and inflammation (for example, rheumatoid arthritis) and disorders primarily associated with joint degeneration (for example, osteoarthritis with some localized inflammation). Refer to Table 12–1 for

TABLE 12-1

Features of Inflammatory and Degenerative Arthritis*

Findings	Degenerative Arthritis (Osteoarthritis)	Inflammatory Arthritis (Rheumatoid Arthritis)
Joints commonly involved	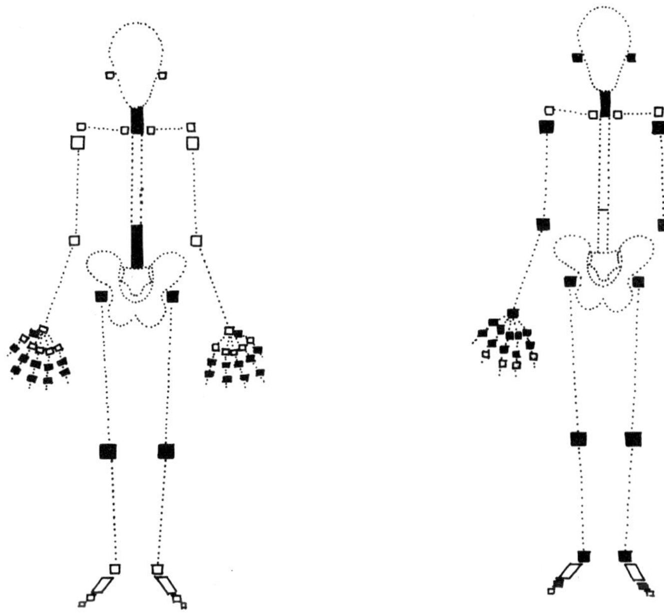	
Joint swelling	Uncommon	Common
Morning stiffness	Minimal	Often greater than 1 hour
Joint changes	Osteophytes	Pannus (synovial membrane proliferation)
Sedimentation rate	Normal or minimally elevated	Elevated
Additional findings	Heberden's and Bouchard's nodes	Rheumatoid nodules Baker's cysts Vasculitis Osteoporosis Peripheral sensory deficit

* Adapted from Katz.[1]

an overview of disease characteristics. The application of thermal agents for each of the two categories will be reviewed separately.

Rheumatoid Arthritis

Rheumatoid arthritis (RA) is a systemic disorder of unknown etiology characterized by articular inflammation.[1,2] There is often a natural course of exacerbations and remissions. The synovial lining cells hypertrophy, forming a vascularized granulation tissue (pannus). Digestants in the synovial fluid and pannus destroy periarticular tissue and articular surfaces. Pannus causes periarticular adhesions as well as weakening of capsular and ligamentous structures. The end result can be hypermobility or hypermobility and deformity. As a result of inflammation, joint temperature is elevated.[3] Treatment including medication, splinting, and thermal agents are aimed at reducing pain and inflammation, and exercise is also important for preserving range of motion and muscle strength.

Other dysfunctions associated with RA include but are not limited to osteoporosis, bursitis, tendinitis, skin breakdown, rheumatoid nodules, and arteritis.

HEAT. The stage of the disease process, particularly with inflammatory arthritis, must be taken into account. A patient with rheumatoid arthritis who has an acutely inflamed joint may find his or her symptoms further exacerbated by heat application. During this time, the application of ice packs may aid in reducing pain and inflammation. If the disease process is in the subacute stage, superficial heat or cold may be equally effective in reducing discomfort and in ultimately improving function.

Superficial heating agents are probably the most commonly applied of the thermal agents for persons with rheumatoid arthritis. The patient will usually report temporary relief of or decrease in pain following such application. Patients can be instructed in the use of hot packs and paraffin for home use allowing carry over from the hospital or clinic setting.

The majority of the studies that investigated superficial heat application measured the effects of an agent on the hands of patients with rheumatoid arthritis (Table 12–2). Harris and Millard[4] reported a slight increase in pain, tenderness, and swelling, and an increase in grip strength, following daily paraffin applied to patients with rheumatoid arthritis. The treatment was given at a temperature of 44°C for a duration of 6 weeks. The results of treatment were not considered to be statistically significant. When they applied paraffin daily for three weeks, no difference was found between treated and untreated groups. Gallagher and associates[5] conducted a study in which the control group was given active range-of-motion (AROM) exercises, while the test group received both paraffin and AROM exercises daily for 10 days. There was no significant difference found between the control and test groups when strength, AROM, pain, stiffness, and functional dexterity were measured. The results of both experiments would suggest that paraffin is of little value in the final outcome when applied for a few weeks or less. Paraffin treatment continues to be one of the most widely recommended[1,6] and employed thermal agents in the management of rheumatoid arthritis. Even though the long-term benefits may not be apparent, clinical experience suggests that heat prior to exercise will relax and psychologically prepare a patient in pain for exericse.

The newest thermal agent, Fluidotherapy, is a useful adjunct in the conservative management of a person with arthritis. Exercise can be performed while the hand or foot is within the heated unit. Finsterwald and associates (unpublished data) have recently compiled information that compares paraffin with Fluidotherapy applied to the hands of persons with

TABLE 12-2
Heat Application to the Hands of Patients with Rheumatoid Arthritis

Investigator	Thermal Agent and Treatment Protocol	Control	Conclusions
Finsterwald (unpublished)	Paraffin on one hand followed by exercise, 10 days, BID Fluidotherapy on other hand, 43.5°C with exercise while in heat unit, 10 days, BID	None	Preliminary results suggest patients with Fluidotherapy showed greater improvement
Gallagher, Eshlemann, and Schumacher[5]	Paraffin followed by AROM, daily for 10 days	AROM	No significant difference between the groups
Harris and Millard[4]	Paraffin daily for 3 weeks; paraffin daily for 6 weeks; both groups did exercises	No treatment	No differences among all groups at 3 weeks, but group treated for 6 weeks was slightly improved at the end of this time
Mainardi and associates[11]	Electric mitten at 40°C, 30 minutes BID for 2 years	Opposite hand received no heat	No further changes on x-ray that could be attributed to heat application

rheumatoid arthritis. Paraffin followed by an exercise regimen was used with one of the patient's hands, while the patient's other hand was treated simultaneously with Fluidotherapy at 43.5°C and exercise. Both treatments were administered two times a day for a total of 20 sessions. Preliminary results suggest that Fluidotherapy provided greater pain relief, increase in strength and range of motion, and improvement in functional skills than did paraffin. In this study, no controls were used. It may be difficult to use control subjects in some clinical settings, such as one where a portion of a treatment regimen is denied to patients. Some research protocols are designed to compare and contrast different treatment techniques used in a particular rehabilitation setting with a single patient population.

There are far fewer studies in the literature on the results of deep heat application to patients with inflammatory arthritis. Soren[7] treated patients with rheumatoid wrists and hips with ultrasound at 2.5 W/cm^2 for eight to 10 treatments, two to three times a week, for a total of 10 to 15 sessions. The findings show that ultrasound produced no improvement in over 60 percent of the 40 patients studied. Pain appeared to be reduced when ultrasound was given to rheumatoid nodules at an intensity of 1.0 to 2.5 W/cm^2 for eight to 10 treatments.[8] No other improvements or changes were noted.

During the last decade, controversy has arisen regarding the long-term effects of heat application to persons with inflammatory arthritis.[9] Persons with active rheumatoid arthritis can have elevated joint temperatures up to 37°C.[3] Normal intra-articular temperature is 3°C to 5°C lower. One could consider that further elevating joint temperature with a thermal agent during the period of acute or subacute inflammation may be additive and thus more detrimental to joint structures. Many of the treatments of rheumatoid arthritis aim to reduce joint temperature by reducing inflammation. Intra-articular corticosteroid administration and splinting of an inflamed joint are examples of two methods that have been used to reduce inflammation within a joint. Concern regarding elevation of joint temperature by a thermal agent in patients with active rheumatoid arthritis probably emerged as a result of laboratory studies conducted in the laboratory of Harris and McCroskery.[10] They demonstrated in an in vitro study that collagen cartilage lysis by rheumatoid synovial collagenase was four times greater when temperatures of the preparation were elevated to 36°C.

A 2-year study was conducted by Mainardi and associates[11] to investigate the long-term results of daily heat application to the hands of persons with rheumatoid arthritis. Heat was applied to one hand through an electric mitten at 40°C for 30 minutes two times a day for 2 years. The other hand of each person served as the control. On x-ray examination, no further evidence of joint destruction could be attributed to the heat treated hands. Therefore, more clinical investigations on the long-term effects of heat therapy to rheumatoid joints seem to be warranted.

HYDROTHERAPY. Hydrotherapy is often recommended for patients with inflammatory and degenerative arthritis for decreasing pain, thus facilitating the ease with which exercises can be performed. An 8-week, biweekly course of hydrotherapy and exercises for patients with rheumatoid arthritis was evaluated by Dial and Windsor.[12] When the patients were evaluated at the end of the program, they demonstrated a significant improvement in range of motion and a decrease in time required to perform functional tasks. By 1 month postprogram, the patients tended to return to preprogram status. The long-term benefits of the program appeared to be the psychosocial improvement expressed by the patients. This can be very important in assisting to improve the self-image of the patient with a chronic disability.

Contrast baths have long been used in arthritis and sports rehabilitation. Documentation of the short- and long-term effectiveness of this treatment is lacking. The studies that have appeared in the literature measured the changes in skin temperature produced by contrast baths in normals and in persons with rheumatoid arthritis.[13–15] The skin temperature changes in those with arthritis were less dramatic than were those with no pathology. Although this may provide some insight into the peripheral vascular status of some arthritic patients, any other clinical correlations do not seem to be apparent.

COLD. Cryotherapy has been gaining increased popularity in arthritis treatment over the last two decades. Ice packs were applied for 20 minutes three times a day, for 1 month, to the knees of patients with rheumatoid arthritis.[16] An increase in ROM and sleep duration and decreases in pain (as measured by a visual analog pain scale) and in oral analgesic intake were reported. There were no changes in synovial fluid composition. In this study, one knee was treated with ice, while the other knee had no cold application, thus serving as a comparison. Pegg, Littler, and Littler[17] used 5-minute ice pack applications and exercise daily for 2 weeks in treating the knees and elbows of rheumatoid patients. Stiffness and pain were reduced in most patients, and ROM improved in 50 percent of the patients. When the same investigators changed treatment to immersing patients' hands in cold water (dipping in and out for 10 minutes), the treatment was less effective.

In a small sampling, Wright and Johns[18] and Backlund and Tiselius[19] found that immersion of the hands in a cold bath *increased* the stiffness of finger joints. Studies by Kirk and Kersley,[20] in which cold application to the knees *reduced* stiffness, do not support these findings. In the case of cold application to the knee, the temperature of the joint structures was probably not lowered, whereas cold application to the hands may have lowered the temperature of the joint capsule, thus increasing elastic stiffness. This may account for the differences reported by the investigators. Some patients with inflammatory arthritis will not tolerate cold application, particularly those with cryoglobulinemia and cold hypersensitivity syndromes.[21]

HEAT VERSUS COLD. Heat and cold both seem to be valuable adjuncts in the rehabilitation of persons with rheumatoid arthritis. Logically, the next subject to be addressed is the comparison of heat and cold. Two studies compared ice pack with hot pack application to the knees of rheumatoid arthritis patients. Kirk and Kersley[20] reported that 60 percent of their subjects preferred cold applications. Both groups improved in range of motion without one being more statistically significant than the other. All patients were on a standard exercise program.

Utsinger and associates[22] compared 1 week of ice packs (two times a day) with 1 week of hot packs (three times a day) applied to the same patients on alternating weeks. Fifty percent preferred hot packs to cold and 18 percent had no preference of one over the other. All patients showed improvement in some of the measured variables (sleep duration, pain, timed functional tests). In those patients who preferred cold, naloxone was administered prior to a subsequent cold application. In most of these patients, after the administration of naloxone, cold was no longer effective in reducing pain. The investigators suggest that cold may be effective in reducing pain by facilitating activation of endorphins.

If the disease process is chronic with no active joint inflammation and if the patient has soft tissue tightness secondary to lack of active mobility or to immobilization, a more vigorous approach is suggested. A deep heat in conjunction with a slow, gentle stretch may be most beneficial.[23] Suggestions for patient positioning for stretching are elaborated on in an article by Kottke and associates.[24] Caution must be used in considering a stretch to an unstable joint (such as medial and lateral) or in a patient with osteoporosis. Prior to attempting stretching or splinting of hypomobile joints, x-ray findings should be reviewed to help the therapist determine if it will be realistic to expect an increase in range of motion.

Thermal agents should be used very cautiously in patients with vasculitis or skin ulceration.

Osteoarthritis

Osteoarthritis is characterized by joint cartilage destruction with subsequent osteophyte spur formation at joint margins.[2] Associated synovitis can occur with advanced disease. Acute inflammatory flareups may be induced by trauma. Pain is present on passive motion and during weight bearing. The course of this disorder appears to be exacerbated by abnormal stresses, such as those caused by obesity, placed on joints (see Table 12–1).

HEAT. In degenerative arthritis, pain and limited range of motion, rather than joint inflammation, are the primary problems. Heating, then, may be more vigorous in treating this patient population. Often, the patient with a osteoarthritis will be obese. If this is the case, diathermy, particularly capacitance SWD, may be contraindicated or may be used only with extreme precaution.[25] Elderly patients with the disease, women more likely than men, may have osteoporosis. Again, caution should be used when having these patients perform a stretch to increase their range of motion; active motion may be a more appropriate choice.

Hot packs are routinely used to relieve the symptoms of pain and muscle spasm in patients with inflammatory and degenerative rheumatic diseases. There is a dearth of literature supporting the effectiveness of such treatment. Hot pack application was shown to reduce muscle spasm and provide analgesia in patients with "neck and shoulder syndromes."[26]

Hamilton and Bywaters[27] compared superficial heating agents with deep heating agents in patients with inflammatory and degenerative joint diseases. All patients in the study received each of the four treatments reported, for a duration of 1 month. Although most of the patients showed improvement in stair-walking time, range of motion, and strength, no single treatment was shown to be significantly better than any other. The treatments performed included short-wave diathermy, infrared, paraffin, and "cold" short-wave diathermy (as the control group). Each of these agents was incorporated into a complete rehabilitation program. It is interesting to note that those patients who received a dose of thermal energy fared no better than did those receiving the "control" treatment.

If the therapist or physician determines that it may be more advantageous to heat deep structures to accomplish treatment goals (for example, to elevate the temperature of the knee joint capsule structures), then diathermy or continuous wave ultrasound would be selected as the heating agent. More clinical investigations have been made about the effects of deep heat on osteoarthritis than the effects of deep heat on rheumatoid arthritis.

DePreux[28] administered ultrasound to patients' hips and reported a decrease in pain and an improvement in gait. Ultrasound was delivered at an intensity of 1.5 to 2.0 W/cm^2, 10 minutes per field, for a total of 10 to 20 sessions. Unfortunately, no control group was used against which to compare the efficacy of this treatment. When Aldes and Jadeson[29] administered ultrasound to the cervical and lumbar spines of 311 elderly patients, range of motion was improved and pain was reduced in 70 percent. A sham ultrasound group was compared with the ultrasound-treated group, which received 8 to 12 treatments at an intensity of 1.3 to 11.9 watts for 3 to 10 minutes.

Intra-articular steroid injections, nonsteroidal anti-inflammatory drugs (NSAID), and thermal agents have all been used in the management of osteoarthritis of the knee. Wright[30] compared the effects of (1) a placebo pill (one tablet, two times a day); (2) a placebo injection (intra-articular normal saline, a total of four injections over an 8-week period); (3) and short-wave diathermy (SWD), three times a week for 6 weeks. Both the group receiving SWD and the group receiving a placebo injection improved in walking time, had a decrease in pain, and required fewer oral analgesics. These two groups showed a greater improvement than did those who had taken the placebo pill.

Deep heat in conjunction with exercise has been used to increase range of motion in patients with soft tissue contractures secondary to arthritis. But a decrease in range of motion at the knee was reported by Vanharanta[31] following SWD given to rabbits who had "experimentally induced" osteoarthritis. Immobilization of the knee was the model used to produce soft tissue tightness in the rabbits' knees. SWD applied over an 11-week period was felt by the investigator to have been additive to the effects of immobilization. In this study, no exercise was used in conjunction with the heat treatments. Conversely, Gibson, Winter, and Grahame[32] reported an increase in knee flexion and decrease in pain when SWD was used in combination with exercise in patients with osteoarthritis of the knee. The treatment was given three times a week for 2 weeks.

Many patients with degenerative arthritis, often have the same functional limitation of motion (owing to soft tissue tightness) as do patients with periarthritis, an inflammation of structures around the joint. Therefore, results of treatment of patients with periarthritis could be related to the results of physical management of patients with osteoarthritis. Lehmann and associates,[33] studying patients with periarthritis of the shoulder, reported a greater increase in range of motion using ultrasound and exercise than using a combination of microwave diathermy (MWD) and exercise. Both ultrasound and MWD were given daily for 8 days. When Mueller and associates[34] compared sham ultrasound treatment to ultrasound at 2.0 W/cm^2 in a similar group of patients for the same duration of treatment as the study by Lehmann and associates, no difference in function was found between the two groups. Again, these two studies are representative of the conflicting results found in the literature.

HEAT VERSUS COLD. A comparison among the effects of untuned SWD, SWD, and ice on the knees of patients with osteoarthritis, was made by Clarke and associates.[35] Each treatment was given three times a day for 3 weeks. Most patients showed improvement on evaluation 3 months post-onset of treatment, but those receiving ice showed early progress in pain reduction. Results of this study suggest that cold may be valuable in decreasing pain, thus facilitating the ease with which exercise can be performed. A summary of studies that compare heat with cold can be found in Table 12–3.

FACTORS INFLUENCING THE OUTCOME OF TREATMENT

The results of treatment techniques for persons with rheumatic diseases are varied. A number of factors can obscure the outcome of a particular treatment or combination of therapeutic modalities. The *natural course of the disease,* often associated with spontaneous exacerbations and remissions, has been mentioned earlier in this chapter. Because of the *variable course* of inflammatory arthritis, including its exacerbations and remissions, it may be difficult to claim the effectiveness of one particular treatment modality.

The *stage of the disease* is also important to consider. Decreasing pain and improving functional level may be much more realistic in someone with early RA and minimal x-ray changes than in a patient with severe joint destruction and muscle atrophy.

Concurrent use of medications with physical therapy management and/or changes in medication can change the patient's response to treatment. For example, numerous NSAIDs are currently in use. Although many of these have similar actions, including reduction of inflammation and pain,[36] a patient may respond more favorably to one than to another. So, if there is a change in the NSAID or other medication taken by the patient during the course of physical therapy, the patient may improve owing to the new medication. If one is not aware of this change in medication, one may be tempted to attribute the improvement to the physical therapy program. Conversely, a poor response to a change in medication may be erroneously interpreted as a poor response to a program of heat and exercise. It may be difficult to weigh the individual components of a total management program to evaluate the efficacy of each. Patients who are taking pain-relieving medications for their arthritis or who are recovering from arthritis surgery may be mildly obtunded as a side effect. Their abilities to participate in their therapy or to provide information about the treatment may be altered.

Pain management in arthritis is particularly difficult to effect and assess. Common methods of pain management used in arthritis therapy include heat, cold, electrotherapy, EMG biofeedback, relaxation and imagery, and

TABLE 12-3
Summary of Clinical Studies That Compared Heat Versus Cold in Arthritis Management

Investigator	Subjects Treated	Heat Agent	Cold Agent	Control Group	Conclusions
Clarke and associates[25]	Osteoarthritic knees	SWD, t.i.w., 3 weeks	Ice packs, t.i.w., 3 weeks	Untuned SWD	Patients with cold made better early progress; no long-term (3 months later) differences among 3 groups
Hamer and Kirk[37]	Frozen shoulders not due to primary joint disease	US at 0.5 W/cm^2 for 5–8 min; Codman's exercises	Iced towels for 15 minutes; Codman's exercises	None	Both decreased pain and in conjunction with exercise increased ROM; no significant advantage of one over the other
Kirk and Kersley[20]	Rheumatoid arthritic knees	Hot packs daily for 5 days; standard exercise	Ice packs daily for 5 days; standard exercise	Comparison of hot packs and cold packs alternated for 1 week at a time	60% preferred cold; ROM improved with both treatments
Utsinger, Bonner, and Hogan[22]	Rheumatoid arthritic knees	Hot packs TID, 1 week	Ice packs TID, 1 week	Comparison of hot packs to cold packs on same patient	50% preferred HP; naloxone blocked efficacy of cold

medications. If the pain associated with rheumatic diseases was easy to manage, there would not be so many different treatment modes used. The pain associated with arthritis can be chronic. Therefore, psychosocial reactions to pain can compound the physiologic changes.

The variables of pain from patient to patient must be considered. All patients react differently to pain, owing to psychosocial and other factors. This observation may make it more difficult for the therapist or physician to evaluate a patient's pain. Many different methods have been used with patients with arthritis and those with other particular dysfunctions, to assess

TABLE 12-4
Pain Assessment Pre- and Post-Thermal Agent

Investigator	Thermal Agent	Diagnosis	Pain Assessment
Clark and associates[35]	Ice or SWD	Osteoarthritis of knee	Maximum pain score of 17 could be gained by 0 = nil, 1 = slight, 2 = moderate, 3 = severe (pain at rest, with walking, overall pain with other activities); night pain, preventing onset of sleep = 1, occasionally awakening person from a sleep = 1, night pain every night = 2
Hamer and Kirk[37]	Ice or US	Frozen shoulder	Graded on a 5-point scale; 0 = painless, 2, 3 = spontaneous night pain disturbing sleep, 4, 5 = severe distressing night and day pain
Hogan, Lockard, Utsinger (reported by Kangilaski)[16]	Ice packs	Rheumatoid arthritis (knees)	Visual analogue pain scales (VAPS); sleep duration
Mainardi and associates[11]	Electric mitten (heat)	Rheumatoid arthritis (hands)	Joint tenderness and swelling assessed by same observer: 0 = none, 1 = mild, 2 = moderate, 3 = severe

the effectiveness of a thermal agent (Table 12–4). In addition, an evaluation of patients' functional status and range of motion (ROM) may or will give you a better idea of their pain status than use of only a subjective scale will. Therefore, an idea of the pain level and a more objective evaluation of ROM and function can all be used in the total evaluation of treatment efficacy.

Many of the patients with rheumatic diseases that a therapist or physician will see have been through a *multitude of treatments* during the course of their disease. They may be discouraged by the numbers of types of treatments they have undergone. They also may have feelings of *frustration and depression* secondary to the chronic nature of their disorder.

In addition to the patients' having undergone a number of pain-reducing modalities and exercise techniques, the *technique of application* of the particular modalities may have varied. It is important for the therapist to be as thorough as possible when obtaining information about past treatments: How often was the treatment given? If hot packs were given, for example, over what body surface were they applied? Were the hot packs followed by exercise or positioning? Was relief obtained? For how long?

Some patients may come for one treatment and then may fail to keep subsequent appointments. Would you, as a therapist, assume they did not return because they improved? They may not return because they felt their symptoms were exacerbated by the therapy given.

EVALUATION OF TREATMENT RESULTS

Objective measurements are required when assessing the outcome of a rehabilitation program. Subjective impressions by the patient or therapist may be useful in identifying the patients' impression of the treatment but will not be helpful in documentation of the validity of a certain regimen. Three general areas should be assessed: (1) pain; (2) ROM and muscle strength; and (3) functional skills.

An objective measurement of pain is difficult to perform. Some investigators[4,37] have relied on the subjective response of the patient to determine if pain has remained the same, has increased, or has decreased. Others[11] determined pain status by the impression of the evaluator. More useful information can be obtained from other measures such as a visual analog pain scale (McGill Pain Questionnaire), sleep duration, and expression of pain during different activities (that is, pain at rest, pain with activity) (see Table 11–2).

The clinical tool available for evaluating range of motion is the goniometer. With the arthritis patient, however, the level of function and ability to perform activities of daily living may not be predictable from goniometric findings. The patient who has a chronic disease, such as rheumatoid arthritis most likely will have adapted to that loss of motion by the use of substitute motions and adaptive devices. Muscle strength can be evaluated by a manual muscle test, isokinetic testing, and measurements of grip and pinch strength.

Functional skills can be evaluated by the use of timed functional tests.[5,22,36] Recording the time it takes a patient to walk a designated distance on a level surface or to climb stairs and measures that can be duplicated in subsequent test sessions.

Some of the objective measurements are difficult and unrealistic to perform in a clinical setting. Special techniques have been used in research facilities and clinical laboratories. A list of suggested clinical and laboratory tests can be found in Table 12–5.

Time of evaluation should be documented. Was the treatment applied and the evaluation performed at the same time each day? This would be of particular importance in the patient with rheumatoid arthritis, who would most likely have a decreased performance early in the day owing to morning stiffness. The time, dosage, and name of medication intake should be recorded.

TABLE 12-5

Assessment Techniques Used for Patients With Rheumatic Diseases

Clinical	Research Facility/Laboratory
Amount and frequency of analgesic intake	Gait analysis (using force plates, EMG, high-speed photography)
Duration of morning stiffness	Joint fluid analysis
Goniometric measurements	Sodium clearance
Gait analysis (stride length, step length, step width)	Joint stiffness
Isokinetic testing	
Joint circumference	
Hand grip strength	
Manual muscle test	
Sleep duration	
Timed functional tests	
Visual analogue pain scales	
Walking time	

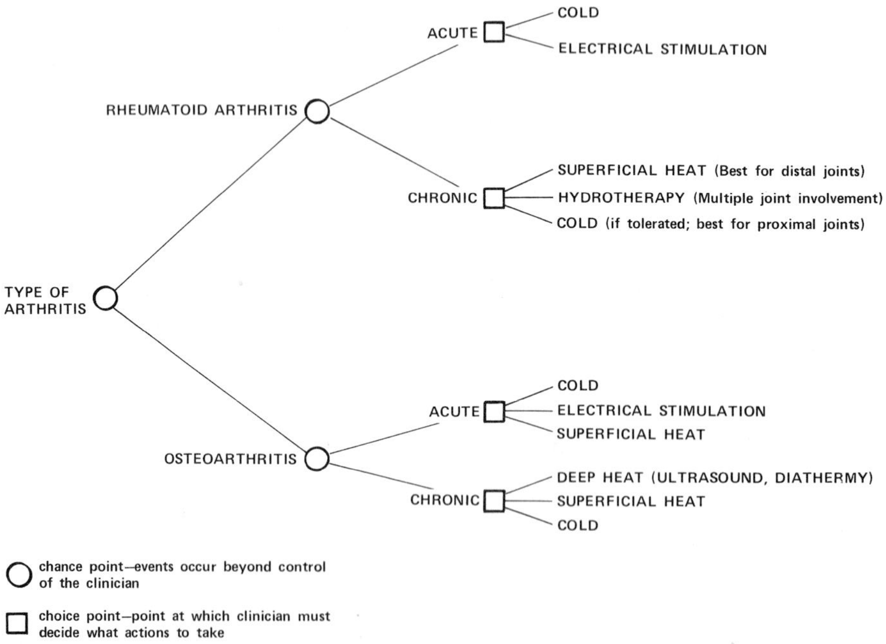

FIGURE 12-2

Clinical decision-making flow chart for application of thermal agents in arthritis. For all cases, the best choice also depends on whether the patient will be using the modality at home. If so, ease of application must be considered. (Courtesy of Bette Ann Harris, M.S., P.T., Boston, MA.)

SUMMARY

Treating the patient who has a rheumatic disease can be both a rewarding and a challenging experience. Treatment regimens and goals must be tailored to the needs of the patient with a chronic dysfunction. Guidelines for the choice of thermal agent in the patient population with arthritis are outlined in Figure 12–2. The evaluation of short- and long-term efficacy of thermal agents applied to the patient with rheumatic disease seems to require further investigation. It was our intention in this chapter to point out problems specific to patients with arthritis, to review studies that have been reported in the literature, and to suggest guidelines for integration of thermal agents into a total treatment program.

REFERENCES

1. Katz, WA: *Rheumatic Diseases: Diagnosis and Management.* JB Lippincott, Philadelphia, 1977.
2. Rodnan, GP, Schumacher, HR (eds): *Primer on the Rheumatic Diseases,* ed 8. Arthritis Foundation, Atlanta, 1983, p 12.
3. Hollander, JL and Horvath, SM: *Intra-articular temperature as a measure of joint reaction.* J Clin Invest 28:469, 1949.
4. Harris, R and Millard, JB: *Paraffin-wax baths in the treatment of rheumatoid arthritis.* Ann Rheum Dis 14:278, 1955.
5. Gallagher, LA, Eshleman, JK, and Schumacher, HR: *A controlled study of the effects of paraffin bath on the rheumatoid hand.* Presented at Arthritis Health Professionals Meeting at the National Arthritis Foundation Meetings, Atlanta, 1980.
6. Policoff, LD: *Physical medicine and rehabilitation in the management of the arthritic patient.* In Katz, WA: *Rheumatic Diseases: Diagnosis and Management.* JB Lippincott, Philadelphia, 1977.
7. Soren, A: *Evaluation of ultrasound treatment in musculoskeletal disorders.* Physiotherapy 51:214, 1965.
8. Clarke, GR and Stenner, L: *Use of therapeutic ultrasound.* Physiotherapy 62:185, 1976.
9. Feibel, A and Fast, A: *Deep heating of joints: a reconsideration.* Arch Phys Med Rehabil 57:513, 1976.
10. Harris, ED and McCroskery, PA: *The influence of temperature and fibril stability on degradation of cartilage collagen by rheumatoid synovial collagenase.* N Engl J Med 290:1, 1974.
11. Mainardi, CL, et al: *Rheumatoid arthritis: failure of daily heat therapy to affect its progression.* Arch Phys Med Rehabil 60:390, 1979.
12. Dial, CA and Windsor, RA: *A pilot study of the impact of a water exercise program for rheumatoid arthritis.* Presented at Arthritis Health Professionals Meetings, Arthritis Foundational Annual Conference, Atlanta, 1980.
13. Woodmansey, A, Collins, DH, and Ernst, MM: *Vascular reactions to contrast both in health and in rheumatoid arthritis.* Lancet 2:1350, 1938.
14. Martin, GM, et al: *Cutaneous temperatures of the extremities of normal subjects and of patients with rheumatoid arthritis.* Arch Phys Med 27:665, 1946.
15. Fricke, EJ and Gersten, JW: *Effect of contrast baths on the vasomotor response of rheumatoid arthritis patients.* Arch Phys Med 33:210, 1952.
16. Kangilaski, J: *Baggie therapy: Simple relief for arthritic knees.* JAMA 247:317, 1981.
17. Pegg, SMH, Littler, TR, and Littler, EN: *A trial of ice therapy and exercise in chronic arthritis.* Physiotherapy 55:51, 1969.
18. Wright, V and Johns, RJ: *Physical factors concerned with the stiffness of normal and diseased joints.* Bull Johns Hopkins Hosp 106:215, 1960.

19. Backlund, L and Tiselius, P: *Objective measurement of joint stiffness in rheumatoid arthritis.* Acta Rheum Scand 13:275, 1967.
20. Kirk, JA and Kersley, GD: *Heat and cold in the physical treatment of rheumatoid arthritis of the knee—A controlled clinical trial.* Ann Phys Med 9:270, 1968.
21. Ritzmann, SE and Levin, WC: *Cryopathies: A review.* Arch Intern Med 107:754, 1961.
22. Utsinger, PD, Bonner, F, and Hogan, N: *Efficacy of cryotherapy and thermotherapy in the management of rheumatoid arthritis pain: Evidence for endorphin effect* (abstr). Arth Rheum 25:S113, 1982.
23. Warren, CG, Lehmann, JD and Koblanski, JN: *Heat and stretch procedures: an evaluation using rat tail tendon.* Arch Phys Med Rehabil 52:465, 1971.
24. Kottke, FJ, Pauley, DL, and Ptak, RA: *The rationale for prolonged stretching for correction of shortening connective tissues.* Arch Phys Med Rehabil 47:345, 1966.
25. Lehmann, JD (ed): *Therapeutic Heat and Cold.* Williams & Wilkins, Baltimore, 1982.
26. Cordray, YN and Kruen, EM: *Use of hydrocollator packs in the treatment of neck and shoulder pains.* Arch Phys Med Rehabil 39:105, 1959.
27. Hamilton, DE and Bywaters, EGL: *A controlled trial of various forms of physiotherapy in arthritis.* Br Med J 1:542, 1959.
28. DePreux, T: *Ultrasonic wave therapy in osteoarthritis of the hip joint.* Br J Phys Med 15:14, 1952.
29. Aldes, JH and Jadeson, WJ: *Ultrasonic therapy in the treatment of hypertrophic arthritis in elderly patients.* Ann W Med Surg 6:525, 1952.
30. Wright, V: *Treatment of osteoarthritis of the knees.* Ann Rheum Dis 23:389, 1964.
31. Vanharanta, H: *Effect of shortwave diathermy on mobility and radiologic stage of the knee in the development of experimental osteoarthritis.* Am J Phys Med 61:59, 1982.
32. Gibson, T, Winter, PJ, and Grahame, R: *Radiotherapy in the treatment of osteoarthritis of the knee.* Rheumatol Rehabil 12;42, 1973.
33. Lehmann, JF, et al: *Comparison of ultrasonic and microwave diathermy in the physical treatment of periarthritis of the shoulder.* Arch Phys Med Rehabil 35:627, 1954.
34. Mueller, EE, et al: *A placebo-controlled study of ultrasound treatment for periarthritis.* Am J Phys Med 33:31, 1954.
35. Clarke, GR, et al: *Evaluation of physiotherapy in the treatment of osteoarthrosis of the knee.* Rheum Rehabil 13:190, 1974.
36. Melvin, JL: *Rheumatic Disease: Occupational Therapy and Rehabilitation,* ed 2. FA Davis, Philadelphia, 1982.
37. Hamer, J and Kirk, JA: *Physiotherapy and the frozen shoulder: A comparative trial of ice and ultrasonic therapy.* NZ Med J 83:191, 1976.

TEMPERATURE CONVERSIONS FOR FAHRENHEIT AND CENTIGRADE

To convert Centigrade to Fahrenheit: $\frac{9}{5}C + 32$

°C	°F	°C	°F
46	114.8	22	71.6
45	113.0	21	69.8
44	111.2	20	68.0
43	109.4	19	66.2
42	107.6	18	64.4
41	105.8	17	62.6
40	104.0	16	60.8
39	102.2	15	59.0
38	100.4	14	57.2
37	98.6	13	55.4
36	96.8	12	53.6
35	95.0	11	51.8
34	93.2	10	50.0
33	91.4	9	48.2
32	89.6	8	46.4
31	87.8	7	44.6
30	86.0	6	42.8
29	84.2	5	41.0
28	82.4	4	39.2
27	80.6	3	37.4
26	78.8	2	35.6
25	77.0	1	33.8
24	75.2	0	32.0
23	73.4		

To convert Fahrenheit to Centigrade: $\frac{5}{9}$ (F − 32)

°F	°C
120	48.9
119	48.3
118	47.8
117	47.2
116	46.7
115	46.1
114	45.6
113	45.0
112	44.4
111	43.9
110	43.3
109	42.8
108	42.2
107	41.7
106	41.1
105	40.5
104	40.0
103	39.9
102	38.8
101	38.3
100	37.8
99	37.2
98	36.7
97	36.1
96	35.5
95	35.0
94	34.4
93	33.9
92	33.3
91	32.8
90	32.2
89	31.7
88	31.1
87	30.6
86	30.0
85	29.4
84	28.9
83	28.3
82	27.8
81	27.2
80	26.7
79	26.1
78	25.6
77	25.0

°F	°C
76	24.4
75	23.9
74	23.3
73	22.7
72	22.2
71	21.7
70	21.1
69	20.6
68	20.0
67	19.4
66	18.9
65	18.3
64	17.8
63	17.2
62	16.7
61	16.1
60	15.5
59	15.0
58	14.4
57	13.9
56	13.3
55	12.8
54	12.2
53	11.7
52	11.1
51	10.6
50	10.0
49	9.4
48	8.9
47	8.3
46	7.8
45	7.2
44	6.6
43	6.1
42	5.6
41	5.0
40	4.4
39	3.9
38	3.3
37	2.8
36	2.2
35	1.7
34	1.1
33	0.6
32	0

MANUFACTURERS OF HEAT, COLD, AND LASER PRODUCTS

This appendix is designed to assist the consumer of heat, cold, and laser products by including sources of reference for these products and by listing the manufacturers of some of them. Inclusion of a product in the list does not indicate endorsement of that product by the editors, authors, or publishers.

SOURCES THAT PROVIDE LISTING OF EQUIPMENT MANUFACTURERS

Center for Devices and Radiological Health
Food and Drug Administration
8757 Georgia Avenue
Silver Spring, MD 20910
Phone: (301) 427-8200
Toll-free: (800) 638-6725

Health Devices Sourcebook
ECRI
5200 Butler Pike
Plymouth Meeting, PA 19462
Phone: (215) 825-6000

Hospital Product Comparison System
(from ECRI in conjunction with McGraw-Hill Publishers)
Available on whirlpools, diathermy, and ultrasound.

Medical Device Register
P.O. Box 50
Smithtown, NY 11787
Phone: (516) 265-3140

Rx Homecare Buyers Guide
825 Barrington Avenue
Los Angeles, CA 90049
Phone: (213) 826-8388

EQUIPMENT MANUFACTURERS

(Addresses of companies are listed after all product categories.)

Cold Therapy: Cooling Units

Chattanooga Corporation
J.A. Preston Corporation

Heat Therapy: Heating Units

Chattanooga Corporation
J.A. Preston Corporation

Fluidotherapy

Fluidotherapy Corporation

Infrared Lamps

Brandt Industries, Inc.
Graham-Field Surgical Company, Inc.

Paraffin Baths

Clinical Models
- Ferno Ille
- Thermo-Electric Company

Home Models
- BernLit Enterprises, Inc.
- Maddak, Inc.
- Talcott Laboratories, Inc.
- WR Medical Electronics Company

Hydrotherapy

Arjo Hospital Equipment, Inc.
Ferno Ille
Jacuzzi
Logan, Inc.
Whitehall Electro Medical Company, Inc.

Shortwave Diathermy

Birtcher Corporation
Elmed, Inc.
Fluidotherapy Corporation
International Medical Electronics Ltd.
J.A. Preston Corporation
Mettler Electronics Corporation
Rich-Mar Corporation

Microwave Diathermy

Elmed, Inc.
Tag Med

Therapeutic Ultrasound

Amrex-Zetron Electronics, Inc.
Birtcher Corporation
Chattanooga Corporation
DynaWave Corporation
Medco Products Co., Inc.
Mettler Electronics Corporation
Rich-Mar Corporation

Low-Power Laser

(NOTE: At this time laser is still considered by the FDA as a Class III device and can be used only for investigational purposes with an Investigational Device Exemption [IDE])

Dynatronics
Physio Technology, Inc.

EQUIPMENT MANUFACTURERS ADDRESSES

Amrex-Zetron Electronics, Inc.
12583 Crenshaw Boulevard
Hawthorn, CA
Phone: (213) 973-5165

Arjo Hospital Equipment, Inc.
6380 Oakton Street
Morton Grove, IL 60053
Phone: (312) 967-0360
Toll-free: (800) 323-1245

BernLit Enterprises, Inc.
5800 Ellwood Avenue
Bristol, PA 19007-3498
Phone: (215) 781-9522

Birtcher Corporation
4501 North Arden Drive
El Monte, CA 91731
Phone: (818) 575-8144
Toll-free: (800) 423-4889

Brandt Industries, Inc.
4461 Bronx Boulevard
Bronx, NY 10470
Phone: (212) 994-0800

Chattanooga Corporation
101 Memorial Drive
P.O. Box 4287
Chattanooga, TN 37405
Phone: (615) 870-2261
Toll-free: (800) 592-7329

Dynatronics
326 South Redwood Road
Salt Lake City, UT 84104
Phone: (801) 974-5109
Toll-free: (800) 874-6251

DynaWave Corporation
2520 Kaneville Road
Geneva, IL 60134
Phone: (312) 232-4945

Elmed, Inc.
60 West Fay Avenue
Addison, IL 60101
Phone: (312) 543-2792

Ferno Ille
P.O. Box 3007
Williamsport, PA 17701-0007
Phone: (717) 323-9491

Fluidotherapy Corporation
Henley International, Inc.
6113 Aletha Lane
Houston, TX 77081
Phone: (713) 776-0443
Toll-free: (800) 222-1537

Graham-Field Surgical Company, Inc.
415 Second Avenue
New Hyde Park, NY 11040
Phone: (516) 328-0500
Toll-free: (800) 645-8146

International Medical Electronics Ltd.
2805 Main
Kansas City, MO 64108
Phone: (816) 221-0115

Jacuzzi
298 North Wiget Lane
P.O. Drawer J
Walnut Creek, CA 94596
Phone: (415) 938-7070
Toll-free: (800) 227-0710

J.A. Preston Corporation
60 Page Road
Clifton, NJ 07012
Phone: (201) 777-2700
Toll-free: (800) 631-7277

Logan, Inc.
3041 S. Shannon St.
Santa Ana, CA 92704
Phone: (714) 556-6441

Maddak, Inc.
Pequannock, NJ 07440-1993
Phone: (201) 694-0500

Medco Products Co., Inc.
P.O. Box E
31 Park Road
Tinton Falls, NJ 07724
Phone: (201) 389-1700

Mettler Electronics Corporation
1333 S. Claudina Street
Anaheim, CA 92805
Phone: (714) 533-2221

Physio Technology, Inc.
1925 West Sixth Street
Topeka, KS 66606
Toll-free: (800) 255-3554

Rich-Mar Corporation
P.O. Box 879
Inola, OK 74036
Phone: (918) 543-2222

Tag Med
6595 Odell Place
Suite B
Boulder, CO 80201
Phone: (303) 530-3845

Talcott Laboratories, Inc.
301 East Barr Street
McDonald, PA 15057
Phone: (412) 926-3011

Thermo-Electric Company
1948 Columbus Road
Cleveland, OH 44113
Phone: (216) 621-7095
Toll-free: (800) 821-9188

Whitehall Electro Medical Company, Inc.
100 Temple Avenue
P.O. Box 701
Hackensack, NJ 07602-0701
Phone: (201) 488-6888

WR Medical Electronics Company
1995 West County Road B2
St. Paul, MN 55113
Phone: (612) 633-8471

INDEX

Numbers in *italics* indicate figures; numbers followed by a "t" indicate tables.